Shoulder Arthroplasty

Shoulder Arthroplasty

Gary M. Gartsman, MD

Attending Shoulder Surgeon
Fondren Orthopedic Group, LLP
Texas Orthopedic Hospital
Clinical Professor
Department of Orthopaedic Surgery
Director, Shoulder and Elbow Fellowship
University of Texas Health Sciences Center at Houston
Houston, Texas

T. Bradley Edwards, MD

Attending Shoulder Surgeon
Fondren Orthopedic Group, LLP
Texas Orthopedic Hospital
Clinical Instructor
Department of Orthopaedic Surgery
Shoulder and Elbow Fellowship
University of Texas Health Sciences Center at Houston
Houston, Texas

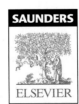

SAUNDERS

ELSEVIER

SAUNDERS
ELSEVIER

1600 John F. Kennedy Blvd.
Ste 1800
Philadelphia, PA 19103-2899

SHOULDER ARTHROPLASTY   ISBN: 978-1-4160-3857-3

Notice

Knowledge and best practice in this field are constantly changing. As new research and
experience broaden our knowledge, changes in practice, treatment and drug therapy may
become necessary or appropriate. Readers are advised to check the most current
information provided (i) on procedures featured or (ii) by the manufacturer of each
product to be administered, to verify the recommended dose or formula, the method and
duration of administration, and contraindications. It is the responsibility of the
practitioner, relying on their own experience and knowledge of the patient, to make
diagnoses, to determine dosages and the best treatment for each individual patient, and to
take all appropriate safety precautions. To the fullest extent of the law, neither the
Publisher nor the Authors assume any liability for any injury and/or damage to persons
or property arising out of or related to any use of the material contained in this
book.

The Publisher

Library of Congress Cataloging-in-Publication Data
Gartsman, Gary M.
    Shoulder arthroplasty / Gary M. Gartsman, T. Bradley Edwards.—1st ed.
      p. ; cm.
    Includes bibliographical references.
    ISBN 978-1-4160-3857-3
  1. Shoulder joint—Endoscopic surgery. I. Edwards, T. Bradley. II. Title.
    [DNLM: 1. Arthroplasty—methods. 2. Shoulder Joint—surgery. WE 810 G2436s 2008]
    RD557.5.G377 2008
    617.5′720597—dc22

2008000952

Acquisitions Editor: Emily Christie
Developmental Editor: Julia Bartz
Publishing Services Manager: Tina Rebane
Project Manager: Amy Norwitz
Design Direction: Louis Forgione
Illustrator: Mike de La Flor
Marketing Manager: Catalina Nolte

Printed in China

Last digit is the print number: 9 8 7 6 5 4 3 2 1

To Carol, whose love and understanding make it all worthwhile.

GMG

To my family: my wife, Elizabeth; my son, Cooper; and my daughter, Anne-Claire. You are truly the best part of my life.

TBE

PREFACE

Shoulder arthroplasty has been in a near-constant state of evolution since the first operation by Jules Emile Péan in 1893. We are indebted to Dr. Charles Neer for his pioneering work with unconstrained shoulder arthroplasty, used first for proximal humeral fracture and later for glenohumeral arthritis. Glenoid resurfacing was added to humeral head replacement and is recognized to provide results superior to those of isolated humeral arthroplasty for many diagnoses. From Dr. Neer's foundation, unconstrained humeral prosthetic design advanced to include modularity and anatomic adaptability. The reintroduction of reverse shoulder arthroplasty, initially in Europe and later in North America, has given patients a more predictable outcome when dealing with the difficult problems of massive rotator cuff deficiency. Surgical techniques advanced simultaneously with the evolution of shoulder prostheses, providing surgeons with well-described surgical approaches that reliably allowed glenoid exposure and soft tissue balancing. Implant fixation techniques, particularly for the glenoid component, help make arthroplasty failure a rarity.

With these evolving technologies and techniques comes a responsibility to employ these powerful tools wisely. As the number of shoulder arthroplasties performed worldwide continues to grow, surgeons will require more education in shoulder arthroplasty.

Shoulder Arthroplasty shows in detail how we approach all aspects of shoulder replacement in our practice. Our goal was to put these ideas into a simple, user-friendly format to allow practical application by the shoulder surgeon.

GARY M. GARTSMAN
T. BRADLEY EDWARDS

CONTENTS

DVD CONTENTS

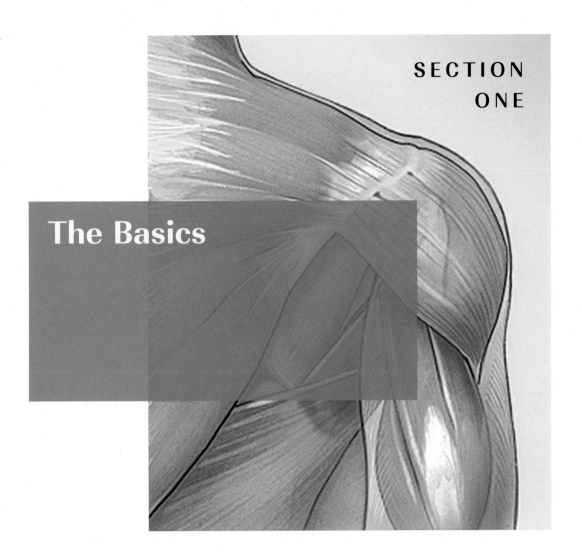

SECTION
ONE

The Basics

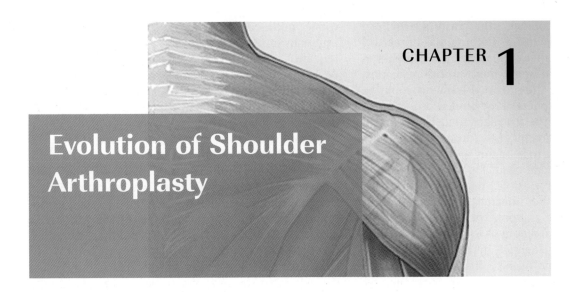

CHAPTER 1

Evolution of Shoulder Arthroplasty

FIRST SHOULDER ARTHROPLASTY

Although Jules Emile Péan is credited with performing the first shoulder arthroplasty, it was probably Themistocles Gluck who first recognized prosthetic replacement as a potential treatment option in the shoulder.[1] Gluck, a Romanian who studied in Germany in the second half of the 19th century, pioneered joint replacement for the treatment of tuberculosis infection. Gluck reported on his design of an ivory shoulder replacement but never documented its use in a living human subject.

The first recorded shoulder arthroplasty was performed in 1893 by Péan, a Parisian surgeon who replaced the shoulder of a patient suffering from tuberculous arthropathy who had refused amputation.[2] Péan implanted a shoulder prosthesis designed and constructed by J. Porter Michaels, a Parisian dentist; the prosthesis consisted of a rubber humeral head that had been boiled in paraffin to harden it and was attached to a platinum shaft via a metal wire. A second metal wire attached the implant to the glenoid. The patient initially "did well" after the surgery before ultimately requiring removal of the prosthesis for recurrence of infection 2 years later.

FIRST-GENERATION SHOULDER ARTHROPLASTY

The first shoulder arthroplasty using a prosthesis with an anatomic design was performed in 1950 by Frederick Krueger.[3] Krueger used a Vitallium implant created by molding proximal humeri obtained from cadavers. He successfully implanted this prosthesis in

a young patient with osteonecrosis of the humeral head. The modern era of shoulder arthroplasty, however, was pioneered by Dr. Charles Neer. Neer originally performed hemiarthroplasty to treat complex proximal humeral fractures starting in 1953.[4] Nearly 20 years later he would report on the use of shoulder replacement for the treatment of glenohumeral arthritis.[5] Neer originally used a monoblock implant; however, variations in humeral head size among patients led to the concept of modularity, which allowed the use of variable humeral head diameters in shoulder arthroplasty. Monoblock implants are now commonly referred to as first-generation shoulder arthroplasty.

SECOND-GENERATION SHOULDER ARTHROPLASTY

The introduction of modular humeral head arthroplasty with variable diameter gave rise to the second generation of shoulder arthroplasty. Although these designs appeared to be an improvement over the earlier monoblock designs, they did not seem to optimally fit all patients. Additionally, not all patients had the good and excellent clinical results reported by Neer after shoulder arthroplasty with first- and second-generation designs.

THIRD-GENERATION SHOULDER ARTHROPLASTY

In the late 1980s Boileau and Walch hypothesized that variations in anatomy prevented current first- and second-generation shoulder arthroplasty stems from achieving optimal fit within the proximal humerus.[6] They undertook an anatomic study of the proximal humerus that yielded some important conclusions. They discovered that the proximal humerus could be modeled by using a sphere and cylinder. A portion of the sphere represents the articular surface of the proximal humerus. The diameter of the humeral head articular surface was found to be highly variable, as was the thickness of the humeral head. Thickness and diameter were found to have a fixed relationship and correlated with one another linearly. They further found the inclination of the anatomic neck of the humerus relative to the humeral diaphysis to be highly variable. Humeral retroversion, defined by the relationship of the humeral anatomic neck to the transepicondylar axis of the elbow, was found to vary by more than 50 degrees. Finally, the sphere (humeral head) was discovered to be offset, usually posteriorly and medially, from the cylinder (humeral diaphysis). These relationships are summarized in Table 1-1.

The anatomic studies of Boileau and Walch gave rise to the third generation of shoulder arthroplasty: the anatomic (adaptable) prosthesis. The concept behind third-generation implants is to adapt the prosthesis to the individual patient's anatomy instead of trying to force the anatomy to adapt to the prosthesis. Anatomic shoulder arthroplasty stems rely on an anatomic neck cut to replicate the patient's normal humeral retroversion. Multiple humeral head diameters are available. The prosthetic stem has a variable neck shaft (inclination) angle, and the head can be placed in varying degrees of posterior and medial offset, thereby allowing nearly perfect replication of the patient's native anatomy.

Several laboratory studies have demonstrated the clinical relevance of advances in design imposed by third-generation humeral implants. Harryman and colleagues demonstrated how placing too thick a humeral component had detrimental effects on glenohumeral motion,[7] whereas Jobe and Iannotti found a decrease in the arc of available glenohumeral motion when using too thin a humeral head component.[8] In an eloquent computer model, Pearl and Kurutz demonstrated the necessity of being able to vary the humeral head diameter, humeral head offset, and neck inclination angle of a humeral prosthesis to replicate the patient's native anatomy (Fig. 1-1).[9]

GLENOID RESURFACING

Neer first reported on the use of a glenoid component in unconstrained shoulder arthroplasty for the treatment of glenohumeral arthritis in 1974.[5] Neer's original implant was a keeled cemented rectangular component (the same anterior-to-posterior diameter superiorly and inferiorly) with a radius of curvature matching the humeral head component.

Advances in glenoid resurfacing have occurred in component design and implantation techniques. Different component designs commonly used include cemented polyethylene keeled convex-back designs, cemented polyethylene keeled flat-back designs, cemented polyethylene pegged convex-back designs, and metal-backed designs. Convex-back designs have been shown experimentally to resist sheer forces better than flat-back designs do, and this has translated into fewer radiolucent lines around the glenoid component in the clinical scenario.[10-12] The larger debate exists over whether to use a keeled or a pegged component. Laboratory studies have demonstrated less micromotion with pegged implants.[13] Clinical studies, however, have reported both the superiority of pegs and the superiority of keels.[14,15] Because radiographic comparison of these two types of implant is difficult, this debate remains unsolved at present. The original metal-backed designs consisted of a metal base plate secured with a screw-type mechanism and a modular polyethylene liner. The thickness of the metal often required that the polyethylene insert be very thin to avoid placing excessive tension on the gleno-

Table 1-1   ANATOMIC VARIABILITY OF THE PROXIMAL HUMERUS

Dimension	Mean	Range
Humeral head diameter	46.2 mm	37.1 to 56.9 mm
Articular surface diameter	43.3 mm	36.5 to 51.7 mm
Articular surface thickness	15.2 mm	12.1 to 18.2 mm
Inclination	129.6 degrees	123.2 to 135.8 degrees
Retroversion	17.9 degrees	–6.7 to 47.5 degrees
Posterior offset	2.6 mm	–0.8 to 6.1 mm
Medial offset	6.9 mm	2.9 to 10.8 mm

From Boileau P, Walch G: Anatomical study of the proximal humerus: Surgical technique consideration and prosthetic design rationale. In Walch G, Boileau P (eds): Shoulder Arthroplasty. Berlin, Springer, 1999, pp 69-82.

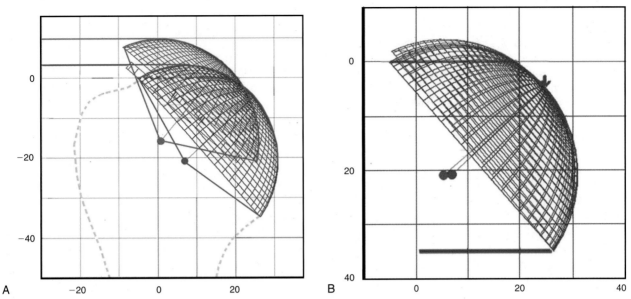

Figure 1-1 **A,** Inability to reproduce the native anatomy with a prosthesis that has a fixed inclination angle. The native anatomy is depicted in blue, and the closest prosthetic fit is depicted in red. **B,** Nearly perfect replication of the native anatomy after variable inclination is introduced into the prosthetic system. (From Pearl ML, Kurutz S: Geometric analysis of commonly used prosthetic systems for proximal humeral replacement. J Bone Joint Surg Am 1999;81:660-671.)

humeral soft tissues. This thinness resulted in poor wear characteristics of the polyethylene and caused implant failure.[16] Many early metal-backed designs have been abandoned; however, implantation of a glenoid component without the use of cement is still appealing, especially in revision surgery, which may involve compromised glenoid bone stock. Research is ongoing in the development of new and improved metal-backed glenoid designs.

One of the most recent and significant advances in glenoid component design is recognition of the significance of glenohumeral prosthetic mismatch. Mismatch is defined as the difference in radius of curvature between the humeral head and glenoid component. Congruent articulations (mismatch = 0) allow optimal surface contact, minimize the risk of surface wear of the glenoid component, and contribute to increased joint stability. However, with these advantages comes a lack of obligate translation (translation between the articular surfaces that normally occurs with shoulder mobility and is absorbed by elastic deformation of the articular cartilage and the glenoid labrum). Lack of obligate translation may lead to loosening of the glenoid component by increasing the stress developed at the implant fixation site. Alternatively, noncongruent articulations (larger glenoid than humeral radius of curvature) allow obligate translation between the humeral head and the glenoid, thereby potentially decreasing the stress observed at the glenoid implant

fixation site. Glenoid component wear and joint stability remain a concern in noncongruent articulations. Laboratory investigations have yielded some insight into appropriate mismatch in shoulder arthroplasty, including studies demonstrating that a 4-mm mismatch is necessary to best replicate normal shoulder mobility, and studies showing that mismatch in excess of 10 mm risks fracture of the polyethylene component.[17,18] The clinical relevance of these laboratory studies was not clear, however, until Walch and coworkers reported on the influence of glenohumeral prosthetic mismatch on radiolucent lines occurring around the glenoid component.[19] This study found that fewer radiolucent lines occurred at minimum 2-year follow-up when a radial mismatch of at least 6 mm was used during performance of total shoulder arthroplasty. An upper limit of mismatch was not established, however, thus prompting ongoing studies to discover the ideal glenohumeral prosthetic mismatch.

Another aspect of glenoid resurfacing that has evolved is the implantation technique of glenoid components. Neer originally recommended preparation of a keel slot with a curette to remove a large amount of bone and create a large cement mantle.[5] More recently, Gazielly and colleagues introduced the bone compaction technique for implantation of keeled glenoid components.[20] Radiolucent lines around glenoid components appear on the initial postoperative radiographs in many cases and have been attributed to technical deficiencies.[21] The compaction technique of bone preparation addresses radiolucent lines in three ways. First, compaction of cancellous bone in the glenoid provides a more stable base for the glenoid component than does bone removal via curettage. Second, a compacted bone slot that has the same dimensions as the component keel allows a primary "press-fit" fixation that should help prevent micromotion of the component as the cement polymerizes. Third, the compaction technique uses a smaller amount of cement, which may decrease thermal necrosis of the adjacent glenoid bone. Clinically, a comparison of the curettage technique with the compaction technique has shown superiority of the compaction technique in minimizing radiolucent lines on immediate and 2-year postoperative radiographs.[22]

ARTHROPLASTY FOR FRACTURE

Neer's original indication for shoulder arthroplasty—complex fractures of the proximal humerus—remains the most difficult diagnosis for which shoulder arthroplasty is used. Performance of shoulder arthroplasty for fracture is fraught with potential complications and often results in disappointing outcomes. The majority of these poor outcomes are related to nonunion or malunion of the greater and lesser tuberosities after arthroplasty. Boileau and associates have identified four potential causes of tuberosity complications after shoulder arthroplasty for fracture.[23] First, improper positioning of the prosthesis may lead to nonunion of the tuberosities by placing undue tension on the rotator cuff, specifically if the prosthesis is implanted proud or in excessive retroversion (Fig. 1-2). Second, the osteopenic nature of the tuberosities in this patient population makes healing of the tuberosities difficult to achieve. Third, fixation of the tuberosities around the prosthesis is difficult, and passing sutures through holes in the prosthetic stem often results in suture breakage and migration of the tuberosities.[24] Fourth, the large amount of proximal metal used in conventional humeral arthroplasties may act as a hindrance to healing of the tuberosities.

Arthroplasty for fracture has evolved specifically to address these issues of tuberosity complications. First, ancillary instrumentation has been developed to allow

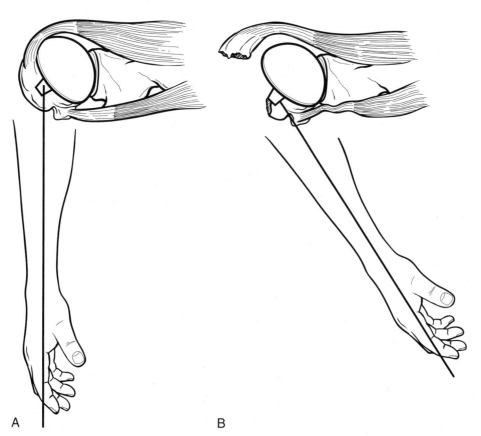

A   B

Figure 1-2   A and **B,** Illustration showing how excessive humeral retroversion can cause tuberosity migration.

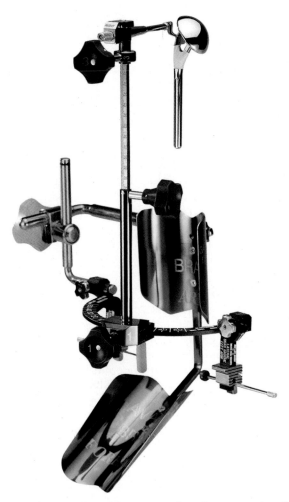

Figure 1-3 Ancillary instrumentation for approximating correct prosthetic height and version.

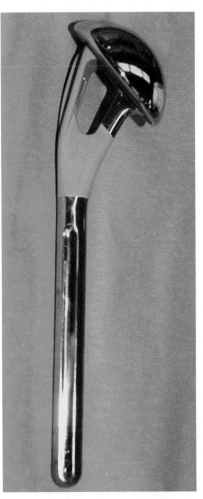

Figure 1-4 Humeral stem specifically designed for use in fracture cases. Note the lower profile proximally and the fenestration to allow bone grafting and promotion of tuberosity healing.

more reliable placement and testing of the humeral implant before definitive cementation (Fig. 1-3). Second, the interface between the greater and lesser tuberosities and the interface between the tuberosities and the native humerus is routinely bone-grafted with autogenous bone from the fractured humeral head. Third, a reproducible, biomechanically stable tuberosity fixation technique has been developed that avoids passage of suture through a metallic implant. Fourth, new implants with less metallic bulk proximally and with metaphyseal fenestrations to promote healing of the tuberosities are available for use in fracture cases (Fig. 1-4). Boileau and colleagues reported on the clinical implications of the use of an arthroplasty system designed for the treatment of proximal humeral fractures and found that tuberosity complications decreased from 49% in procedures involving conventional hemiarthroplasty to 25% in procedures that used a hemiarthroplasty designed for fracture cases.[23]

CONSTRAINED AND SEMICONSTRAINED SHOULDER ARTHROPLASTY

Constrained and semiconstrained arthroplasty were initially introduced in the 1960s to treat patients with glenohumeral arthritis and massive rotator cuff tears. The concept of these devices is to resolve upward migration of the humeral head and thereby restore the normal deltoid moment arm and allow active elevation of the arm powered by the deltoid. Reverse designs, with a sphere fixated to the glenoid and a cup secured to the proximal humerus, were introduced in the past to accomplish this goal. The problem with these early designs was early loosening of the glenoid caused by deltoid forces acting on the laterally offset center of glenohumeral rotation (Fig. 1-5). Such failures eventually resulted in abandonment of these early prosthetic designs.

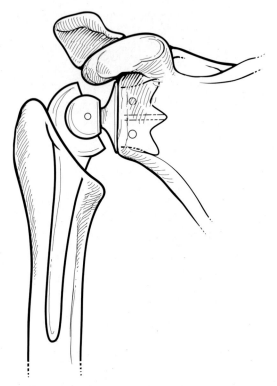

Figure 1-5 The laterally located center of rotation of early reverse-design prostheses caused early loosening.

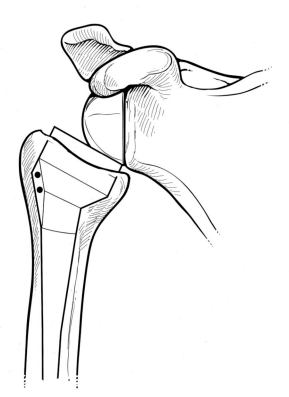

Figure 1-6 The center of rotation of the Grammont prosthesis is within the scapular bone, thus theoretically decreasing the potential for loosening.

In 1987, Paul Grammont introduced a new reverse-design prosthesis in an effort to overcome the failures that had plagued earlier attempts. This new prosthesis uses a "glenosphere" component fixated over the scapular neck and places the center of glenohumeral rotation within the bone of the glenoid instead of lateral to it (Fig. 1-6).[25] This prosthesis now has up to 15 years' follow-up in Europe, and glenoid failure rates have not exceeded those of unconstrained total shoulder prostheses in patients with a competent rotator cuff.[26,27] Additionally, although pain relief has been equivalent to that seen with humeral head replacement, postoperative active shoulder elevation has far exceeded the elevation that can be expected after hemiarthroplasty.

REFERENCES

1. Gluck T: Referat über die Durch das moderne chirurgishe Experiment gewonnenen positiven Resultate betreffend die Nacht und den Ersatz von defecten hoherer Gewebe sowie über die Verwertung resorbirbarer und lebendiger Tamons in der Chirurgie. Arch Klin Chir 1891;41:187-239.
2. Lugli T: Artificial shoulder joint by Péan (1893). The facts of an exceptional intervention and the prosthetic method. Clin Orthop 1978;133:215-218.
3. Krueger FJ: A Vitallium replica arthroplasty on the shoulder: A case report of aseptic necrosis of the proximal end of the humerus. Surgery 1951;30:1005-1011.
4. Neer CS: Articular replacement for the humeral head. J Bone Joint Surg Am 1955;37:215-228.
5. Neer CS: Replacement arthroplasty for glenohumeral osteoarthritis. J Bone Joint Surg Am 1974;56:1-13.
6. Boileau P, Walch G: Anatomical study of the proximal humerus: Surgical technique consideration and prosthetic design rationale. In Walch G, Boileau P (eds): Shoulder Arthroplasty. Berlin, Springer, 1999, pp 69-82.
7. Harryman DT, Sidles JA, Harris SL, et al: The effect of articular conformity and the size of the humeral head component on laxity and motion after glenohumeral arthroplasty: A study in cadavera. J Bone Joint Surg Am 1995;77:555-563.
8. Jobe CM, Iannotti JP: Limits imposed on glenohumeral motion by joint geometry. J Shoulder Elbow Surg 1995;4:281-285.
9. Pearl ML, Kurutz S: Geometric analysis of commonly used prosthetic systems for proximal humeral replacement. J Bone Joint Surg Am 1999;81:660-671.
10. Anglin C, Wyss UP, Pichora DR: Mechanical testing of shoulder prostheses and recommendations for glenoid design. J Shoulder Elbow Surg 2000;9:323-331.
11. Lacaze F, Kempf JF, Bonnomet F, et al: Primary fixation of glenoid implants: An in vitro study. In Walch G, Boileau P (eds): Shoulder Arthroplasty. Berlin, Springer, 1999, pp 141-146.

12. Szabo I, Buscayret F, Walch G, et al: Radiographic comparison of flat back and convex back polyethylene glenoid components in total shoulder arthroplasty. Paper presented at the 16th Annual Meeting of the Société Européenne de Chirurgie de l'Epaule et du Coude, September 2002, Budapest.

13. Anglin C, Wyss UP, Nyffeler RW, Gerber C: Loosening performance of cemented glenoid prosthesis design pairs. Clin Biomech 2001;16:144-150.

14. Gartsman GM, Elkousy HA, Warnock KM, et al: Radiographic comparison of pegged and keeled glenoid components. J Shoulder Elbow Surg 2005;14:252-257.

15. Gazielly D, El-Abiad R: Comparative results of three types of polyethylene cemented glenoid components. In Walch G, Boileau P, Molé D (eds): 2000 Prosthèses d'Epaule . . . Recul de 2 à 10 Ans. Paris, Sauramps Medical, 2001, pp 483-488.

16. Boileau P, Avidor C, Krishnan SG, et al: Cemented polyethylene versus uncemented metal-backed glenoid components in total shoulder arthroplasty: A prospective, double-blind, randomized study. J Shoulder Elbow Surg 2002;11:351-359.

17. Karduna AR, Williams GR, Williams JL, Iannotti JP: Joint stability after total shoulder arthroplasty in a cadaver model. J Shoulder Elbow Surg 1997;6:506-511.

18. Friedman RJ, An YH, Draughn RA: Glenohumeral congruence in total shoulder arthroplasty. Orthop Trans 1997,21.17.

19. Walch G, Edwards TB, Boulahia A, et al: The influence of glenohumeral prosthetic mismatch on glenoid radiolucent lines: Results of a multicentric study. J Bone Joint Surg Am 2002;84:2186-2191.

20. Gazielly DF, Allende C, Pamelin E: Results of cancellous compaction technique for glenoid resurfacing. Paper presented at the 9th International Congress on Surgery of the Shoulder, May 2004, Washington, DC.

21. Brems J: The glenoid component in total shoulder arthroplasty. J Shoulder Elbow Surg 1993;2:47-54.

22. Szabo I, Buscayret F, Edwards TB, et al: Radiographic comparison of two different glenoid preparation techniques in total shoulder arthroplasty. Clin Orthop Relat Res 2005;431:104-110.

23. Boileau P, Coste JS, Ahrens PM, Staccini P: Prosthetic shoulder replacement for fracture: Results of the multicentre study. In Walch G, Boileau P, Molé D (eds): 2000 Prosthèses d'Epaule . . . Recul de 2 à 10 Ans. Paris, Sauramps Medical, 2001, pp 561-578.

24. Gerber C, Wahlström P, Nyffeler R: Suture failure caused by suboptimal prosthetic design may cause secondary tuberosity displacement. Paper presented at the 8th International Congress on Surgery of the Shoulder, April 2001, Cape Town, South Africa.

25. Grammont PM, Baulot E: Delta shoulder prosthesis for rotator cuff rupture. Orthopedics 1993;16:65-68.

26. Favard L, Nové-Josserand L, Levigne C, et al: Anatomical arthroplasty versus reverse arthroplasty in treatment of cuff tear arthropathy. Paper presented at the 14th Annual Meeting of the Société Européenne de Chirurgie de l'Epaule et du Coude, September 2000, Lisbon, Portugal.

27. Bouttens D, Nérot C: Cuff tear arthropathy: Mid term results with the delta prosthesis. Paper presented at the 14th Annual Meeting of the Société Européenne de Chirurgie de l'Epaule et du Coude, September 2000, Lisbon, Portugal.

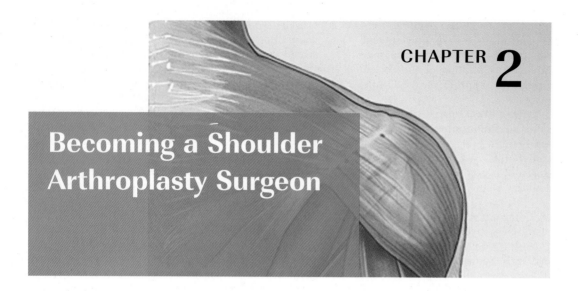

CHAPTER 2

Becoming a Shoulder Arthroplasty Surgeon

Shoulder arthroplasty is much less frequently performed than hip and knee arthroplasty and accounts for only 3.1% of inpatient joint replacements in the United States,[1] largely because hip and knee arthrosis is much more common than glenohumeral arthrosis. Additionally, patients with glenohumeral arthrosis tolerate the symptoms better than those with hip and knee arthrosis because they do not rely on their shoulders for locomotion. Consequently, a busy general orthopedic surgeon may easily perform more than 100 hip and knee replacements in a given year and yet see fewer than five patients who are candidates for shoulder replacement during that same period. Moreover, most orthopedic residencies offer the same lower extremity–focused arthroplasty experience. This has been confirmed by our shoulder fellows, most of whom have seen fewer than five total shoulder arthroplasties during a 4-year orthopedic residency.

The desire and necessity to perform shoulder arthroplasty have evolved from advances made in the field of shoulder surgery during the last 2 decades. Shoulder arthroscopy has developed from a solely diagnostic procedure to a part of the surgical armamentarium that allows treatment of nearly every shoulder problem formerly treated by open surgery. As a result, many orthopedists, largely through technique-driven courses, have become proficient at arthroscopic shoulder procedures, including but not limited to rotator cuff and labral repair. As these same surgeons develop a practice in which an increasing number of patients with shoulder problems are treated, it becomes inevitable that they will encounter diagnoses not amenable to arthroscopic treatment, specifically, diagnoses best treated by shoulder arthroplasty. An aging population that is living longer and remaining more active has

contributed to the increasing number of shoulder arthroplasties performed annually as well. In the United States alone, 28,742 shoulder arthroplasties were performed in 2003, a 14.4% increase over the previous year.[1] This chapter reviews some basic concepts that must be understood when an orthopedic surgeon decides to become a shoulder arthroplasty surgeon.

ANATOMY

An exhaustive review of shoulder anatomy is beyond the scope of this textbook; however, an understanding of open shoulder anatomy is imperative for performing shoulder arthroplasty. Most shoulder arthroplasties are performed through a deltopectoral approach. This section reviews the surgically important anatomic facets of this approach.

Cutaneous

The palpable coracoid process marks the proximal extent of the skin incision for the deltopectoral approach. In thin patients, the deltopectoral interval may be palpable to better assist in directing the skin incision (Fig. 2-1). In revision cases, the skin incision may be extended distally along the lateral aspect of the biceps brachii muscle, which is also palpable (Fig. 2-2).

Subcutaneous

The deltopectoral interval is marked by the cephalic vein. This vein has many small branches, most of

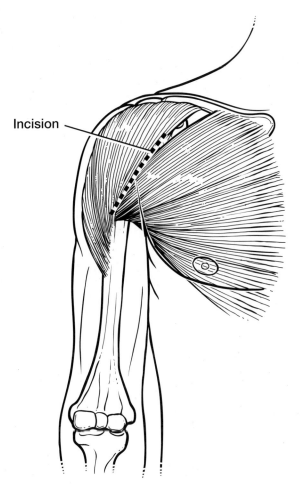

Figure 2-1   Skin incision for the deltopectoral approach to the shoulder.

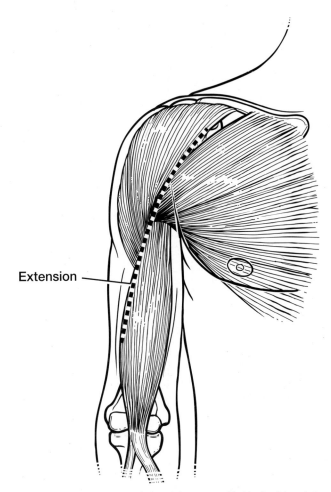

Figure 2-2   Extension of the deltopectoral skin incision into an anterolateral approach to the humeral shaft.

which enter the deltoid muscle (Fig. 2-3). The deltoid has attachments at the acromion and the deltoid tuberosity of the humerus. The pectoralis major has attachments at the clavicle, the sternum, and the humerus just lateral to the long head of the biceps brachii tendon (Fig. 2-4).

Coracoid/Conjoined Tendon

Immediately deep to the deltoid and pectoralis major muscles is the conjoined tendon of the coracobrachialis and the short head of the biceps brachii (Fig. 2-5). This structure passes from the tip of the coracoid process (the proximal extent of dissection) to the anterior humeral shaft. The coracoid process also serves as the point of attachment of the coracoacromial ligament laterally and the pectoralis minor tendon medially (Fig. 2-6).

Neurovascular Structures

As the conjoined tendon is retracted medially, the anterior humeral circumflex vessels can be seen passing along the inferior border of the subscapularis tendon (Fig. 2-7). The axillary nerve may be visualized inferior to the anterior humeral circumflex vessels during dissection with the arm held in a forward-flexed and slightly internally rotated position (Fig. 2-8). The musculocutaneous nerve may be visualized as it enters the coracobrachialis and the short head of the biceps brachii, although it is not routinely exposed during shoulder arthroplasty (Fig. 2-9).

Subscapularis, Rotator Interval, and Biceps

The subscapularis tendon is readily visible just deep to the conjoined tendon as it inserts into the lesser

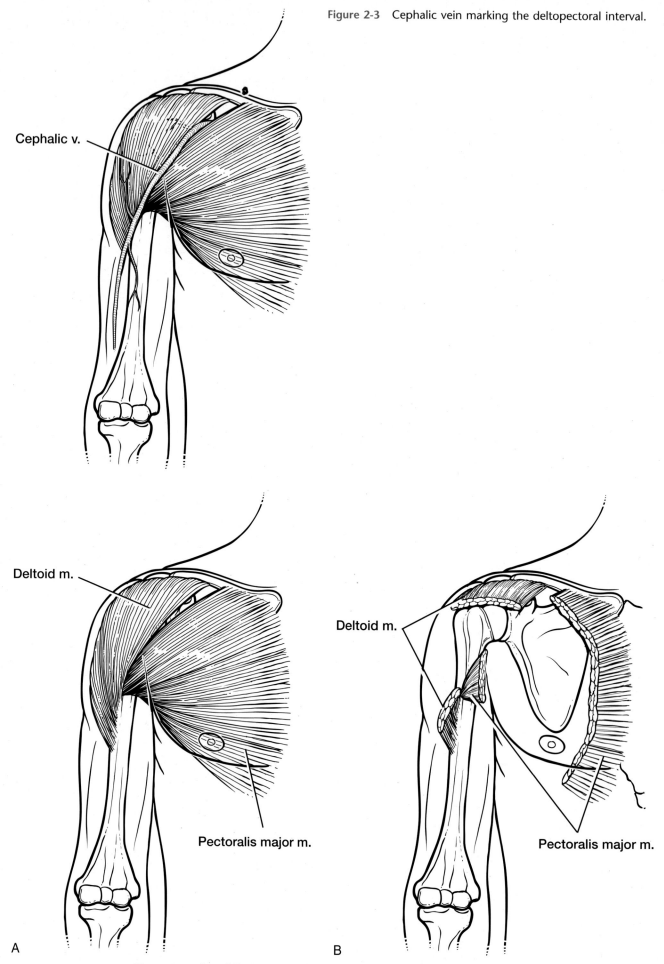

Figure 2-3   Cephalic vein marking the deltopectoral interval.

Cephalic v.

Deltoid m.

Pectoralis major m.

Deltoid m.

Pectoralis major m.

A

B

Figure 2-4   **A** and **B,** Anatomy of the deltoid and pectoralis major muscles.

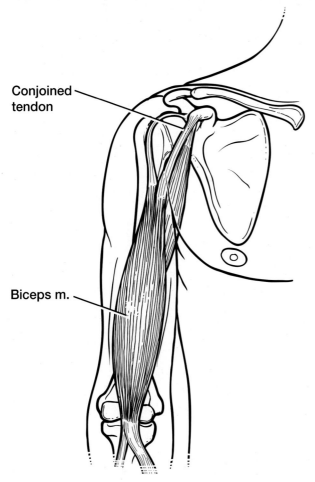

Figure 2-5   Anatomy of the conjoined tendon.

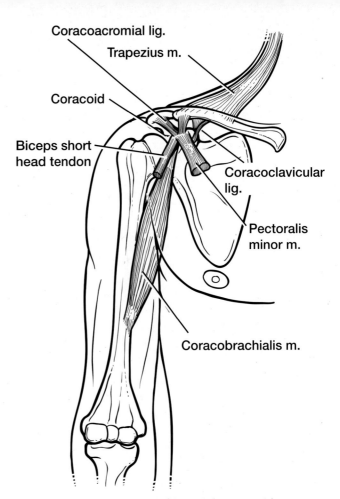

Figure 2-6   Structures attaching to the coracoid process.

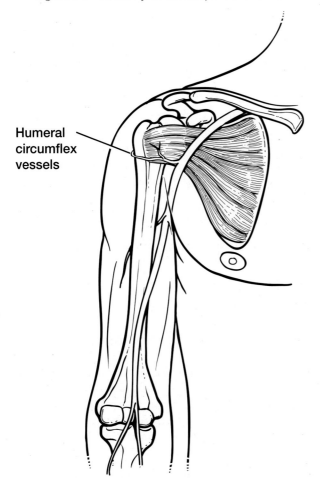

Figure 2-7   Anterior humeral circumflex vessels passing over the inferior aspect of the subscapularis.

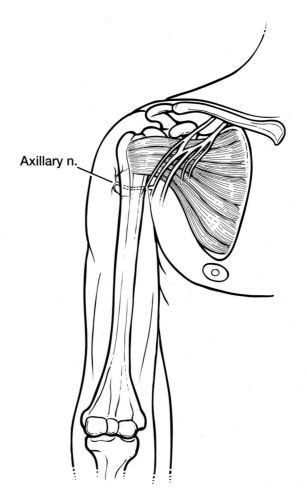

Figure 2-8   The axillary nerve.

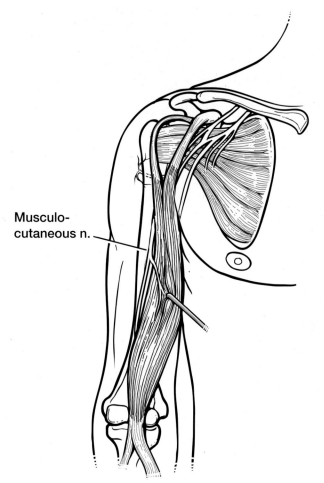

Figure 2-9   The musculocutaneous nerve.

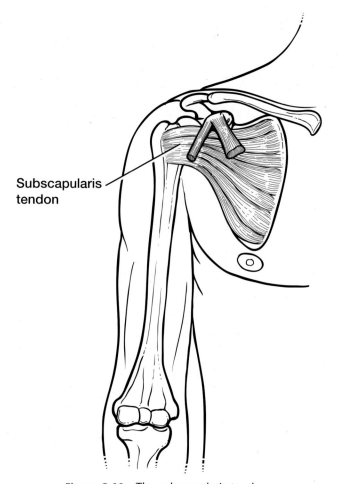

Figure 2-10   The subscapularis tendon.

tuberosity of the humerus (Fig. 2-10). The rotator interval is palpable just superior to the subscapularis tendon and is the site for the initial arthrotomy during shoulder arthroplasty (Fig. 2-11). The long head of the biceps brachii exits the bicipital groove of the humerus, traverses the rotator interval, and inserts on the superior glenoid labrum and supraglenoid tubercle.

Glenohumeral Ligaments and Capsule

After a subscapularis tenotomy, the superior, middle, and inferior glenohumeral ligaments may be visualized, as well as the inferior joint capsule (Fig. 2-12). The posterior joint capsule is more readily visualized after the humeral head is resected (Fig. 2-13).

Rotator Cuff

After dislocation of the humeral head, the articular surface of posterior superior rotator cuff is visible. The "bare area" of the humeral head marks the insertion

of the infraspinatus, with the supraspinatus inserting superior and anterior to the bare area. The teres minor inserts immediately inferior to the infraspinatus and is not readily distinguishable as a distinct tendon separate from the infraspinatus (Fig. 2-14).

Osseous Structures

Relevant osseous anatomy consists of the proximal humerus and glenoid. The native anatomy of both these structures can be distorted by arthritic changes or fractures (Fig. 2-15).

IMPLANTS AND TECHNIQUES

When performing shoulder arthroplasty, it is important to realize that "the shoulder is not the hip." Although some of the implant research and development pertaining to hip arthroplasty is applicable to the shoulder, much of it is not. Similarly, technical

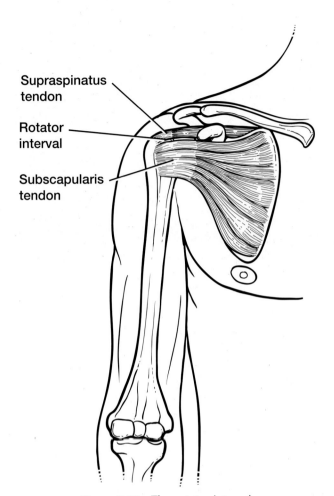

Figure 2-11   The rotator interval.

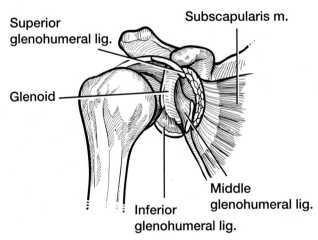

Figure 2-12   Glenohumeral ligaments and joint capsule as visualized through the deltopectoral approach.

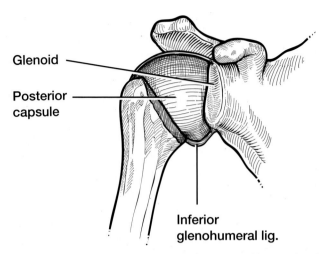

Figure 2-13   The posterior joint capsule is readily visualized after resection of the humeral head.

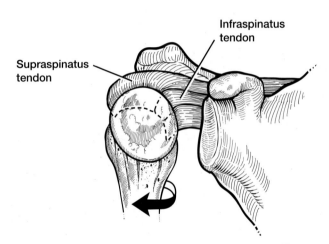

Figure 2-14   The posterior superior rotator cuff.

points of paramount importance during hip arthroplasty are inconsequential in shoulder arthroplasty. Although large forces cross the shoulder during activity, the fact that the shoulder is not a weight-bearing joint accounts for many of these differences.

In total hip arthroplasty, femoral stem loosening has been a problem. Innovations in implants and in insertion techniques have minimized many of these problems. Conversely, the rate of humeral stem loosening is exceptionally low. This low rate of failure has been observed with both cemented and press-fit stems. No single stem type, regardless of fixation or finish type, has proved superior to other types with respect to prosthetic loosening. Additionally, although "third-generation" cementing techniques have proved efficacious in hip arthroplasty, humeral stem loosening is no more prevalent with "finger packing" of cement than with instrumented pressurization.

In contrast to hip arthroplasty, the "socket side" of shoulder arthroplasty has most commonly been the site of failure. Although metal-backed acetabular components in hip arthroplasty have been considered an

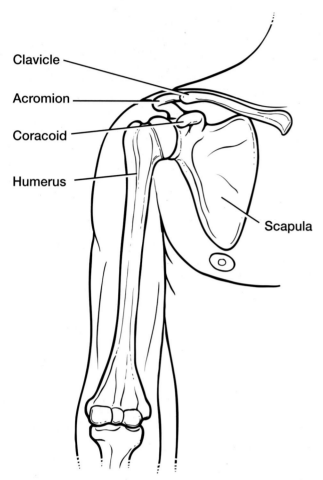

Clavicle

Acromion

Coracoid

Humerus

Scapula

Figure 2-15   Osseous anatomy of the shoulder girdle.

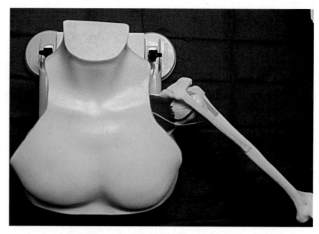

Figure 2-16   Model used for teaching the technique of shoulder arthroplasty at the Joe W. King Invitational Advanced Shoulder Arthroplasty Course.

advance, most metal-backed glenoid components have been disappointing in unconstrained total shoulder arthroplasty.

Overall, it is important for the shoulder arthroplasty surgeon to recognize that the shoulder is a unique joint and that techniques and implants for shoulder arthroplasty are specific to this procedure, not merely extrapolated from those used for lower extremity arthroplasty.

RESOURCES FOR BECOMING A SHOULDER ARTHROPLASTY SURGEON

Many resources are available that attempt to teach shoulder arthroplasty, including courses, instructional videos, textbooks, and Internet resources. Educational courses that aim to teach shoulder arthroplasty, both diverse and specific, are frequently offered by organizations such as the American Academy of Orthopaedic Surgeons (AAOS) and the American Shoulder and Elbow Surgeons (ASES). Additionally, many of the

implant manufacturers offer periodic courses in the use of their implants. Many of these courses provide instruction through lecture and laboratory sessions. Unfortunately, the laboratory sessions of most of these courses provide the surgeon a single opportunity to perform shoulder arthroplasty on a cadaver forequarter or multiple opportunities to perform shoulder arthroplasty on synthetic bones devoid of soft tissue. In our experience, these scenarios are insufficient to adequately teach shoulder arthroplasty. We believe that the best way to learn a skill is by repetition, and performance of a single arthroplasty on a forequarter that is usually poorly held by a metal clamp is suboptimal. We further believe shoulder arthroplasty to be largely a soft tissue operation, thus limiting the usefulness of practice with synthetic bone devoid of soft tissue. To combat these obstacles, in 2004 we began the Joe W. King Invitational Advanced Shoulder Arthroplasty Course. A specially designed shoulder arthroplasty model that includes soft tissues is used to teach by repetition in this course (Fig. 2-16). In addition, after mastering the surgical techniques with the model, each participant performs a shoulder arthroplasty on a full cadaver positioned on an operating table to better replicate reality.

Many instructional videos on shoulder arthroplasty are exhibited each year at the annual meeting of the AAOS. These videos demonstrate a variety of shoulder arthroplasty techniques and are available for purchase through the AAOS. Technical videos demonstrating our preferred techniques are provided with this textbook on a DVD.

Many textbooks contain sections on shoulder arthroplasty, including multiple-volume general orthopedic textbooks, textbooks focusing on the shoulder, and textbooks limited to shoulder arthroplasty. This textbook, modeled after *Shoulder Arthroscopy* by Gartsman, was born out of the practical needs we observed while teaching a course in shoulder arthroplasty. This textbook eliminates much of the theoretical discussion of shoulder arthroplasty in favor of providing practical information that actually assists the surgeon in the technical part of the procedure and postoperative care.

REFERENCE

1. Mendenhall Associates, Inc: A shoulder implant update. Orthopedic News Network 2005;16:11-13.

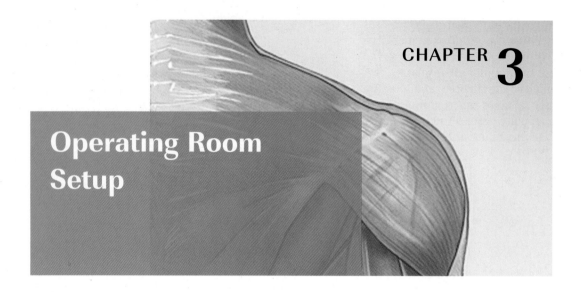

CHAPTER 3

Operating Room Setup

This chapter outlines the organization of the operating room used for shoulder arthroplasty. Organization of the arthroplasty surgical suite focuses on the correct position of equipment, staff, and lights. In addition, all necessary surgical instrumentation must be available.

OPERATING ROOM LAYOUT

A large operating room is preferable when performing shoulder arthroplasty. Larger operating rooms allow a complete set of implants to be stored in the room on a mobile shelving unit to minimize traffic in and out of the operating suite. Our operating suite has two doors: one main door from the hall through which the patient is transported and a second door going into the substerile area. After the patient is placed on the operating table, the main door is locked to further minimize traffic. A view box is used to display radiographs and secondary imaging studies during the procedure so that they can be referenced quickly if necessary (Fig. 3-1).

An overview of the operating room layout is shown in Figure 3-2. The operating table is placed directly under the operating lights and is not angled within the room. Anesthesia equipment is located at the head of the operating table. The electrocautery unit and power source (saw/drill/reamer) are placed on a mobile cart at the foot of the operating table. A Mayo stand is positioned over the patient's lower extremities and comes in from the nonoperative side. Two back tables of equipment are placed on the nonoperative side. The cord for the electrocautery handpiece and the tubing for suction are passed off the foot of the operating

table. Mobile shelving units containing a full set of implants are placed against a wall of the operating room.

STAFF POSITIONING

Figure 3-2 shows the location of each member of the operative team. The operating surgeon stands facing the patient's axilla. The first assistant stands just behind the operative shoulder, facing the surgeon. If available, a second assistant stands on the opposite side of the operating table from the surgeon. The position of the second assistant serves dual purposes: first, it allows the assistant to perform retraction without "crowding" the surgeon, and second, if any observers are present, this allows them to have an unhindered view of the procedure. The surgical technician stands on the nonoperative side of the patient between the back tables and the operating table. If needed in the absence of a second assistant, the surgical technician can use one hand to hold a retractor during selected portions of the procedure.

OVERHEAD LIGHTING

Lighting is critical when performing shoulder arthroplasty. Although some surgeons use accessory lighting (i.e., headlamps) for open shoulder surgery, we have found that proper positioning of the overhead lights precludes the need for such devices. Figure 3-3 demonstrates proper light positioning during shoulder arthroplasty performed by a right hand–dominant surgeon. The main operating room light is positioned

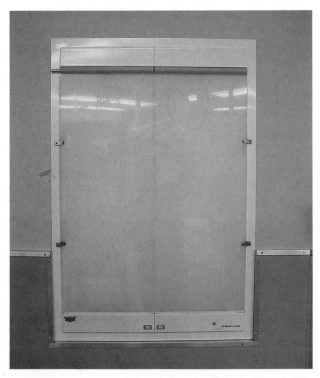

Figure 3-1 Typical radiographic view box available in the operating suite.

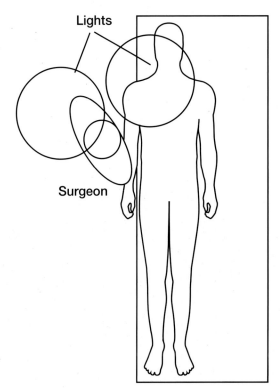

Figure 3-3 Position of the overhead lighting for a right hand–dominant surgeon.

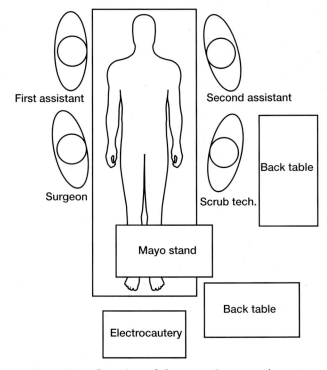

Figure 3-2 Overview of the operating room layout.

just above the surgeon's left shoulder to prevent the surgeon's operating hand from interfering with the light path. The secondary light is positioned on the surgeon's right side more cephalic than the main light. These relationships are reversed for a left hand–dominant surgeon.

SURGICAL INSTRUMENTATION

Figure 3-4 shows the arrangement of instruments placed on the Mayo stand during shoulder arthroplasty. Figures 3-5 and 3-6 show the arrangement of instruments on the back tables. Table 3-1 lists all instruments in our shoulder arthroplasty set along with their use during the procedure. Table 3-2 lists the sutures and disposable instruments that we have available during shoulder arthroplasty. Table 3-3 lists the specific product sets that we use during shoulder arthroplasty.

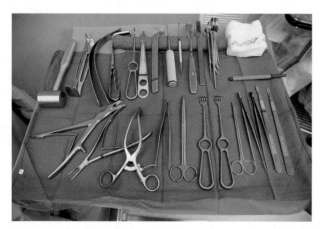

Figure 3-4 Arrangement of instruments placed on the Mayo stand during surgery.

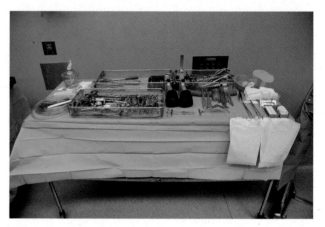

Figure 3-5 Arrangement of instruments on one of the back tables.

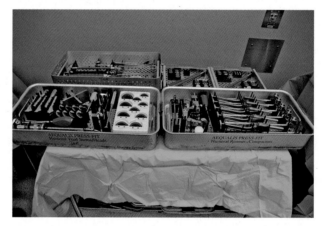

Figure 3-6 Arrangement of instruments on the other back table.

Table 3-1   INSTRUMENTS USED DURING SHOULDER ARTHROPLASTY

Instrument	Quantity	Use	Figure
Forceps			
Vascular forceps	2	Dissection	3-7
Ferris-Smith forceps	2	Dissection	3-8
Adson forceps with teeth	1	Skin closure	3-9
Scissors			
Long curved Metzenbaum scissors	1	Dissection, subscapularis release	3-10
Long curved Mayo scissors	1	Dissection	3-11
Straight Mayo scissors	1	Cutting suture	3-12
Bandage scissors	1	Removal of draping	3-13
Retractors			
Medium skin rake	2	Skin retraction	3-14
Army-Navy retractor	2	Deltopectoral retraction	3-15
Cerebellar retractor	2	Deltopectoral retraction	3-16
Hohmann retractor	4	Proximal retraction, humeral retraction, glenoid retraction	3-17
Narrow Richardson retractor	1	Conjoined tendon retraction	3-18
Small glenoid rim retractor	1	Anterior glenoid retraction	3-19B
Trillat humeral head retractor	1	Humeral retraction during glenoid exposure	3-20
Fukuda humeral head retractor	1	Humeral retraction during glenoid exposure	3-21
Large glenoid rim retractor	1	Humeral retraction during glenoid exposure	3-19A
Special Hohmann retractor	1	Inferior medial humeral retraction during humeral preparation	3-22
Double-pointed Hohmann retractor	1	Inferior glenoid retraction	3-23
Clamps			
Kocher hemostat	2	Sponge removal	3-24A
Kelly hemostat	2	Tagging stay sutures	3-24B
Standard hemostat	6	Tagging stay sutures	3-24C
Mosquito hemostat	2	Tagging stay sutures	3-24D
Lahey clamp	1	Handling of tuberosities during fracture cases	3-25
Towel clips	2	Creation of bone tunnels through hard bone (lesser tuberosity)	3-26
Power Equipment			
Battery-powered sagittal saw	1	Humeral head osteotomy, humeral shaft osteotomy in revision	3-27
Battery-powered drill/reamer	1	Glenoid preparation	3-28

Table 3-1 INSTRUMENTS USED DURING SHOULDER ARTHROPLASTY—cont'd			
Instrument	**Quantity**	**Use**	**Figure**
Miscellaneous			
Long no. 3 knife handle	2	Skin incision, subscapularis tenotomy, biceps tenotomy	3-29
8-Inch Mayo needle holder	2	Suture passage	3-30
Cobb elevator	1	Inferior capsular retraction during inferior capsular release	3-31
$^1/_2$-Inch straight osteotome	1	Removal of humeral osteophytes	3-32
Mallet	1	Removal of humeral osteophytes, insertion of implants	3-33
1-Inch straight osteotome	1	Iliac crest bone graft harvest for glenoid revision	3-34
Freer elevator	1	Removal of excess cement	3-35
$^3/_4$-Inch curved osteotome	1	Iliac crest bone graft harvest for glenoid revision	3-36
Small bone tamp	1	Impaction of bone graft	3-37 *top*
Large bone tamp	1	Impaction of bone graft	3-37 *bottom*
Bone hook	1	Dislocation of proximal humerus after glenoid preparation	3-38
Lamina spreader	1	Distraction between humerus and glenoid for posterior capsule exposure	3-39
Large rongeur	1	Osteophyte removal	3-40A
Small rongeur	1	Osteophyte removal	3-40B
Heavy needle holder	1	Suture passage through hard bone (lesser tuberosity)	3-41
Vise grip pliers with slap hammer	1	Prosthetic removal during revision	3-42
Large Cobb elevator	1	Prosthetic removal during revision	3-43

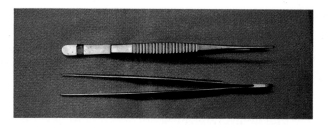

Figure 3-7   Vascular forceps.

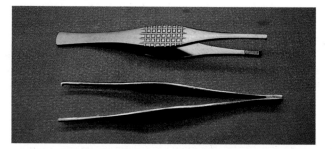

Figure 3-8   Ferris-Smith forceps.

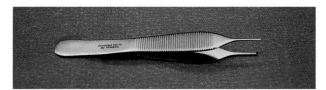

Figure 3-9   Adson forceps with teeth.

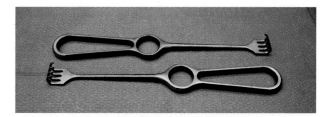

Figure 3-14   Medium skin rake.

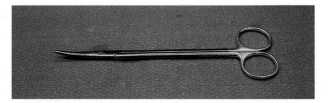

Figure 3-10   Long curved Metzenbaum scissors.

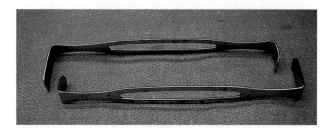

Figure 3-15   Army-Navy retractor.

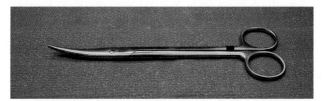

Figure 3-11   Long curved Mayo scissors.

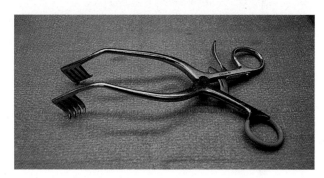

Figure 3-16   Cerebellar retractor.

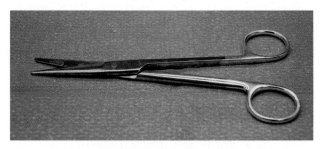

Figure 3-12   Straight Mayo scissors.

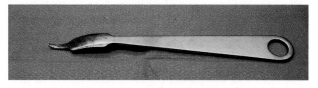

Figure 3-17   Hohmann retractor.

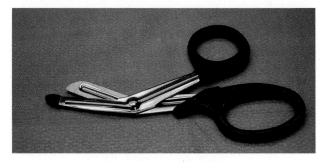

Figure 3-13   Bandage scissors.

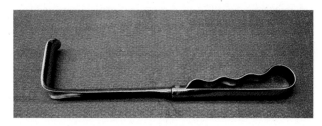

Figure 3-18   Narrow Richardson retractor.

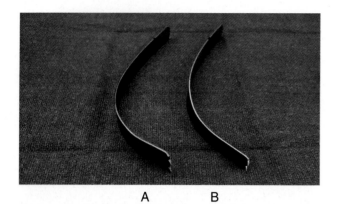

A   B

Figure 3-19   Large glenoid rim retractor **(A)** and small glenoid rim retractor **(B)**.

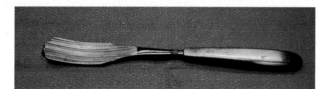

Figure 3-20   Trillat humeral head retractor.

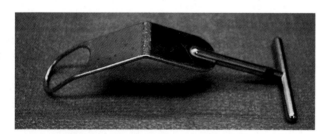

Figure 3-21   Fukuda humeral head retractor.

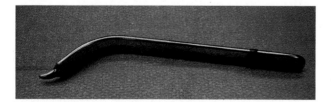

Figure 3-22   Special Hohmann retractor.

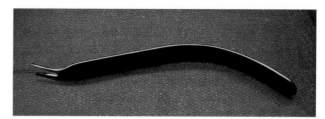

Figure 3-23   Double-pointed Hohmann retractor.

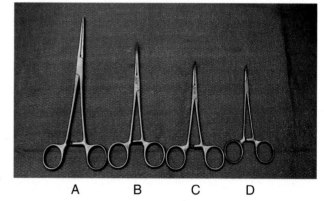

A   B   C   D

Figure 3-24 **A,** Kocher hemostat. **B,** Kelly hemostat. **C,** Standard hemostat. **D,** Mosquito hemostat.

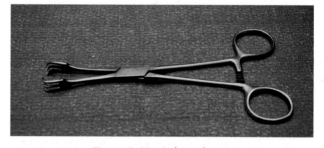

Figure 3-25   Lahey clamp.

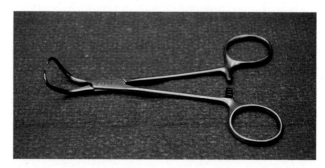

Figure 3-26   Towel clips.

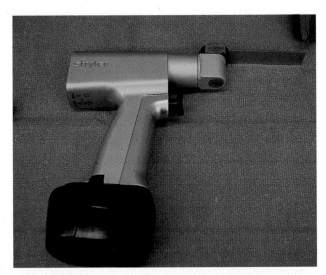

Figure 3-27   Battery-powered sagittal saw.

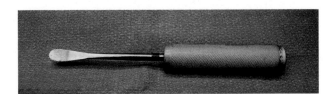

Figure 3-31   Cobb elevator.

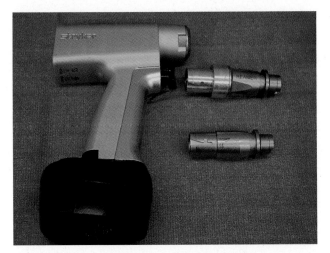

Figure 3-28   Battery-powered drill/reamer.

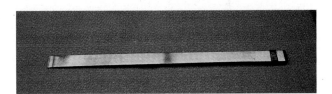

Figure 3-32   ¹/₂-Inch straight osteotome.

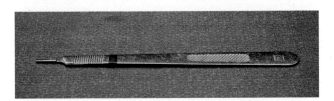

Figure 3-29   Long no. 3 knife handle.

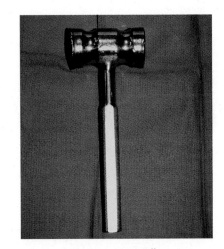

Figure 3-33   Mallet.

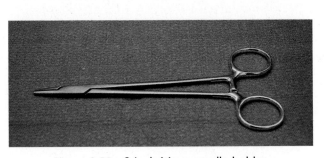

Figure 3-30   8-Inch Mayo needle holder.

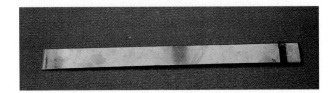

Figure 3-34   1-Inch straight osteotome.

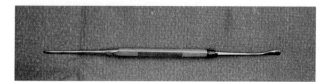

Figure 3-35 Freer elevator.

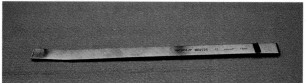

Figure 3-36 ³/₄-Inch curved osteotome.

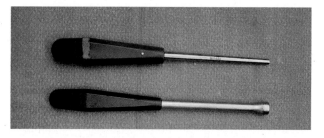

Figure 3-37 Small bone tamp (*top*) and large bone tamp (*bottom*).

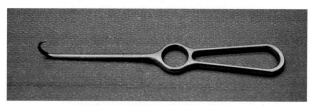

Figure 3-38 Bone hook.

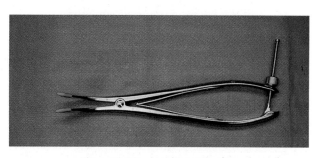

Figure 3-39 Lamina spreader.

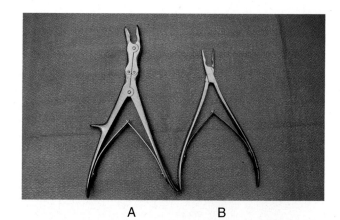

A   B

Figure 3-40 Large rongeur **(A)** and small rongeur **(B)**.

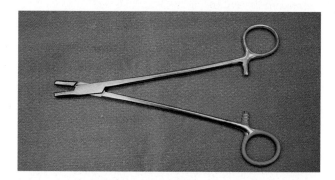

Figure 3-41 Heavy needle holder.

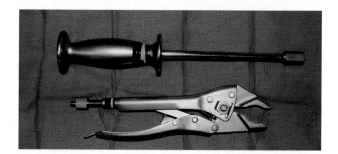

Figure 3-42 Vise grip pliers with slap hammer.

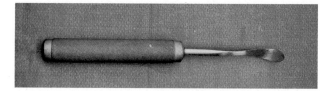

Figure 3-43 Large Cobb elevator.

Table 3-2 DISPOSABLE INSTRUMENTS AND SUTURE USED DURING SHOULDER ARTHROPLASTY

Instrument	Quantity	Use	Figure
Suture			
No. 0 Vicryl (taper needle)	3	Hemostasis, wound closure	3-44
No. 2 Ethibond (taper needle)	1-7	Subscapularis stay suture, fixation of biologic glenoid resurfacing	3-44
No. 2 Fiberwire (taper needle)	3-6	Subscapularis closure, tuberosity fixation	3-44
No. 1 Vicryl (taper needle)	1-4	Subscapularis closure, posterior capsulorrhaphy	3-44
2-0 Vicryl	1	Wound closure	3-44
3-0 PDS	1	Wound closure	3-44
Skin stapler	1	Wound closure (revision cases)	3-45
Miscellaneous			
Saw blade	1	Humeral head osteotomy	3-46
Electrocautery with needle tip	1	Hemostasis, dissection	3-47
Suction tip with tubing	1	Visualization	3-48
Bulb syringe	1	Irrigation	3-49
Catheter tip 60-mL syringe	1	Cement application	3-50

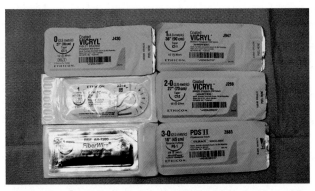

Figure 3-44   Suture packages.

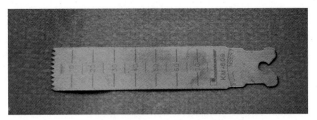

Figure 3-46   Saw blade.

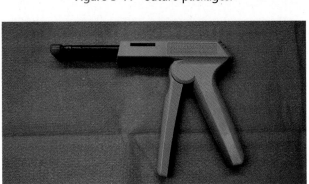

Figure 3-45   Skin stapler.

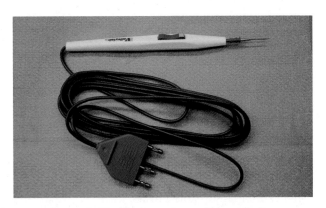

Figure 3-47   Electrocautery with needle tip.

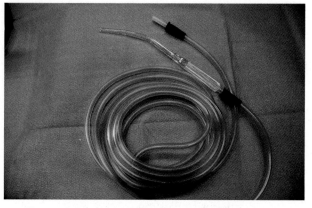

Figure 3-48 Suction tip with tubing.

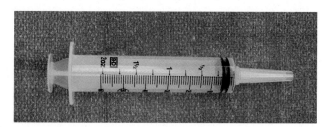

Figure 3-50 Catheter tip 60-mL syringe.

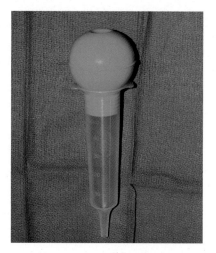

Figure 3-49 Bulb syringe.

Table 3-3	SPECIFIC INSTRUMENT SETS AVAILABLE DURING SHOULDER ARTHROPLASTY		
Set	**Manufacturer**	**Use**	**Figure**
Press-fit unconstrained humeral head replacement set	Tornier	Unconstrained shoulder arthroplasty	3-51
Keel/peg glenoid set	Tornier	Unconstrained shoulder arthroplasty	3-52
Cemented unconstrained humeral head replacement set	Tornier	Unconstrained shoulder arthroplasty	3-53
Reverse shoulder arthroplasty set	Tornier	Semiconstrained shoulder arthroplasty	3-54
Fracture arthroplasty set	Tornier	Unconstrained shoulder arthroplasty for fracture	3-55
Long-stem fracture arthroplasty set	Tornier	Unconstrained revision shoulder arthroplasty	3-56
Long-stem reverse shoulder arthroplasty set	Tornier	Semiconstrained revision shoulder arthroplasty	3-57
Cerclage cable set	Kinamed	Fixation of humeral osteotomy during revision	3-58
4.0-mm cannulated screw set	Synthese	Fixation of bone graft in uncontained glenoid defect	3-59
SmartPin bioabsorbable pin set	Linvatec	Fixation of bone graft in uncontained glenoid defect	3-60

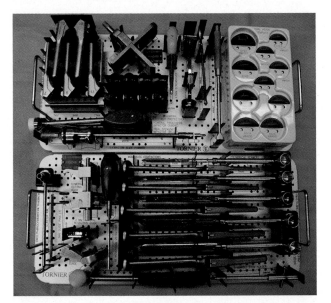

Figure 3-51 Press-fit unconstrained humeral head replacement set.

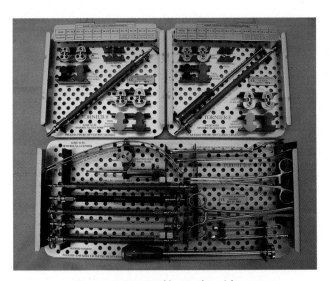

Figure 3-52 Keel/peg glenoid set.

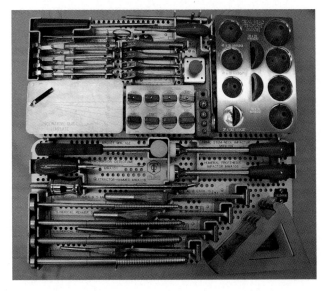

Figure 3-53 Cemented unconstrained humeral head replacement set.

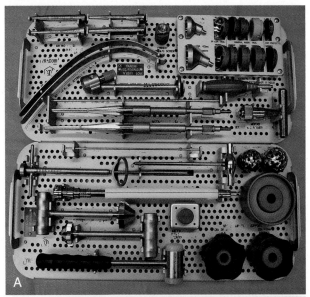

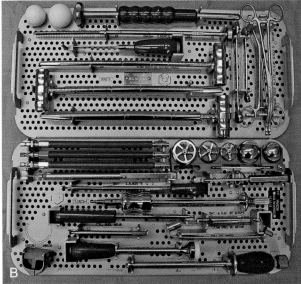

Figure 3-54 Reverse shoulder arthroplasty set.

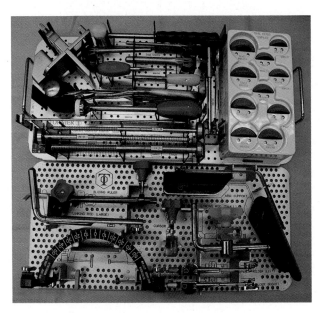

Figure 3-55 Fracture arthroplasty set.

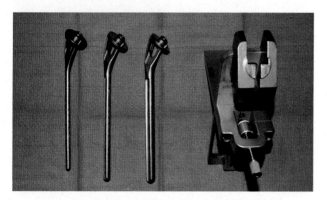

Figure 3-56 Long-stem fracture arthroplasty set.

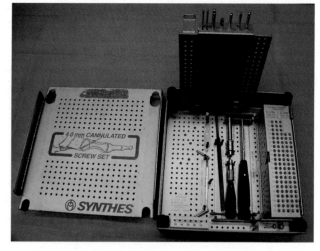

Figure 3-59 4.0-mm cannulated screw set.

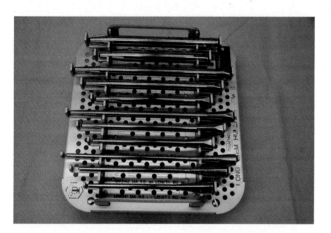

Figure 3-57 Long-stem reverse shoulder arthroplasty set.

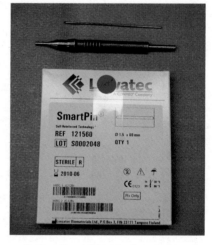

Figure 3-60 SmartPin bioabsorbable pin set.

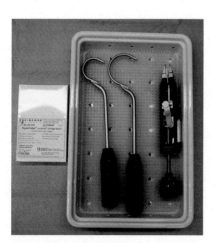

Figure 3-58 Cerclage cable set.

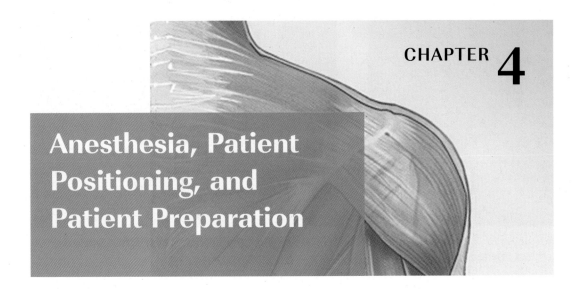

CHAPTER **4**

Anesthesia, Patient Positioning, and Patient Preparation

This chapter reviews the anesthesia used for shoulder replacement surgery. Additionally, proper patient positioning and surgical preparation and draping are described.

ANESTHESIA*

Provided that no contraindication exists, all of our shoulder arthroplasty patients undergo a preoperative interscalene block administered in the preoperative holding area by an anesthesiologist. The interscalene block serves two purposes. First, use of the block minimizes the amount of general anesthetic needed during surgery, and second, it aids in postoperative pain management. Our anesthesiologists use a posterior approach and insert an indwelling brachial plexus catheter that is maintained for up to 48 hours after surgery (Fig. 4-1).[1] General anesthesia, as well as neuromuscular paralytic agents, is then administered to all patients. Neuromuscular paralysis greatly facilitates exposure during glenoid resurfacing and can be discontinued after implantation of the glenoid component.

*The authors would like to acknowledge and thank Gurunath Sigireddi, MD, and Steve T. Boozalis, MD, of Greater Houston Anesthesiology and the Department of Anesthesiology at Texas Orthopedic Hospital, for their assistance with the Anesthesia section of this chapter.

PATIENT POSITIONING

Proper patient positioning is crucial during shoulder arthroplasty. We use a standard operating table with the patient positioned sufficiently to the operative side to allow extension of the arm (Fig. 4-2). A rolled sheet is placed between the scapulae to slightly elevate the shoulder off the operating table and allow proper surgical preparation of the posterior aspect of the shoulder (Fig. 4-3). The use of certain types of operating tables developed for shoulder arthroscopy, in which the portion of the table posterior to the scapula is removed, is discouraged because these tables inhibit control of the scapula and thus make glenoid exposure difficult.

The patient is placed in the modified beach chair position. To obtain the proper position, the operating table is first reflexed (Fig. 4-4) and the patient's knees are flexed (Fig. 4-5). The patient is then placed in a slight Trendelenburg position to prevent sliding inferiorly on the operating table (Fig. 4-6). Finally, the back of the operating table is elevated approximately 45 to 60 degrees relative to the floor (Fig. 4-7). The position of the patient's head and neck is checked to ensure neutral alignment. Occasionally, it is necessary to slightly flex the head portion of the operating table to eliminate cervical extension. Once cervical alignment and the head position are acceptable, the forehead and chin are secured with 1-inch silk adhesive tape as shown in Figure 4-8. In patients with fragile skin, a dry gauze pad is used to minimize tape contact

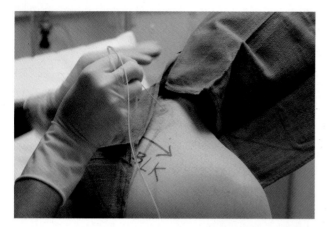

Figure 4-1 Patient undergoing a preoperative brachial plexus block with the catheter inserted through a posterior approach.

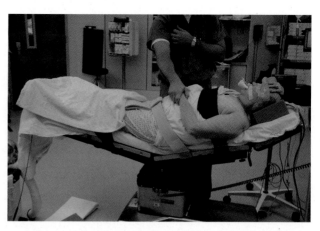

Figure 4-4 The operating table is first reflexed.

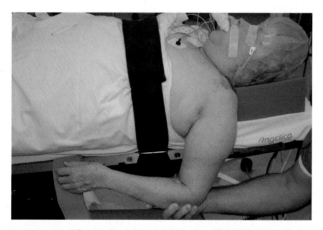

Figure 4-2 The patient is positioned sufficiently laterally on the operating table to allow full arm extension.

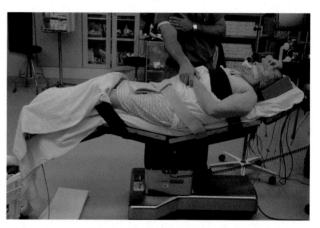

Figure 4-5 The patient's knees are flexed.

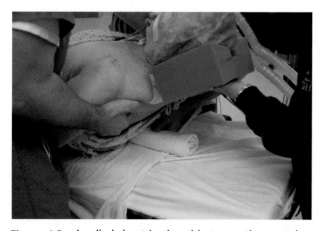

Figure 4-3 A rolled sheet is placed between the scapulae.

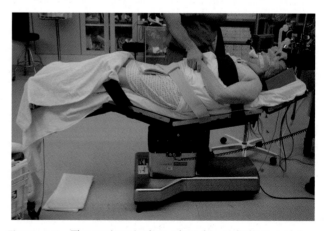

Figure 4-6 The patient is then placed in a slight Trendelenburg position to prevent sliding inferiorly on the operating table.

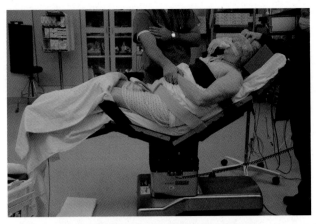

Figure 4-7 The back of the operating table is elevated approximately 45 to 60 degrees with respect to the floor.

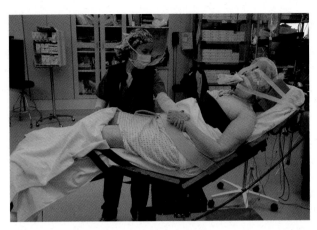

Figure 4-9 Final patient position before skin preparation.

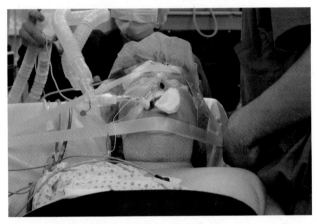

Figure 4-8 The forehead and chin are secured with 1-inch silk adhesive tape.

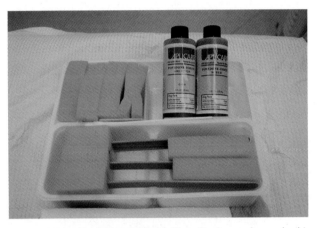

Figure 4-10 Povidone-iodine (Betadine) scrub and skin preparation.

and prevent skin tears. Care should be taken to pad and protect bony prominences and sites of subcutaneous vulnerable nerves near the elbow (ulnar) and knee (peroneal). Figure 4-9 shows the final position of the patient before skin preparation.

SURGICAL PREPARATION AND DRAPING

Skin preparation begins the day before surgery. We advise the patient to shave the affected shoulder girdle and axilla; it is not necessary to shave the arm below the elbow. Shaving the surgical area a day in advance allows any skin irritation caused by shaving to subside. Patients are also advised to bathe with an antibacterial soap the morning of surgery before coming to the hospital. Once in the operating room, the skin of the affected upper extremity and shoulder girdle is cleaned

with isopropyl alcohol. A povidone-iodine (Betadine) scrub is then performed. The surgical area is dried with towels and painted with a Betadine solution (Fig. 4-10). In patients with allergy or hypersensitivity to Betadine, a scrub with 4% chlorhexidine gluconate solution (Betasept) is performed (Fig. 4-11). The scrub solution is removed with sterile water and an isopropyl alcohol preparation is applied. The area included in the surgical preparation extends medially to the midline, distally to the level of the nipple, and proximally to the level of the mandible and encompasses the entire upper extremity, including the hand (Fig. 4-12).

Draping is initiated by the assistant's draping the patient's hand with an impermeable stockinet (Fig. 4-13). A reinforced disposable paper drape is placed from the inferior aspect of the surgical field and extended over the torso and lower extremities to

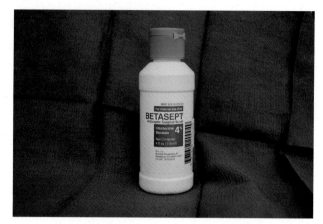

Figure 4-11 Chlorhexidine gluconate (Betasept) solution used for surgical scrub in patients with an allergy or hypersensitivity to Betadine.

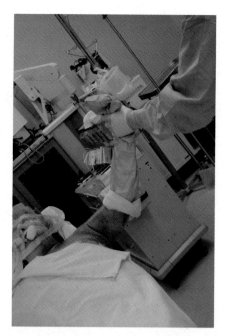

Figure 4-13   Placement of an impermeable stockinet.

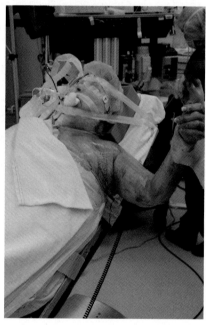

Figure 4-12 Completed skin preparation extending medially to the midline, distally to the level of the nipple, proximally to the level of the mandible, and including the entire upper extremity.

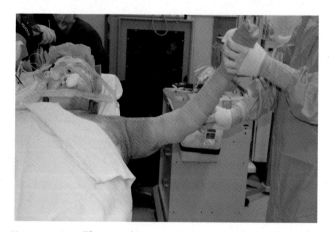

Figure 4-14 The stockinet is secured with a disposable elastic wrap.

prevent contamination of the operative team during the remainder of the draping. The stockinet is rolled proximally, past the elbow in most cases, and is covered and secured with disposable elastic wrap (Fig. 4-14). In cases in which direct palpation of the humeral epicondyles is necessary, such as hemiarthroplasty with a fracture jig, the stockinet covers only the hand and forearm. A towel is used to dry an area circumferentially around the shoulder to allow the ensuing "U" drapes to adhere to the skin (Fig. 4-15). A disposable

impermeable "U" drape is placed inferiorly to superiorly, with the two limbs of the drape meeting superiorly (Fig. 4-16). A large disposable reinforced paper "U" drape is applied inferiorly to superiorly (Fig. 4-17). A smaller disposable paper "U" drape is placed superiorly to inferiorly (Fig. 4-18). The remaining exposed skin in the surgical field, including the axillary skin, is dried with a towel. In patients with previous surgical incisions, skin scars are marked with a skin-marking pen (Fig. 4-19). An occlusive adhesive drape is applied to the shoulder to effectively remove the axilla from the surgical field. We prefer the occlusive drape to be impregnated with Betadine; however, in patients with

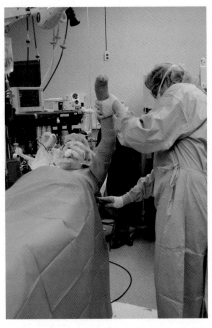

Figure 4-15 The area around the shoulder is dried to allow adhesion of the operative drapes.

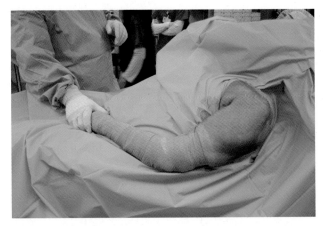

Figure 4-16 A disposable impermeable "U" drape is placed inferiorly to superiorly with the two limbs of the drape meeting superiorly.

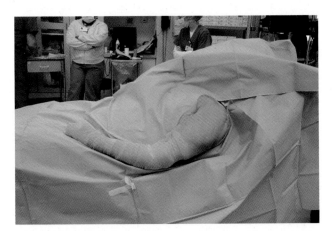

Figure 4-17 A large disposable reinforced paper "U" drape is applied inferiorly to superiorly.

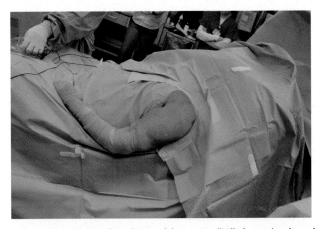

Figure 4-18 A smaller disposable paper "U" drape is placed superiorly to inferiorly.

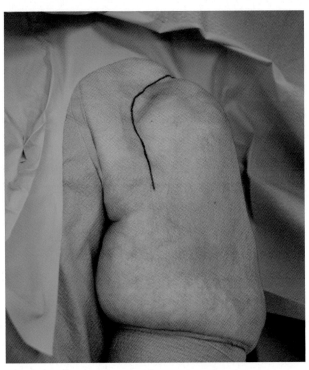

Figure 4-19 Previous incisions are marked with a sterile marking pen.

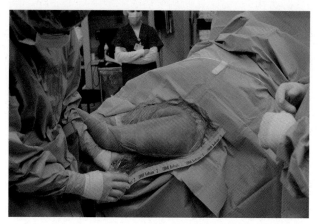

Figure 4-20   Placement of an occlusive adhesive drape with the arm abducted to allow isolation of the axilla from the operative field.

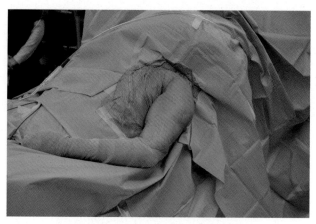

Figure 4-21   Final draping.

Betadine allergy or hypersensitivity, we use a non–Betadine-impregnated version of the same drape. The occlusive drape is applied by first securing the drape to the posterior aspect of the shoulder. The arm is then abducted and externally rotated as the occlusive drape is placed anteriorly initially and then around the arm to cover the axilla (Fig. 4-20). Final patient positioning and draping are shown in Figure 4-21.

REFERENCE

1. Sandefo I, Iohom G, Van Elstraete A, et al: Clinical efficacy of the brachial plexus block via the posterior approach. Reg Anesth Pain Med 2005;30:238-242.

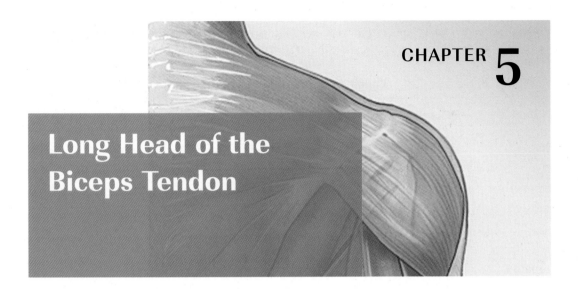

CHAPTER 5

Long Head of the Biceps Tendon

Historically, the functional role of the long head of the biceps tendon has been controversial. Viewpoints have ranged from the biceps' being a critical structural restraint to superior migration of the humeral head, to its being a vestigial structure that has little if any functional role in the shoulder. More recently, the long head of the biceps has been implicated as a source of pain in patients with rotator cuff tears and in those with continued pain after shoulder arthroplasty performed for a proximal humeral fracture.[1,2]

In our patients undergoing shoulder arthroplasty, we have noted gross abnormalities of the long head of the biceps tendon in 61%. Table 5-1 details bicipital abnormalities observed at the time of shoulder arthroplasty by diagnosis.

Handling of the long head of the biceps tendon during shoulder arthroplasty has ranged from systematic preservation to systematic tenotomy or tenodesis regardless of its condition. In a series of 688 shoulder arthroplasties performed for primary osteoarthritis, concomitant biceps tenodesis or tenotomy was shown to improve outcomes. In this series, 121 shoulders underwent biceps tenodesis or tenotomy at the time of shoulder arthroplasty, independent of the condition of the biceps. These patients demonstrated a significantly higher postoperative mean activity score, mean mobility score, mean total Constant score, mean active anterior elevation, and mean active external rotation and better subjective results than did patients not undergoing concomitant biceps surgery.[3] Fewer radiolucencies were reported around the glenoid component in shoulders that had undergone biceps tenotomy or tenodesis. Importantly, the incidence of complications was not affected by cutting the long head of the biceps tendon.

Based largely on the findings of the aforementioned study, our preference is to systematically remove the intra-articular portion of the biceps tendon at the time of shoulder arthroplasty in all cases. We do not recognize the long head of the biceps tendon as being essential to normal shoulder function after arthroplasty. We view cutting the biceps at the time of shoulder arthroplasty as akin to a general surgeon's performance of appendectomy during another abdominal procedure; even if the structure appears normal, it serves no critical function and could eventually cause a problem, so it is removed.

In our practice, the decision to perform tenodesis or tenotomy of the long head of the biceps is based on patient age, body habitus, and cosmetic concerns. We have anecdotally observed no differences in pain relief or function between tenodesis and tenotomy. In younger patients, thin patients, and those concerned about the appearance of their arm, we opt for biceps tenodesis. In patients not fitting these criteria, biceps tenotomy is sufficient and takes less operative time.

TECHNIQUE FOR HANDLING THE LONG HEAD OF THE BICEPS TENDON

The long head of the biceps tendon may be addressed any time it is visualized during shoulder arthroplasty. In most cases, we remove the intra-articular portion of the biceps just after preparation of the humerus and immediately before preparation of the glenoid because it is easily visualized at this junction of the procedure. Additionally, in some cases the long head of the biceps tendon may be contracted or lacks normal excursion. This could potentially hinder glenoid exposure, so the

Table 5-1   **CONDITION OF THE LONG HEAD OF THE BICEPS TENDON IN CASES OF SHOULDER ARTHROPLASTY PERFORMED AT TEXAS ORTHOPEDIC HOSPITAL FROM 2003 TO 2005**

	Condition of the Long Head of the Biceps Tendon			
Diagnosis	Normal	Rupture	Partial Tear/Synovitis	Spontaneous Tenodesis
Primary osteoarthritis	63	3	41	0
Acute fracture	4	1	14	0
Rotator cuff tear arthropathy	4	31	11	2
Atraumatic osteonecrosis	5	3	3	0
Instability arthropathy	9	2	9	0
Rheumatoid arthritis	1	7	1	0
Post-traumatic arthropathy	10	11	5	0
Revision arthroplasty	3	9	3	1
Miscellaneous diagnoses	4	0	3	1
Total	103	67	90	4

tendon is released before glenoid preparation. However, in fracture cases treated by hemiarthroplasty, the long head of the biceps tendon is left intact as an anatomic point of reference until just before fixation of the tuberosities.

After humeral head resection and proximal humeral preparation, large curved Mayo scissors are placed superior and posterior to the long head of the biceps tendon to allow visualization of the tendon as it enters the bicipital groove (Fig. 5-1). A scalpel is used to transect the tendon at the entrance of the bicipital groove (Fig. 5-2). The tendon is pulled out of the bicipital groove inferiorly and sutured to the pectoralis major tendon with a figure-of-eight no. 1 nonabsorbable braided suture if tenodesis is to be performed (Fig. 5-3). Residual tendon is sharply removed to complete the tenodesis (Fig. 5-4). When the humeral head is retracted posteriorly for glenoid exposure, the remaining intra-articular stump of the long head of the biceps tendon is removed with Mayo scissors (Fig. 5-5). In cases of obvious tenosynovitis, any remaining bicipital sheath is removed as well.

In fracture cases, the long head of the biceps tendon is released from its insertion at the supraglenoid tubercle with curved Mayo scissors just before tuberosity fixation and then undergoes tenodesis, if applicable, via the same technique described earlier.

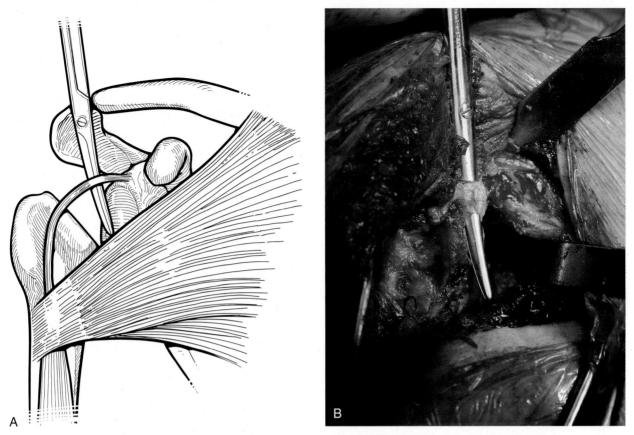

Figure 5-1 **A** and **B,** Large curved Mayo scissors are placed superior and posterior to the long head of the biceps tendon to allow visualization of the tendon as it enters the bicipital groove.

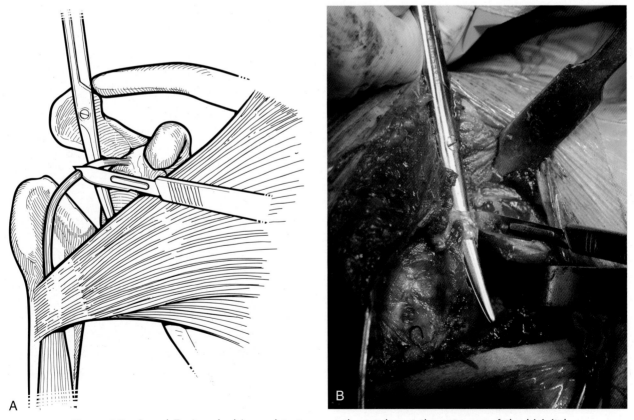

Figure 5-2 **A** and **B,** A scalpel is used to transect the tendon at the entrance of the bicipital groove.

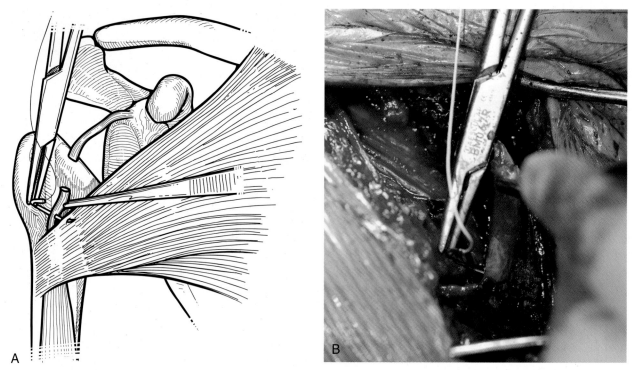

Figure 5-3 **A** and **B,** The long head of the biceps tendon is pulled out of the bicipital groove inferiorly and sutured to the pectoralis major tendon with a figure-of-eight no. 1 nonabsorbable braided suture.

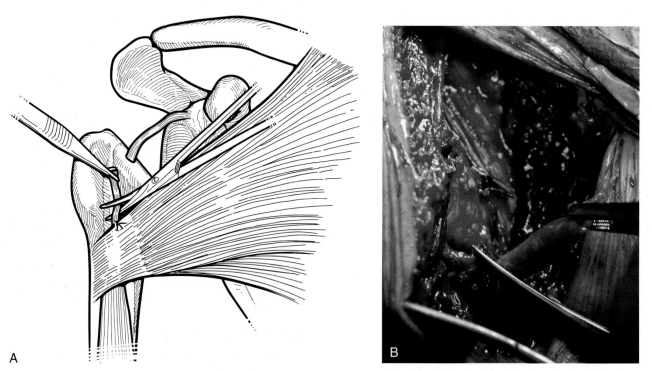

Figure 5-4 **A** and **B,** Residual tendon is sharply removed to complete the tenodesis.

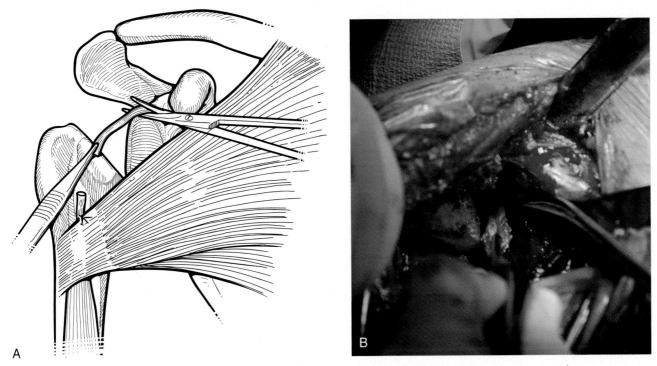

Figure 5-5 **A** and **B,** With the humeral head retracted posteriorly for glenoid exposure, the remaining intra-articular stump of the long head of the biceps tendon is removed with Mayo scissors.

REFERENCES

1. Walch G, Edwards TB, Nové-Josserand L, et al: Arthroscopic tenotomy of the long head of the biceps in the treatment of rotator cuff tears: Clinical and radiographic results of 307 cases. J Shoulder Elbow Surg 2005;14:238-246.
2. Dines D, Hersch J: Long head of the biceps lesions after shoulder arthroplasty. Paper presented at the 8th International Congress on Surgery of the Shoulder, April 2001, Cape Town, South Africa.
3. Fama G, Edwards TB, Boulahia A, et al: The role of concomitant biceps tenodesis in shoulder arthroplasty for primary osteoarthritis: Results of a multicentric study. Orthopedics 2004;27:401-405.

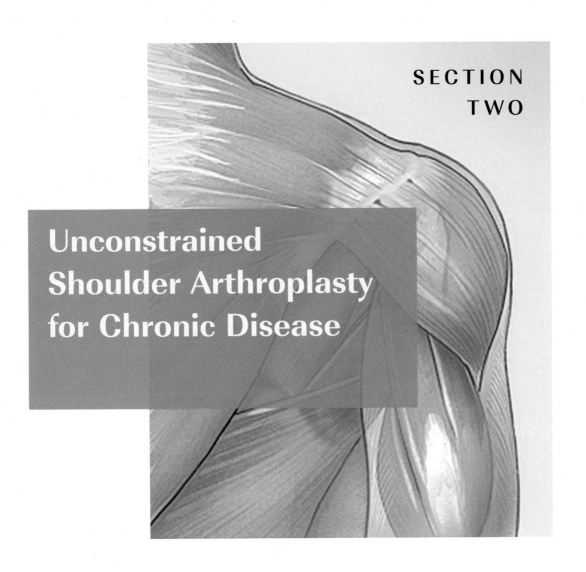

Unconstrained Shoulder Arthroplasty for Chronic Disease

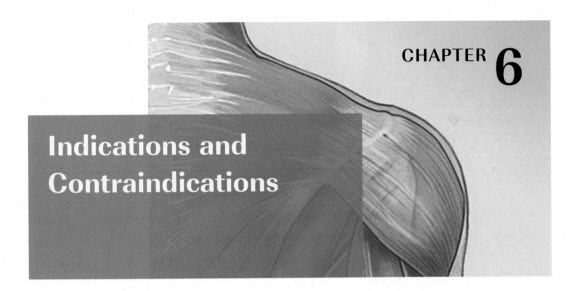

CHAPTER 6

Indications and Contraindications

Indications for unconstrained shoulder arthroplasty can be divided into arthroplasty performed for acute fracture and arthroplasty performed for chronic shoulder disease. This chapter focuses on indications for unconstrained shoulder arthroplasty in patients with chronic shoulder disease. Indications for unconstrained shoulder arthroplasty in patients with an acute fracture are covered in Chapter 17.

Multiple chronic indications for unconstrained shoulder arthroplasty include, but are not limited to, primary osteoarthritis, inflammatory arthropathies, humeral head osteonecrosis, instability arthropathy, post-traumatic arthritis, fixed glenohumeral dislocation, rotator cuff tear arthropathy (glenohumeral arthritis with a massive rotator cuff tear), postinfectious arthropathy, glenohumeral chondrolysis, proximal humeral fracture nonunion, glenohumeral arthritis associated with neurologic pathology, glenohumeral arthritis associated with previous radiation therapy, glenohumeral arthritis associated with skeletal dysplasia, and tumor. This chapter looks at unique characteristics and special considerations for each of these indications. Additionally, indications for total shoulder arthroplasty versus hemiarthroplasty are discussed, and contraindications to unconstrained shoulder arthroplasty are detailed.

HEMIARTHROPLASTY VERSUS TOTAL SHOULDER ARTHROPLASTY: INDICATIONS FOR GLENOID RESURFACING

Indications for glenoid resurfacing in unconstrained shoulder arthroplasty are a much debated topic. We

currently favor total shoulder arthroplasty because the results are superior and the complication rate is equal to or lower than that seen in hemiarthroplasty. Our decision to perform glenoid resurfacing or not is detailed according to diagnosis in the following sections.

Two major requirements exist for performance of glenoid resurfacing in unconstrained shoulder arthroplasty: the glenoid bone must be sufficient to allow implantation of components (judged by preoperative imaging studies; see Chapter 7), and the anterior and posterior rotator cuff must be functioning (judged by clinical examination and preoperative imaging studies; see Chapter 7).[1] Lack of either of these requirements represents an absolute contraindication to glenoid resurfacing. A relative contraindication to glenoid resurfacing is young patient age. A "safe" age at which to implant a polyethylene glenoid component has not been established. Concerns of polyethylene wear are heightened in younger patients because of their residual life expectancy. In general, we favor biologic glenoid resurfacing in patients younger than 40 years in whom total shoulder arthroplasty would otherwise be indicated.

PRIMARY OSTEOARTHRITIS

Primary osteoarthritis was initially described by Neer and is the most common single indication for shoulder arthroplasty in our practice.[2] In a large multicenter study, primary osteoarthritis was the underlying cause in half of the primary shoulder arthroplasties performed.[3]

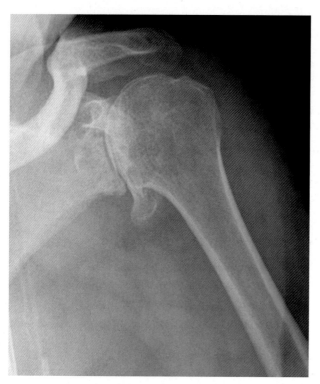

Figure 6-1 Radiograph of primary osteoarthritis showing the typical loss of the glenohumeral joint space and the presence of large humeral osteophytes.

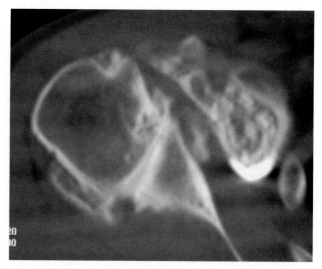

Figure 6-2 Large loose body in the subscapularis fossa in a patient with primary osteoarthritis.

Clinical Findings

Clinical findings in patients with primary osteoarthritis include glenohumeral crepitus and stiffness. Rotator cuff testing may be normal or compromised by pain.

Imaging Findings

Plain radiography demonstrates loss of the normal glenohumeral joint space. Humeral head osteophytes are usually present and may be large (Fig. 6-1). Loose bodies may be apparent on plain radiography, especially in the subscapularis recess (Fig. 6-2).

Secondary imaging studies (computed tomographic arthrography, magnetic resonance imaging) will show the "classic" posterior glenoid erosion with biconcavity in only 20% of cases (Fig. 6-3).[3] Approximately half of patients with primary osteoarthritis will have the humeral head centered within the glenoid, and another 25% will demonstrate posterior subluxation without osseous erosion (Fig. 6-4).[3] Less than 5% of patients with primary osteoarthritis will demonstrate a dysplastic-appearing glenoid morphology (Fig. 6-5).[3]

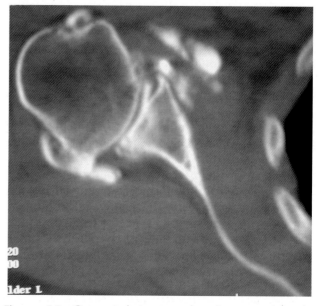

Figure 6-3 Computed tomography demonstrating the "classic" biconcave glenoid seen in primary osteoarthritis.

Seven percent of patients with primary osteoarthritis have a full-thickness rotator cuff tear limited to the supraspinatus, and an additional 7% have a partial-thickness rotator cuff tear.[4] Moreover, moderate to severe fatty infiltration of the infraspinatus or subscapularis (or both) occurs in approximately 20% of patients with primary osteoarthritis.[4]

Special Considerations

We perform total shoulder arthroplasty in nearly all cases of primary osteoarthritis because it has been

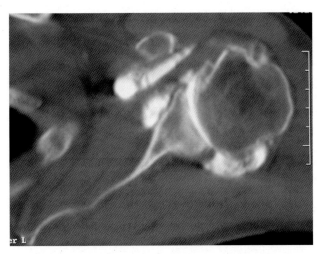

Figure 6-4 Computed tomography showing the more common posterior humeral head subluxation without the osseous glenoid erosion seen in primary osteoarthritis.

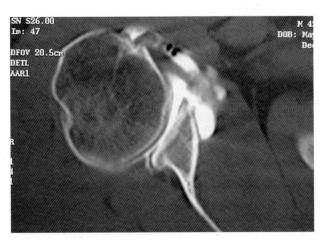

Figure 6-5 Dysplastic glenoid morphology seen rarely in primary osteoarthritis. Note the excessive glenoid retroversion present with a relatively well centered humeral head.

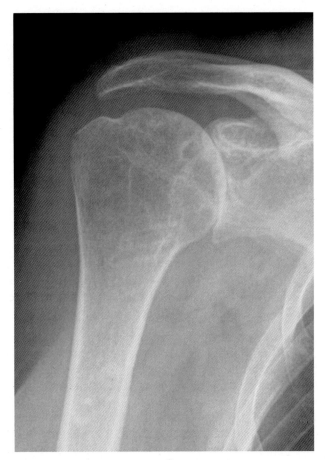

Figure 6-6 Radiograph of rheumatoid arthritis showing the typical loss of the glenohumeral joint space and a paucity of humeral osteophytes.

shown to be superior to hemiarthroplasty without an increased risk of complications or reoperations.[5,6] The only patients with primary osteoarthritis in whom we perform hemiarthroplasty are those with insufficient glenoid bone or anterior or posterior rotator cuff insufficiency. In patients with rotator cuff insufficiency, we usually opt for a reverse-design prosthesis instead of a hemiarthroplasty (see Section Four).

RHEUMATOID ARTHRITIS

Rheumatoid arthritis is the most common inflammatory joint disease. Shoulder manifestations develop in 60% to 90% of patients as their disease progresses. In a large multicenter study, rheumatoid arthritis was the underlying cause in 12% of the primary shoulder arthroplasties performed.[7]

Clinical Findings

Clinical findings in patients with rheumatoid arthritis include glenohumeral crepitus and stiffness. Rotator cuff testing may be normal, compromised by pain, or compromised by a rotator cuff tear.

Imaging Findings

Plain radiography demonstrates loss of the normal glenohumeral joint space. Humeral head osteophytes are rarely present (Fig. 6-6). The humeral head may be centered or statically migrated, depending on the condition of the rotator cuff.

Secondary imaging studies (computed tomographic arthrography, magnetic resonance imaging) may show

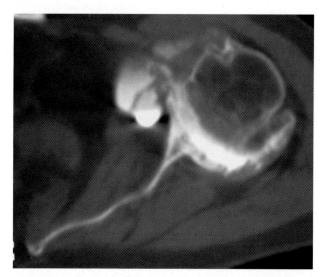

Figure 6-7   Computed tomogram demonstrating a protrusio-type glenoid morphology seen in rheumatoid arthritis.

protrusio-type glenoid morphology (Fig. 6-7). Eight percent of patients with rheumatoid arthritis have a full-thickness rotator cuff tear limited to the supraspinatus, and an additional 9% have a partial-thickness supraspinatus tear.[8] Twelve percent of patients with rheumatoid arthritis have massive rotator cuff tears involving the supraspinatus and infraspinatus tendons.[8] Additionally, moderate to severe fatty infiltration of the infraspinatus or the subscapularis (or both) occurs in approximately 45% of patients with rheumatoid arthritis.[8]

Special Considerations

We perform total shoulder arthroplasty in nearly all cases of rheumatoid arthritis because it has been shown to be superior to hemiarthroplasty.[9] The only patients with rheumatoid arthritis in whom we perform hemiarthroplasty are those with insufficient glenoid bone or anterior or posterior rotator cuff insufficiency. In patients with rotator cuff insufficiency, we usually opt for a reverse-design prosthesis instead of a hemiarthroplasty, provided the patient does not have severe osteopenia (see Section Four).

A rare subtype of rheumatoid arthritis that rarely requires shoulder arthroplasty but merits special consideration is juvenile-onset rheumatoid arthritis. In our limited experience, these patients tend to have severe preoperative stiffness that may require more soft tissue releases than normal, including release of the entire pectoralis major. Additionally, the humerus and glenoid may be exceptionally small and thus necessitate the use of custom-manufactured implants.

OTHER INFLAMMATORY ARTHROPATHIES

Other inflammatory arthropathies affecting the glenohumeral joint sufficiently to require shoulder arthroplasty are rare and include Paget's disease, ankylosing spondylitis, psoriatic arthritis, systemic lupus erythematosus, scleroderma, and polymyalgia rheumatica. Unfortunately, because of the relative rarity of these conditions, little information is available regarding special considerations for these diseases. When any of these conditions evolve to complete loss of articular cartilage and fail reasonable nonoperative treatment, shoulder arthroplasty may be considered. Provided that the rotator cuff is competent and sufficient glenoid bone stock exists, we opt to resurface the glenoid in these patients.

HUMERAL HEAD OSTEONECROSIS

Although humeral head osteonecrosis is rare, it is the most common nontraumatic indication for shoulder hemiarthroplasty in our practice. In a large multicenter study, osteonecrosis was the underlying cause in only 5% of the primary shoulder arthroplasties performed.[10] Many factors have been implicated as contributing to atraumatic osteonecrosis, including corticosteroid use, alcohol abuse, and hematologic disorders. Despite the influence of these factors, most cases of humeral head osteonecrosis are idiopathic.

Clinical Findings

Clinical findings in patients with atraumatic osteonecrosis range from solely subjective complaints of pain to glenohumeral crepitus and stiffness such as seen in primary osteoarthritis. Rotator cuff testing is usually normal but may be compromised by pain, especially in the later stages.

Imaging Findings

Radiographic classification of humeral head osteonecrosis has evolved from that described for the femoral head.[11,12] Stage I is a preradiographic stage that requires diagnosis by magnetic resonance imaging or scintigraphy. Stage II is characterized by a zone of osteopenia surrounding a zone of relatively increased osseous density with the sphericity of the humeral head preserved (Fig. 6-8). Stage III is characterized by the presence of a subchondral fracture (the "crescent sign"); sphericity of the humeral head is preserved (Fig. 6-9). Stage IV corresponds to loss of sphericity of the humeral head as a result of collapse of the necrotic segment

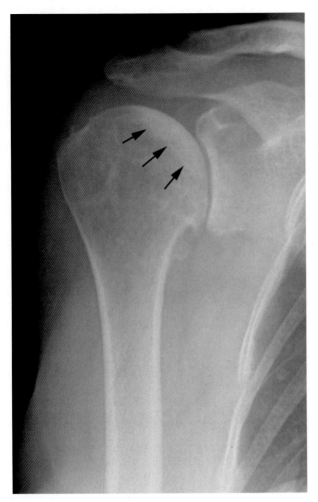

Figure 6-8 Stage II osteonecrosis is characterized by a zone of osteopenia surrounding a zone of relatively increased osseous density (*arrows*), with the sphericity of the humeral head preserved.

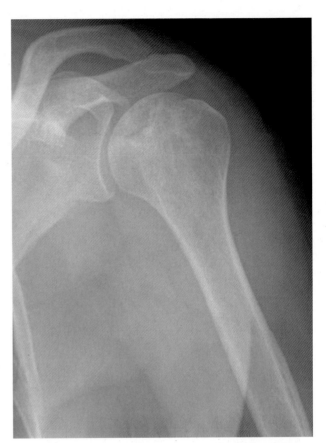

Figure 6-9 Stage III osteonecrosis is characterized by the presence of a subchondral fracture (the "crescent sign"); the sphericity of the humeral head is preserved.

(Fig. 6-10). Stage V is characterized by loss of glenoid articular cartilage with secondary osteoarthritis (Fig. 6-11). Stage VI is characterized by osseous collapse of the humeral head with medialization of the humerus relative to the glenoid (Fig. 6-12).

Magnetic resonance imaging will reliably show the area of osteonecrosis in all except the earliest cases (what has been described as stage 0 in the hip and characterized by increased intraosseous pressure without imaging abnormalities), as shown in Figure 6-13. Secondary imaging studies (computed tomographic arthrography, magnetic resonance imaging) almost always show a concentric glenoid.

The incidence of rotator cuff tears in patients with atraumatic osteonecrosis is similar to that observed in primary osteoarthritis. Conversely, moderate to severe fatty infiltration of the infraspinatus or subscapularis (or both) occurs less frequently than with primary osteoarthritis.[10]

Special Considerations

We perform hemiarthroplasty for stage I, II, III, and IV osteonecrosis because the results have been shown to be equal to those of total shoulder arthroplasty.[12] In patients with stage V and VI osteonecrosis, we perform total shoulder arthroplasty if no contraindications to glenoid resurfacing exist.

INSTABILITY ARTHROPATHY

Instability arthropathy of the shoulder necessitating shoulder arthroplasty is a rare entity; it is seen in less than 5% of unconstrained primary shoulder arthroplasties in our practice. Patients with previous shoulder dislocations treated operatively and nonoperatively are included in this category. Patients usually fall into a bimodal distribution with regard to age at the time

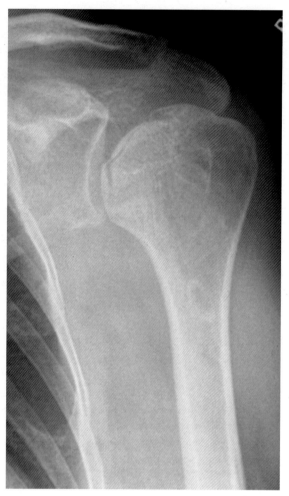

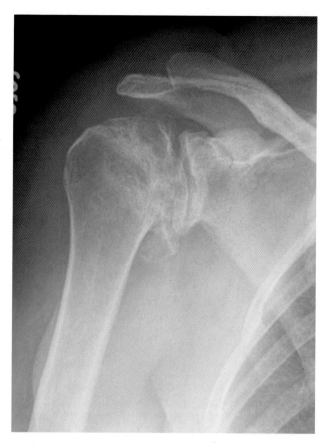

Figure 6-11   Stage V osteonecrosis is characterized by loss of glenoid articular cartilage with secondary osteoarthritis.

Figure 6-10   Stage IV osteonecrosis corresponds to loss of sphericity of the humeral head caused by collapse of the necrotic segment.

of initial dislocation. The first group of patients dislocate their shoulder when they are relatively young, and progressive arthropathy develops over a period of several years. The second group of patients are older (>60 years) at the time of initial dislocation and are prone to a rapidly developing glenohumeral arthritis that may result in a complete loss of articular cartilage within months of the initial dislocation. We have not been able to distinguish between what has previously been termed "capsulorrhaphy arthropathy" and "instability arthropathy" and consequently include these patients in a single entity under the diagnosis of instability arthropathy.[13]

Clinical Findings

Clinical findings in patients with instability arthropathy include glenohumeral crepitus and stiffness.

Rotator cuff testing may be normal or compromised by pain or rotator cuff tearing.

Imaging Findings

Plain radiography demonstrates loss of the normal glenohumeral joint space. In patients with slowly progressing arthropathy, the radiographic changes are very similar to those of primary osteoarthritis and consist of humeral head osteophytes with or without loose bodies (Fig. 6-14). In older patients with rapidly appearing instability arthropathy, loss of the glenohumeral joint space with a paucity of osteophytes is apparent (Fig. 6-15).

Secondary imaging studies (computed tomographic arthrography, magnetic resonance imaging) show posterior subluxation with or without glenoid erosion with biconcavity in 20% of cases, and this finding occurs in both patients who have previously undergone stabilization surgery and those who have not.[13]

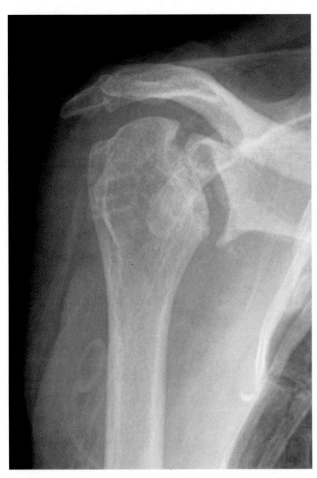

Figure 6-12 Stage VI osteonecrosis is characterized by osseous collapse of the humeral head with medialization of the humerus relative to the glenoid.

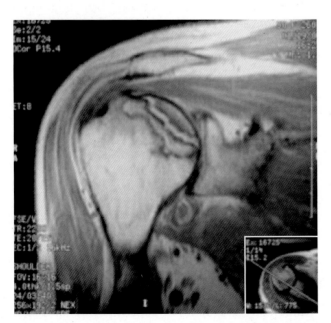

Figure 6-13 Magnetic resonance imaging showing an area of osteonecrosis of the humeral head.

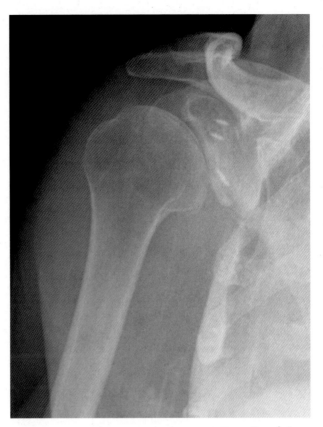

Figure 6-14 Slowly progressing instability arthropathy.

Twenty percent of patients with instability arthropathy have a full-thickness rotator cuff tear, with most being limited to the supraspinatus tendon.[13]

Special Considerations

We perform total shoulder arthroplasty in nearly all cases of instability arthropathy because it has been shown to be superior to hemiarthroplasty and is not associated with an increased risk of complications or reoperations.[13] The only patients with instability arthropathy in whom we perform hemiarthroplasty are those with insufficient glenoid bone or anterior or posterior rotator cuff insufficiency. In patients with rotator cuff insufficiency, we usually opt for a reverse-design prosthesis instead of hemiarthroplasty (see Section Four).

POST-TRAUMATIC ARTHRITIS

Post-traumatic glenohumeral arthritis covers a large spectrum of causes, including chondral damage secondary to blunt trauma and malunion and nonunion

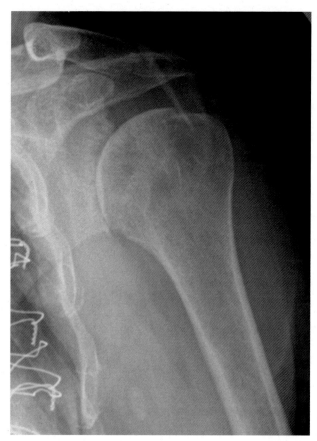

Figure 6-15 Rapidly appearing instability arthropathy in an older patient.

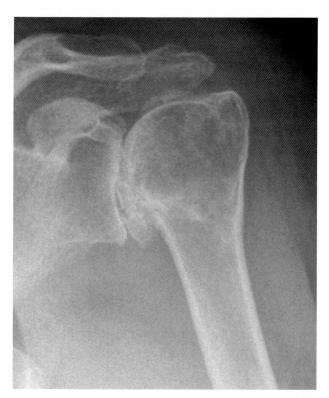

Figure 6-16 Post-traumatic arthritis with minimal residual deformity.

of the proximal humerus after fracture. This diagnosis can be relatively uncomplicated to treat when little glenohumeral osseous deformity is present (Fig. 6-16) or extremely difficult to treat in the case of severe proximal humeral malunion (Fig. 6-17). The integrity of the rotator cuff and the position of the tuberosities are very important when considering a patient for shoulder arthroplasty. If the rotator cuff is largely intact and the tuberosities are acceptably positioned to allow nearly normal rotator cuff function, unconstrained shoulder arthroplasty is our treatment of choice. In situations in which rotator cuff or tuberosity compromise (nonunion, severe malunion) is severe and would require a greater tuberosity osteotomy, we often opt for a reverse-design prosthesis (see Section Four).

Rarely, post-traumatic arthritis will develop after a glenoid fracture (Fig. 6-18). In these cases it is of paramount importance to ensure that the osseous glenoid is sufficient to allow placement of a glenoid component (Fig. 6-19). We prefer computed tomographic arthrography rather than magnetic resonance imaging.

Clinical Findings

Clinical findings in patients with post-traumatic arthritis are variable. Findings in patients with relatively well preserved proximal humeral anatomy are similar to those of primary osteoarthritis with its requisite glenohumeral crepitus and stiffness. In patients with distortion of proximal humeral anatomy as a result of malunion, shoulder stiffness may be exceptionally severe and attributable to mechanical impingement, subdeltoid contracture, and subacromial contracture, in addition to the glenohumeral incongruity and capsular contracture seen in primary osteoarthritis. Rotator cuff testing may be normal or compromised by pain or rotator cuff tearing.

Imaging Findings

Plain radiography demonstrates loss of the normal glenohumeral joint space. Other radiographic findings are variable, as previously mentioned, and depend on the source of the post-traumatic arthritis (chondral injury, malunion, etc.)

Secondary imaging studies (computed tomographic arthrography, magnetic resonance imaging), like plain radiography, show variable findings, depending on the deformity present. We much prefer the use of

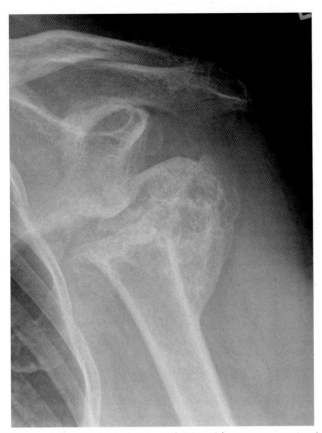

Figure 6-17 Post-traumatic arthritis with severe proximal humeral malunion.

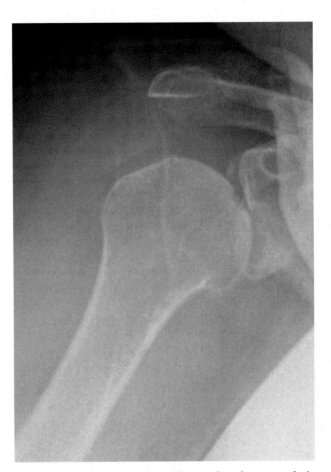

Figure 6-18 Post-traumatic arthritis after fracture of the glenoid.

computed tomographic arthrography over magnetic resonance imaging in this diagnosis for the osseous detail provided.

Special Considerations

We perform total shoulder arthroplasty in nearly all cases of post-traumatic arthritis because it has been shown to be superior to hemiarthroplasty without an increased risk of complications or reoperations.[14] The only patients with post-traumatic arthritis in whom we perform hemiarthroplasty are those with insufficient glenoid bone or anterior or posterior rotator cuff insufficiency. In patients with rotator cuff insufficiency or in those who would require a greater tuberosity osteotomy to perform humeral arthroplasty, we usually opt for a reverse-design prosthesis instead of hemiarthroplasty (see Section Four).

FIXED GLENOHUMERAL DISLOCATION

A distinct subset of patients with glenohumeral instability are those with fixed (chronic) glenohumeral

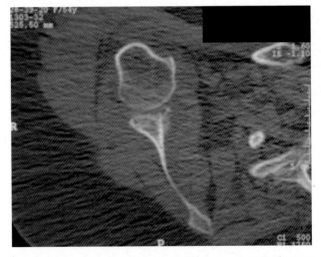

Figure 6-19 Computed tomogram of a patient with post-traumatic arthritis after a glenoid fracture.

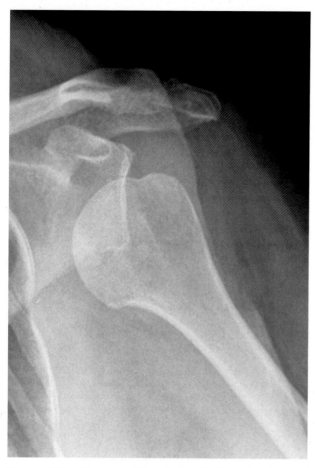

Figure 6-20 Chronic dislocation of the glenohumeral joint.

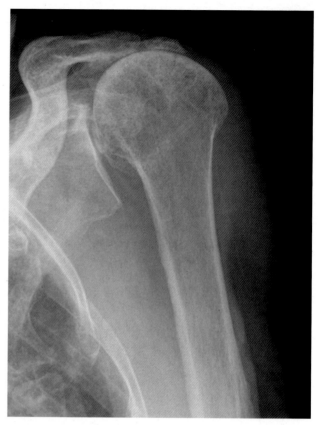

Figure 6-21 Glenohumeral arthritis combined with a massive rotator cuff tear.

dislocations (Fig. 6-20). These dislocations can be anterior or posterior. Long-standing dislocations can result in severe glenohumeral arthritis with complete loss of proximal humeral articular cartilage, especially in older patients. Our results using unconstrained shoulder arthroplasty in this subset of patients have been disappointing.[15] We now use a reverse-design prosthesis in this patient subset (see Section Four).

ROTATOR CUFF TEAR ARTHROPATHY (GLENOHUMERAL OSTEOARTHRITIS WITH A MASSIVE ROTATOR CUFF TEAR)

Historically, hemiarthroplasty has been the operative treatment of choice in patients with osteoarthritis combined with a massive irreparable rotator cuff tear (Fig. 6-21). Unconstrained total shoulder arthroplasty is contraindicated because of the risk of loosening of the glenoid component by eccentric loading of the glenoid component.[1] The results of hemiarthroplasty for this diagnosis, however, have been disappointing,

with most patients achieving only modest improvement postoperatively.[16]

Since its introduction in the United States and because of its superior results, we have used the reverse prosthesis in nearly all cases of osteoarthritis with massive irreparable rotator cuff tears that we have treated operatively.[16] We still consider the use of unconstrained hemiarthroplasty in patients with insufficient glenoid bone stock to support the reverse-prosthesis glenoid component and in elderly patients with severe osteopenia who would seemingly be at increased risk for glenoid failure after the implantation of a reverse-design prosthesis (Fig. 6-22).

POSTINFECTIOUS ARTHROPATHY

Postinfectious arthropathy is a rare and somewhat controversial indication for shoulder arthroplasty. Successful shoulder arthroplasty in these patients depends on complete eradication of the infection before shoulder arthroplasty is undertaken. We use a systematic approach in our workup of these patients preoperatively. We first confirm through review of

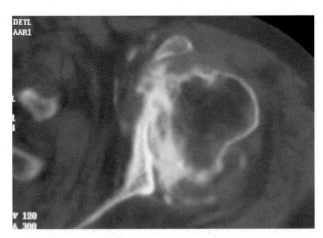

Figure 6-22 Computed tomogram of a patient with rotator cuff tear arthropathy and insufficient glenoid bone stock to allow implantation of a reverse-prosthesis glenoid component.

previous medical records the type of infection (hematogenous versus postoperative, type of organism). We also ensure that the infection was properly and adequately treated. Consultation with an infectious disease specialist is obtained and continued throughout the preoperative workup and the shoulder arthroplasty. Patients are not considered for shoulder arthroplasty for postinfectious arthropathy until they are free of infection for at least 6 months.

Clinical Findings

Clinical findings in patients with postinfectious arthropathy are variable. Most patients demonstrate glenohumeral crepitus and severe stiffness. Rotator cuff testing may be normal but is often compromised because many of these cases are caused by postoperative infections emanating from an attempt at rotator cuff repair.

Imaging Findings

Plain radiography demonstrates loss of the normal glenohumeral joint space in nearly all cases (Fig. 6-23). Humeral head osteophytes may be present if the condition has been long-standing and has progressed over many years. The humeral head may be statically subluxated superiorly or anterosuperiorly in cases of massive rotator cuff tearing (Fig. 6-24).

Secondary imaging studies (computed tomographic arthrography, magnetic resonance imaging) show various findings. The osseous humeral head and glenoid are usually well preserved, although in patients with previous osteomyelitis, substantial bony defi-

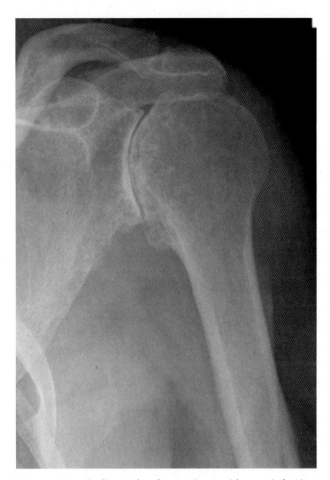

Figure 6-23 Radiograph of a patient with postinfectious arthropathy.

ciency may be present as a result of either the infection or subsequent osseous débridement. The condition of the rotator cuff is variable in postinfectious arthropathy, with patients who have undergone a previous attempt at rotator cuff repair more likely to demonstrate rotator cuff compromise.

Special Considerations

Patients are not considered for arthroplasty until 6 months after their shoulder infection has resolved, and the preoperative infection workup is not initiated until this time. In all patients with postinfectious arthropathy, fluoroscopically guided aspiration of the glenohumeral joint is performed after the patient has been off all antibiotics for at least 2 weeks (even antibiotics used for other conditions such as respiratory infections). The aspirate is cultured for aerobic bacteria, anaerobic bacteria, mycobacteria, and fungi. Serum studies include a complete blood count with differential, a sedimentation rate, and C-reactive protein. At

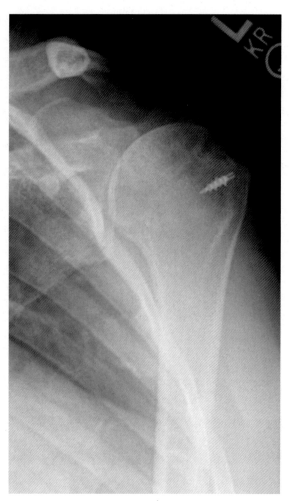

Figure 6-24 Static superior migration of the humeral head in a patient with postinfectious arthropathy after an attempt at rotator cuff repair that became infected.

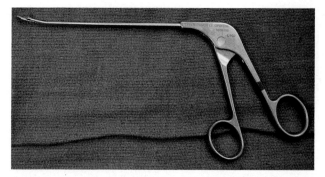

Figure 6-25 Arthroscopic punch used to obtain a synovial biopsy specimen in patients with a previous shoulder infection.

the time of fluoroscopically guided aspiration, patients undergo computed tomographic arthrography or magnetic resonance imaging (if they are allergic to radiographic contrast material).

The patient is considered actively infected if aspirate cultures are positive and is treated as such, with the arthroplasty being delayed indefinitely. If the aspirate demonstrates moderate to many white blood cells or serum testing is highly suggestive of infection (increased white blood cells, increased C-reactive protein), infection is considered possible even in the absence of a positive culture. Isolated elevation of the sedimentation rate is not considered by us a reliable indicator of infection in this patient population.

In all patients with postinfectious arthropathy and negative aspirate cultures, arthroscopic synovial biopsy is performed before arthroplasty. An arthroscopic

punch is used to obtain more than 10 synovial specimens before the administration of perioperative antibiotics (Fig. 6-25); after obtaining the synovial specimens, standard perioperative intravenous antibiotics are administered immediately. These specimens are sent for microscopic analysis by a pathologist and cultured for aerobic bacteria, anaerobic bacteria, mycobacteria, and fungi. If these cultures are positive or if findings of the frozen section are indicative of infection (more than five polymorphonuclear leukocytes per high-power field on five consecutive fields), the patient is considered actively infected and treated as such, and the arthroplasty is delayed indefinitely.[17] If this workup is negative for infection, the patient is a candidate for total shoulder arthroplasty. With these criteria our infection rate has been no higher for this indication than for primary osteoarthritis.

We perform total shoulder arthroplasty in nearly all cases of postinfectious arthropathy. In younger patients (<40 years), we opt for biologic glenoid resurfacing over the use of a conventional polyethylene component. The only patients with postinfectious arthropathy in whom we perform hemiarthroplasty are those with insufficient glenoid bone or anterior or posterior rotator cuff insufficiency. In patients with rotator cuff insufficiency, we usually opt for a reverse-design prosthesis instead of hemiarthroplasty (see Section Four).

GLENOHUMERAL CHONDROLYSIS

A rare but disturbing disease process that we are seeing with increasing frequency is glenohumeral chondrolysis.[18] We have observed this diagnosis in patients in the early portion of their third decade. Nearly all patients have a history of an arthroscopic shoulder stabilization procedure, with or without the use of thermal energy.[18] We have observed a single patient with glenohumeral chondrolysis at age 21 after a single dislocation with no surgery performed. The chondrolysis that occurs is diffuse and affects both the humeral head and glenoid.

Clinical Findings

Clinical findings in patients with glenohumeral chondrolysis include glenohumeral crepitus and stiffness. Rotator cuff testing is usually normal but may be compromised by pain.

Imaging Findings

Plain radiography demonstrates loss of the normal glenohumeral joint space. Humeral head osteophytes are absent (Fig. 6-26).

Secondary imaging studies show concentric loss of glenohumeral articular cartilage. The rotator cuff is

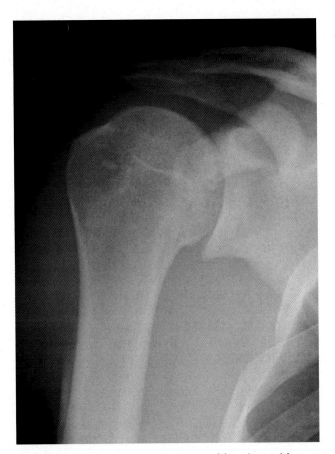

Figure 6-26 Radiograph of a 20-year-old patient with complete glenohumeral chondrolysis after arthroscopic surgery for instability.

generally intact, and any osseous wear is minimal and centrally oriented.

Special Considerations

A major problem in dealing with cases of glenohumeral chondrolysis is young patient age. Because the disease occurs on both the humeral head and the glenoid, we are compelled to address the glenoid pathology and not simply perform a hemiarthroplasty. As a result of the young patient age, we opt for biologic resurfacing of the glenoid combined with either hemiarthroplasty or humeral head resurfacing (see Section Five). Our results with arthrodesis have been disappointing, and hence we avoid this procedure in nearly all cases.

GLENOHUMERAL ARTHRITIS ASSOCIATED WITH NEUROLOGIC PATHOLOGY

Infrequently, we encounter patients with glenohumeral osteoarthritis combined with a systemic neurologic disorder. The most common neurologic disorder in patients with glenohumeral arthritis is Parkinson's disease.[19] Clinically, these patients are usually functioning at a lower level than patients with primary osteoarthritis. Radiographically and on secondary imaging studies, these patients resemble those with primary osteoarthritis (Fig. 6-27).

GLENOHUMERAL ARTHRITIS ASSOCIATED WITH PREVIOUS RADIATION THERAPY

An indication for shoulder arthroplasty that we are seeing less frequently is glenohumeral arthritis after radiation therapy (Fig. 6-28).[20] Most patients in this diagnostic group have undergone radiation therapy for the treatment of breast cancer or lymphoma. Radiographically, some cases resemble aseptic osteonecrosis and other cases resemble inflammatory arthropathy. This indication is becoming less common as radiotherapy technology improves and becomes less toxic.

GLENOHUMERAL ARTHRITIS ASSOCIATED WITH SKELETAL DYSPLASIA

An exceedingly rare indication for unconstrained shoulder arthroplasty is glenohumeral arthritis associ-

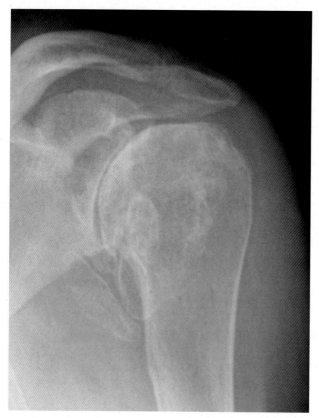

Figure 6-27   Radiograph of a patient with Parkinson's disease and glenohumeral arthritis.

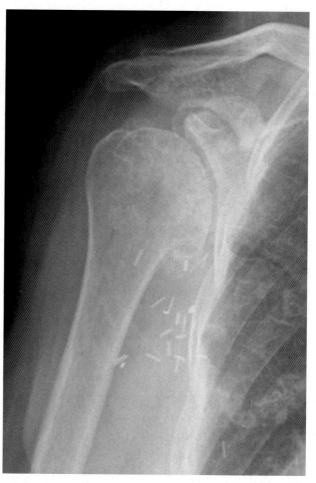

Figure 6-28   Radiograph of a patient with glenohumeral arthritis associated with previous radiation therapy.

ated with skeletal dysplasia. Little is known about this entity. Our limited experience with this indication has led us to treat it like primary osteoarthritis (i.e., perform total shoulder arthroplasty), provided that the anterior and posterior rotator cuff is intact and the osseous glenoid is sufficient. Many of these patients require custom-manufactured implants because of their small size and osseous distortion (Fig. 6-29).

TUMOR

Tumors about the shoulder girdle are an exceptionally rare indication for unconstrained shoulder arthroplasty. In our practice, we infrequently assist in reconstruction of the shoulder after tumor resection by an orthopedic oncologic surgeon. If the resection leaves the rotator cuff and tuberosities intact and attached to the humeral diaphysis, an unconstrained prosthesis can be considered and would usually consist of a hemiarthroplasty. In nearly all cases of shoulder girdle

tumor, however, the rotator cuff is substantially compromised by the resection. In our practice, we opt for use of a reverse-design prosthesis (see Section Four).

CONTRAINDICATIONS TO UNCONSTRAINED SHOULDER ARTHROPLASTY

Contraindications to unconstrained shoulder arthroplasty are listed in Table 6-1. Some of these contraindications are absolute and others are relative. Additionally, some situations are contraindications to glenoid resurfacing with an unconstrained implant but not to unconstrained hemiarthroplasty.

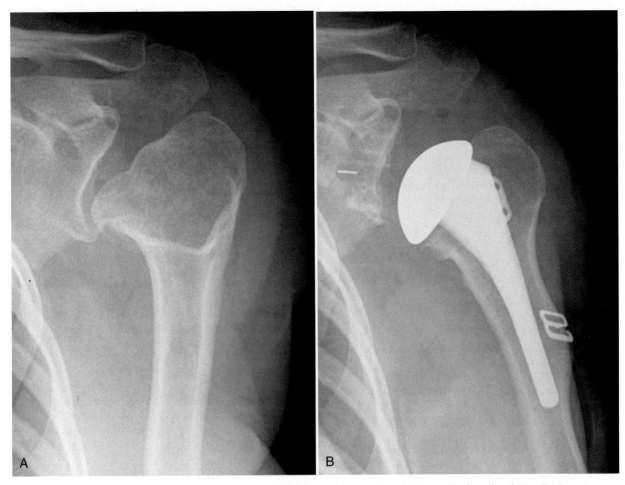

Figure 6-29 **A,** Radiograph of a patient with glenohumeral arthritis and achondroplasia. **B,** A custom-manufactured humeral stem of shorter length was required.

Table 6-1 CONTRAINDICATIONS TO UNCONSTRAINED SHOULDER ARTHROPLASTY

Contraindication	Absolute or Relative	Comments
Poor generalized health	Relative	Appropriate perioperative medical treatment required
Active infection	Absolute	
Axillary nerve palsy	Relative	Probably better suited for resection arthroplasty or arthrodesis
Suprascapular nerve palsy	Relative	Glenoid component contraindicated; better suited for hemiarthroplasty or a reverse prosthesis
Massive rotator cuff tear	Relative	Glenoid component contraindicated; better suited for hemiarthroplasty or a reverse prosthesis
Insufficient humeral bone stock	Absolute	
Insufficient glenoid bone stock	Relative	Glenoid component contraindicated; better suited for hemiarthroplasty
Ankylosed shoulder	Absolute	
Previous shoulder arthrodesis	Absolute	
Upper motor neuron lesion	Relative	Absolute contraindication if the patient has uncontrolled shoulder spasticity
Poor patient motivation	Absolute	

REFERENCES

1. Franklin JL, Barrett WP, Jackins SE, Matsen FA III: Glenoid loosening in total shoulder arthroplasty: Association with rotator cuff deficiency. J Arthroplasty 1988;3: 39-46.
2. Neer CS 2nd: Replacement arthroplasty for glenohumeral osteoarthritis. J Bone Joint Surg Am 1974;56:1-13.
3. Edwards TB: Primary glenohumeral osteoarthritis: Epidemiological, clinical, and radiographic findings in patients undergoing shoulder arthroplasty. In Walch G, Boileau P, Molé D (eds): 2000 Prosthèses d'Epaule . . . Recul de 2 à 10 Ans. Paris, Sauramps Medical, 2001, pp 65-72.
4. Edwards TB, Boulahia A, Kempf JF, et al: The influence of the rotator cuff on the results of shoulder arthroplasty for primary osteoarthritis: Results of a multicenter study. J Bone Joint Surg Am 2002;84:2240-2248.
5. Edwards TB, Kadakia NR, Boulahia A, et al: A comparison of hemiarthroplasty and total shoulder arthroplasty in the treatment of primary glenohumeral osteoarthritis: Results of a multicenter study. J Shoulder Elbow Surg 2003;12:207-213.
6. Gartsman GM, Roddey TS, Hammerman SM: Shoulder arthroplasty with or without resurfacing of the glenoid in patients who have osteoarthritis. J Bone Joint Surg Am 2000;82:26-34.
7. Aswad R, Franceschi JP, Levigne C: Rheumatoid arthritis: Epidemiology and preoperative radiographic assessment. In Walch G, Boileau P, Molé D (eds): 2000 Prosthèses d'Epaule . . . Recul de 2 à 10 Ans. Paris, Sauramps Medical, 2001, pp 159-162.
8. Vandermaren C, Docquier P: Shoulder arthroplasty in rheumatoid arthritis: Influence of the rotator cuff on the results. In Walch G, Boileau P, Molé D (eds): 2000 Prostheses d'Epaule . . . Recul de 2 à 10 Ans. Paris, Sauramps Medical, 2001, pp 177-182.
9. Loehr J, Levigne C: Shoulder arthroplasty in rheumatoid arthritis: Influence of the glenoid on the results. In Walch G, Boileau P, Molé D (eds): 2000 Prosthèses d'Epaule . . . Recul de 2 à 10 Ans. Paris, Sauramps Medical, 2001, pp 171-176.
10. Willems WJ: Atraumatic avascular osteonecrosis of the humeral head: Epidemiology and radiology. In Walch G, Boileau P, Molé D (eds): 2000 Prosthèses d'Epaule . . . Recul de 2 à 10 Ans. Paris, Sauramps Medical, 2001, pp 121-126.
11. Cruess RL: Steroid-induced avascular necrosis of the head of the humerus. J Bone Joint Surg Br 1976;58:313-317.
12. Nové-Josserand L, Basso M: Prosthèses d'épaule sur ostéonécroses avasculaires: Facteurs pronostiques. In Walch G, Boileau P, Molé D (eds): 2000 Prosthèses d'Epaule . . . Recul de 2 à 10 Ans. Paris, Sauramps Medical, 2001, pp 135-142.
13. Matsoukis J, Tabib W, Guiffault P, et al: Shoulder arthroplasty in patients with a prior anterior shoulder dislocation: Results of a multicenter study. J Bone Joint Surg Am 2003;85:1417-1424.
14. Duparc F, Trojani C, Boileau P: Results of shoulder arthroplasty in cephalic collapse or necrosis following proximal humerus fractures (type 1 fracture sequelae). In Walch G, Boileau P, Molé D (eds): 2000 Prosthèses d'Epaule . . . Recul de 2 à 10 Ans. Paris, Sauramps Medical, 2001, pp 279-289.
15. Matsoukis J, Tabib W, Guiffault P, et al: Primary unconstrained shoulder arthroplasty in patients with a fixed anterior glenohumeral dislocation: Results of a multicenter study. J Bone Joint Surg Am 2006;88:547-552.
16. Favard L, Lautmann S, Sirveaux F, et al: Hemiarthroplasty versus reverse shoulder arthroplasty in the treatment of osteoarthritis with massive rotator cuff tear. In Walch G, Boileau P, Molé D (eds): 2000 Prosthèses d'Epaule . . . Recul de 2 à 10 Ans. Paris, Sauramps Medical, 2001, pp 261-268.
17. Feldman DS, Lonner JH, Desai P, Zuckerman JD: The role of intraoperative frozen sections in revision total joint arthroplasty. J Bone Joint Surg Am 1995;77:1807-1813.
18. Larsen MW, Higgins LD, Basamania CJ: Severe glenohumeral chondrolysis following shoulder arthroscopy: A series of 6 cases treated with hemiarthroplasty. Paper presented at the 22nd Open Meeting of the American Shoulder and Elbow Surgeons, March 2006, Chicago.
19. Garreau de Loubresse C: Prothèse d'épaule et affections neurologiques. In Walch G, Boileau P, Molé D (eds): 2000 Prosthèses d'Epaule . . . Recul de 2 à 10 Ans. Paris, Sauramps Medical, 2001, pp 195-203.
20. Godenèche A: Shoulder arthroplasty and previous radiotherapy. In Walch G, Boileau P, Molé D (eds): 2000 Prosthèses d'Epaule . . . Recul de 2 à 10 Ans. Paris, Sauramps Medical, 2001, pp 143-148.

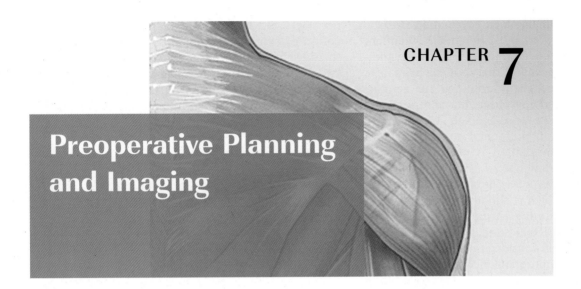

CHAPTER **7**

Preoperative Planning and Imaging

Although the majority of cases of unconstrained shoulder arthroplasty are routine, certain patients have unique characteristics that merit special consideration. Preoperative planning identifies patients who may require deviation from routine unconstrained shoulder arthroplasty. Preoperative planning should be done well in advance of the surgical procedure and not be an afterthought the morning of surgery. The surgeon should review the patient's clinical history and physical examination, radiographs, and any secondary imaging studies. This chapter presents our approach to preoperative planning for unconstrained shoulder arthroplasty.

CLINICAL HISTORY AND EXAMINATION

Although description of a detailed shoulder history and examination are beyond the scope of this textbook, certain aspects of the history and physical examination are important in preoperative planning for unconstrained shoulder arthroplasty. The shoulder-specific complaints of the patient are reviewed, such as the type of symptoms (pain, stiffness, weakness), duration of symptoms (weeks, months, years), and previous treatment (activity modification, nonsteroidal anti-inflammatory medications, corticosteroid injections, viscosupplementary injections, previous surgery). These shoulder-specific complaints help the surgeon decide which patients are candidates for shoulder replacement surgery. A patient with complaints of only mild pain, mild weakness, or mild stiffness (or any combination of these complaints) may initially best be treated with nonoperative (or nonarthroplasty) modalities, even if radiographs demonstrate end-stage glenohumeral arthritis. Similarly, a patient with a sudden onset of symptoms of a short duration to date may be experiencing a transient acute rotator cuff tendinitis concomitantly with chronic glenohumeral arthritis that has been well tolerated. In this situation, a period of nonoperative treatment would certainly be indicated. Special attention is given to factors that could make the operative procedure more difficult. Chronic use of nonsteroidal anti-inflammatory medications can result in excessive operative blood loss, so such drugs should be discontinued the week before surgery.

Any previous surgery merits special consideration. The type of surgery should be noted. Although previous arthroscopic procedures are usually inconsequential to the performance of shoulder arthroplasty, previous open procedures may introduce difficulties. Specifically, previous instability surgery may have resulted in severe stiffness, especially in external rotation, and may have caused excessive scar tissue that will make the surgical approach more difficult. The type of surgical procedure should be elucidated whenever possible. Procedures that alter normal anatomic relationships, such as tendon transfers (subscapularis transfers, i.e., the Magnusson-Stack procedure) and coracoid transfers, are especially important when considering the surgical approach. Previous rotator cuff surgery may focus attention on determining preoperative rotator cuff integrity.

Any symptoms of infection, especially in patients who have previously undergone surgery or injections, should be investigated further. If patients have a history of infection after shoulder surgery or have had symptoms suggestive of infection (systemic fever; shoulder warmth, redness), a preoperative infection workup, including hematologic evaluation with a complete blood cell count and differential, a sedimentation rate, and C-reactive protein, is indicated. Additionally, a fluoroscopically guided shoulder aspirate is obtained and the specimen submitted for aerobic, anaerobic, fungal, and mycobacterial culture. If the findings are suggestive or diagnostic of infection, shoulder arthroplasty is postponed or canceled until infectious disease consultation is obtained and the infection is appropriately treated (Table 7-1).

Any medical history of systemic illness (diabetes mellitus, cardiac problems) should be considered in the preoperative planning. Although these factors may not affect the actual surgical procedure, they may necessitate special considerations in the patient's postoperative care. Appropriate medical consultations should be obtained well in advance of the surgery date. The availability of appropriate care, including consultants for these systemic illnesses, should be confirmed before surgery.

All our patients undergo a thorough shoulder examination. Motion and rotator cuff strength are of critical importance. Both active and passive mobility is recorded. Mobility parameters recorded are elevation in the plane of the scapula (Fig. 7-1), abduction (Fig. 7-2), external rotation with the arm at the side (Fig. 7-3), external rotation with the arm abducted 90 degrees (when possible) (Fig. 7-4), and internal rotation as determined by the vertebral level reached with an outstretched thumb (Fig. 7-5). Any incongruity of the glenohumeral joint as indicated by the presence of glenohumeral crepitus with motion is noted, as is any discrepancy in active and passive mobility.

Rotator cuff examination consists of testing each tendon of the rotator cuff by isolating it as much as possible. Jobe's test is used to test supraspinatus integ-

rity (Fig. 7-6).[1] The external rotation lag sign and evaluation of external rotation strength with the arm at the side are used to test the infraspinatus (Figs. 7-7 and 7-8).[2] The teres minor is tested via the horn blower's sign (Fig. 7-9).[3] The subscapularis is tested with the belly press test and, when mobility allows, the lift-off test (Figs. 7-10 and 7-11).[4]

Table 7-1 **WORKUP FOR INFECTION BEFORE UNCONSTRAINED SHOULDER ARTHROPLASTY**	
Test	**If Abnormal**
White blood cell count with differential	Increase suspicion for infection; consider arthroscopic biopsy
Sedimentation rate	Increase suspicion for infection if combined with an abnormal white blood cell count or C-reactive protein; consider arthroscopic biopsy
C-reactive protein	Increase suspicion for infection; consider arthroscopic biopsy
Fluoroscopically guided aspiration	Consider the shoulder as actively infected and treat as such; arthroscopic biopsy is unnecessary
Arthroscopic biopsy	Consider the shoulder as actively infected and treat as such

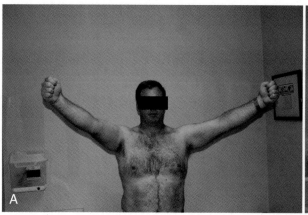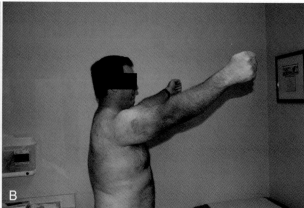

Figure 7-1 **A** and **B,** Elevation in the plane of the scapula.

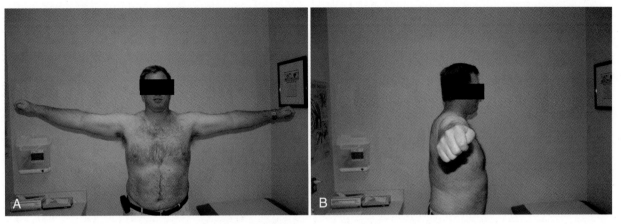

Figure 7-2 **A** and **B,** Abduction. The arm is kept in the coronal plane.

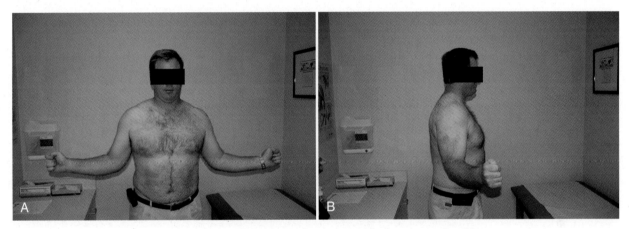

Figure 7-3 **A** and **B,** External rotation with the arm at the side.

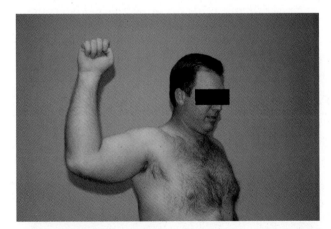

Figure 7-4 External rotation with the arm abducted 90 degrees. Measurement of this mobility parameter is not possible in all patients because of limited mobility in severe cases.

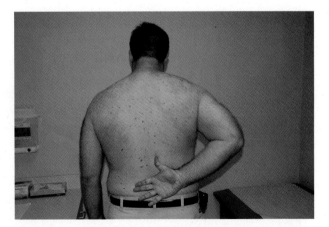

Figure 7-5 Internal rotation as measured by the vertebral level reached with an outstretched thumb.

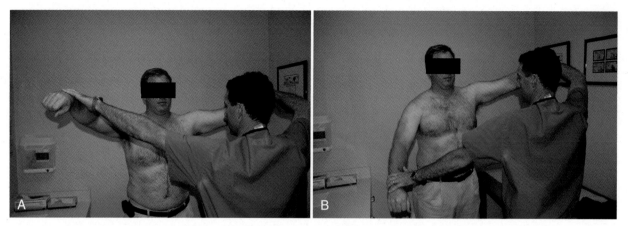

Figure 7-6 **A** and **B,** Jobe's test for supraspinatus integrity. The patient elevates the pronated arm in the plane of the scapula and resists the downward force of the examiner.

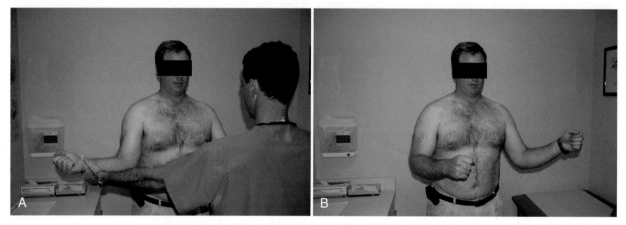

Figure 7-7 **A** and **B,** External rotation lag sign for infraspinatus integrity. The examiner maximally externally rotates the arm at the side and asks the patient to maintain this position. If the patient is unable to maintain this position, the test is considered positive for infraspinatus insufficiency.

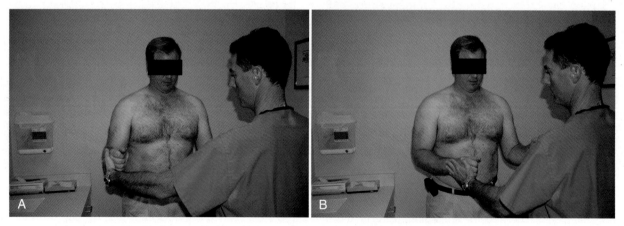

Figure 7-8 **A** and **B,** Evaluation of external rotation strength with the arm at the side. The patient resists the examiner's internally directed force. Weakness in this position may indicate infraspinatus insufficiency.

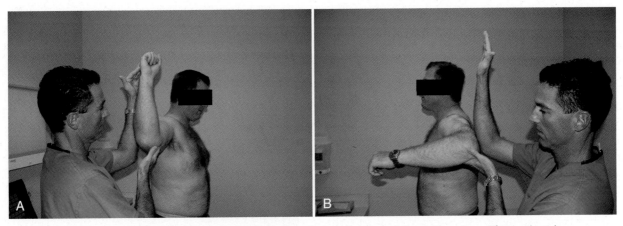

Figure 7-9 **A** and **B,** The horn blower's sign for evaluation of the teres minor. The patient is asked to actively externally rotate the 90-degree abducted arm. Inability to perform this maneuver may indicate teres minor insufficiency.

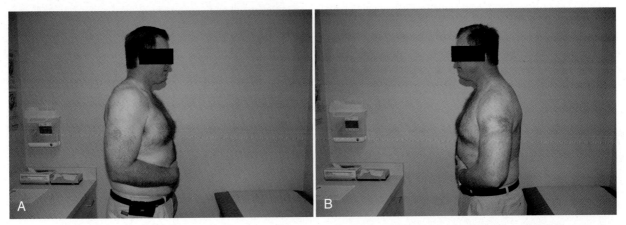

Figure 7-10 Belly press test for subscapularis insufficiency. The test is considered positive if the patient must flex the wrist and extend the arm to press on the abdomen. **A,** Positive test. **B,** Negative test.

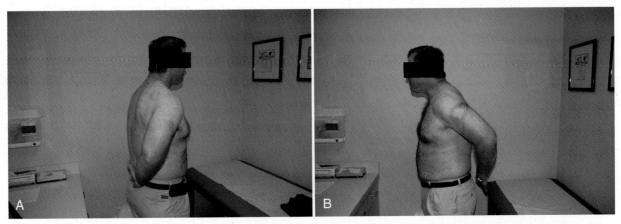

Figure 7-11 The lift-off test for subscapularis insufficiency. The test is considered positive if the patient is unable to lift the hand off the back. **A,** Positive test. **B,** Negative test.

The results of the clinical history and physical examination are documented in the patient's chart and are reviewed well in advance of surgery as part of preoperative planning.

RADIOGRAPHY

Radiographs are obtained in all patients who are candidates for shoulder arthroplasty. We prefer an anteroposterior view of the glenohumeral joint with the arm in neutral rotation (Fig. 7-12), an axillary view (Fig. 7-13), and a scapular outlet view (Fig. 7-14). The anteroposterior radiograph is used to evaluate the glenohumeral joint space, the presence of humeral and glenoid osteophytes, the size of the humeral canal (Fig. 7-15), the presence of any loose bodies (Fig. 7-16), and the presence of any deformity of the humeral shaft (Fig. 7-17) because these factors may all have an impact on the planned procedure. The axillary radiograph is used to evaluate the glenohumeral joint space, the presence of anterior or posterior humeral head subluxation, and the presence of osseous glenoid wear

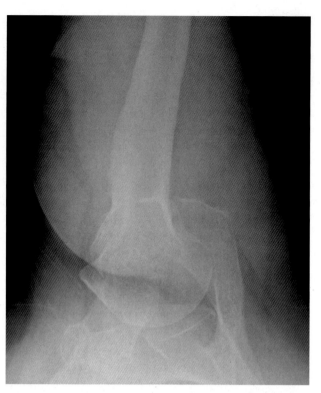

Figure 7-13   Axillary radiograph.

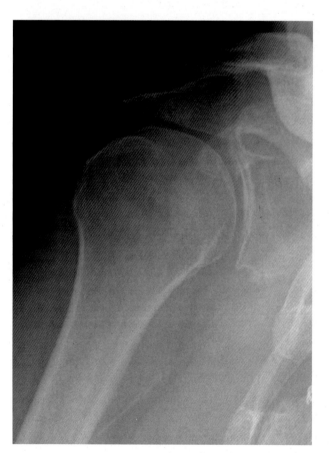

Figure 7-12   Anteroposterior radiograph of the glenohumeral joint with the arm in neutral rotation.

and dysplasia (Fig. 7-18). The scapular outlet radiograph is used to evaluate the presence of anterior or posterior humeral head subluxation (Fig. 7-19), the presence of loose bodies in the subscapularis recess, and any deformity of the humeral shaft. Findings on these radiographs assist the surgeon in predicting the need for custom implants (proximal humeral deformity), predicting the need to remove large loose bodies in the subscapularis recess that may not be visible at the time of surgery, and predicting cases in which the glenoid portion of the procedure may be exceptionally difficult.

Ideally, these radiographs are taken with magnification under fluoroscopic control to allow accurate assessment of the glenohumeral joint space and an accurate measure of the acromiohumeral interval, an important predictor of static humeral subluxation resulting from rotator cuff insufficiency. Some patients arrive at our clinic with radiographs taken by a referring physician. If these radiographs are judged to be of sufficient quality and less than 6 months old and no unusual circumstances (excessively small humeral intramedullary canal) exist, radiographs are not repeated. In all other cases, radiographs are repeated with magnification and fluoroscopically controlled techniques.

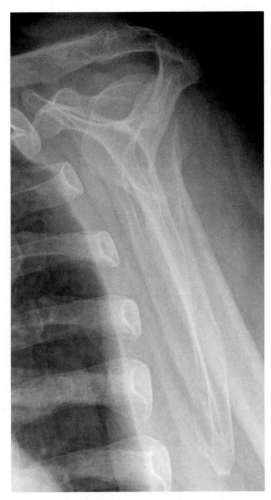

Figure 7-14   Scapular outlet radiograph.

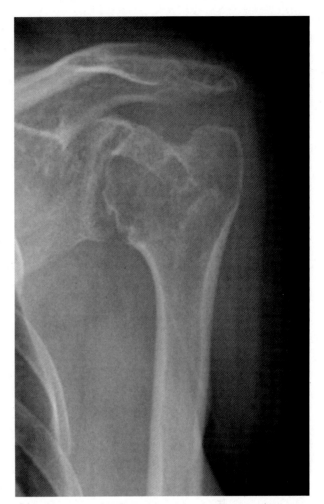

Figure 7-15   Anterior posterior radiograph of a patient with juvenile rheumatoid arthritis and an exceptionally small humeral intramedullary canal. A standard humeral component is too large for this patient, so a custom-manufactured stem is required.

Most shoulder arthroplasty prosthetic systems have radiographic templates available for preoperative planning (Fig. 7-20). Use of an adaptable, anatomic prosthetic system minimizes the need for radiographic templates in most cases because humeral stem size, humeral head size and position, and glenoid size will be determined intraoperatively. In select cases, such as patients with substantial deformity of the proximal humerus (Fig. 7-21) or an excessively small humeral canal, use of radiographic templates preoperatively is mandatory. We use these templates to determine whether existing prefabricated implants are sufficient or a custom-manufactured implant is required.

SECONDARY IMAGING

A secondary imaging study is obtained in all patients before unconstrained shoulder arthroplasty to evaluate the rotator cuff and, more importantly, glenoid morphology. Our preferred secondary imaging modality is computed tomographic arthrography. We find that it provides the greatest osseous detail and allows concomitant evaluation of the rotator cuff tendons and musculature. Some patients come to our clinic with a magnetic resonance imaging scan. If the scan allows sufficient evaluation of the osseous structures and rotator cuff and is less than 6 months old, we will not order additional secondary imaging.

Glenoid morphology is classified by computed tomography (or magnetic resonance imaging) according to the system of Walch and colleagues (Fig. 7-22).[5] In type A, or concentric glenoid morphology, the humeral head is centered, and loads are equally

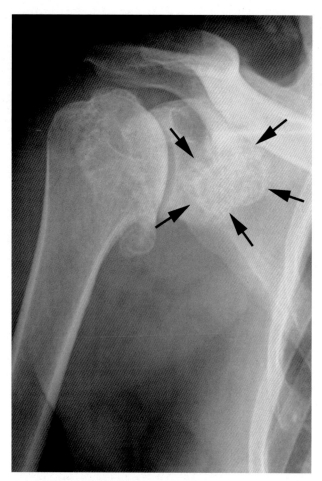

Figure 7-16   Large loose body (*arrows*) in the subscapularis recess identified on an anteroposterior radiograph. It should be removed at the time of arthroplasty.

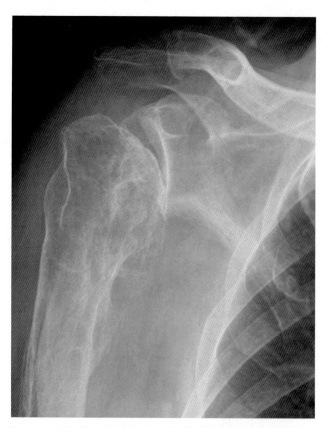

Figure 7-17   Proximal humeral diaphyseal malunion in a patient with glenohumeral arthritis. A standard uncemented humeral stem should not be used in this patient.

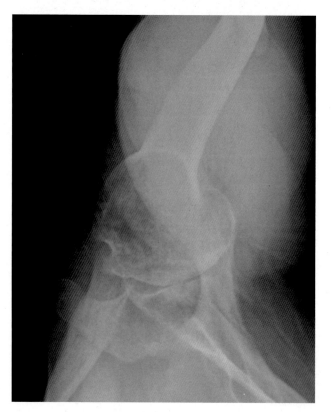

Figure 7-18   Posterior glenoid wear with posterior humeral head subluxation identified on an axillary radiograph.

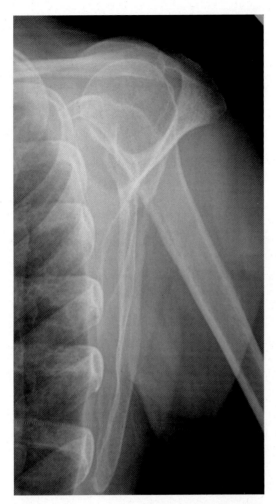

Figure 7-19 Anterior humeral head subluxation with coracohumeral impingement identified on a scapular outlet radiograph.

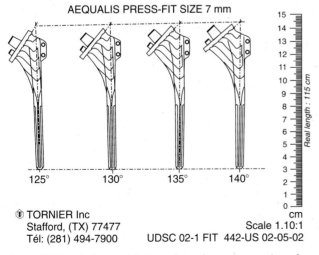

AEQUALIS PRESS-FIT SIZE 7 mm

125°   130°   135°   140°

15
14
13
12
11
10
9
8
7
6
5
4
3
2
1
0

Real length : 115 cm

cm

Ⓣ TORNIER Inc
Stafford, (TX) 77477
Tél: (281) 494-7900

Scale 1.10:1

UDSC 02-1 FIT 442-US 02-05-02

Figure 7-20 Radiographic templates for preoperative planning for unconstrained shoulder arthroplasty.

distributed on the glenoid. Glenoid osseous erosion may be minor, type A1, or major, type A2. Type B, or nonconcentric glenoid morphology, is characterized by a posteriorly subluxated humeral head and asymmetric loads across the glenoid. Type B1 shows narrowing of the posterior joint space, subchondral sclerosis, and osteophytes, and type B2 demonstrates a biconcave glenoid resulting from posterior osseous erosion. The final glenoid morphology, type C or dysplastic, is defined by glenoid retroversion greater than 25 degrees and a centered or only slightly subluxated humeral head. Classification of glenoid morphology is critical in two scenarios when performing unconstrained shoulder arthroplasty. First, in a patient with severe glenoid erosion (A2 and B2) or severe dysplasia (C), insufficient glenoid bone stock may prohibit implantation of a standard glenoid component (Fig. 7-23). In this case the surgeon must opt for hemiarthroplasty or choose to alter the glenoid component (i.e., shorten the keel or pegs). Second, in cases of posterior humeral head subluxation and a biconcave glenoid (B2), posterior capsulorrhaphy may be required at the time of shoulder arthroplasty. When these cases are identified by preoperative secondary imaging, an additional step of testing glenohumeral stability with the trial components is included as part of the surgical technique (Chapter 13).

The rotator cuff is next evaluated with secondary imaging modalities, including assessment of tendon integrity and evaluation of muscle quality (fatty infiltration). In addition, the condition of the long head of the biceps tendon is noted, particularly its position (centered, subluxated, dislocated, ruptured) to assist in identifying it at the time of surgery. Although full-thickness rotator cuff tears limited to the supraspinatus tendon may not change the operative plan, tears of the supraspinatus combined with either posterior (infraspinatus) or anterior (subscapularis) rotator cuff tears are contraindications to glenoid resurfacing and may best be treated with a reverse-design prosthesis (Fig. 7-24).[6] The degree of fatty infiltration of the supraspinatus and infraspinatus musculature has been shown to influence the results of unconstrained shoulder arthroplasty in patients with primary osteoarthritis.[6] Although we do not necessarily change our operative plan based on fatty infiltration, we routinely classify the degree of fatty infiltration of these muscles by using a three-tiered modification of the Goutallier classification to assist in determining the patient's postoperative prognosis.[7] The soft tissue axial sections of a computed tomogram or the T1-weighted axial sections of magnetic resonance imaging are used to classify fatty infiltration (Fig. 7-25).

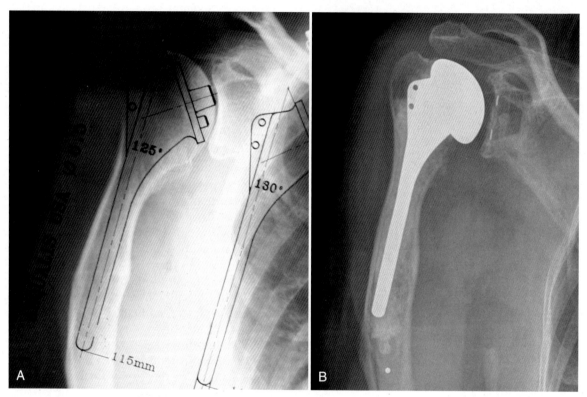

Figure 7-21 A, Preoperative radiographic templating in a patient with a proximal humeral diaphyseal malunion. **B,** In this case, a small prefabricated cemented humeral stem was selected and successfully implanted.

Figure 7-22 Schematic of glenoid morphology as described by Walch and colleagues. **A,** Type A1 glenoid with concentric loading. **B,** Type A2 glenoid with concentric loading and excessive central wear. **C,** Type B1 glenoid with eccentric loading causing posterior subluxation of the humeral head. **D,** Type B2 glenoid with eccentric loading, posterior subluxation of the humeral head, and excessive posterior glenoid wear (biconcave glenoid). **E,** Type C glenoid representing glenoid dysplasia.

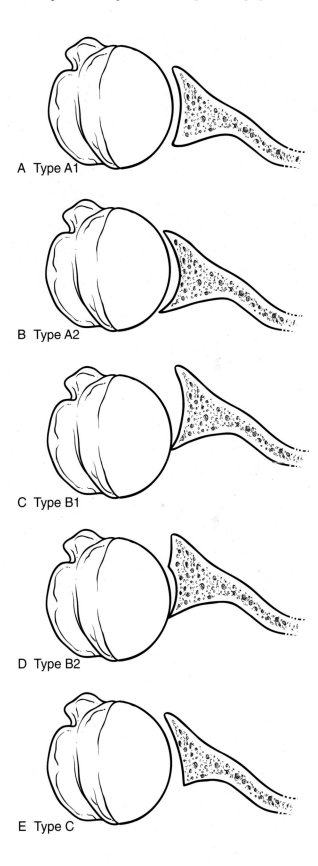

A Type A1

B Type A2

C Type B1

D Type B2

E Type C

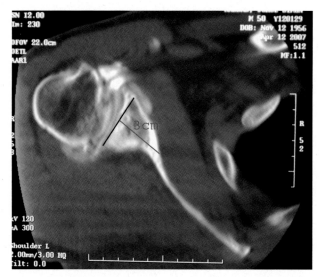

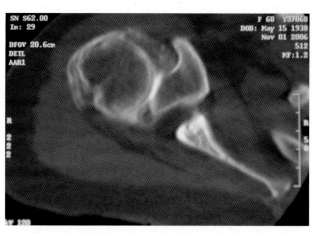

Figure 7-23 Measurement of the depth of the glenoid vault with a computed tomogram preoperatively to determine whether a standard glenoid implant may be used in this case.

Figure 7-24 Computed tomographic arthrography demonstrating a large tear of the rotator cuff involving the supraspinatus and infraspinatus, for which unconstrained total shoulder arthroplasty is contraindicated. In this case either a semiconstrained reverse-design prosthesis (preferable) or hemiarthroplasty should be used.

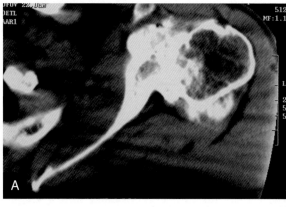

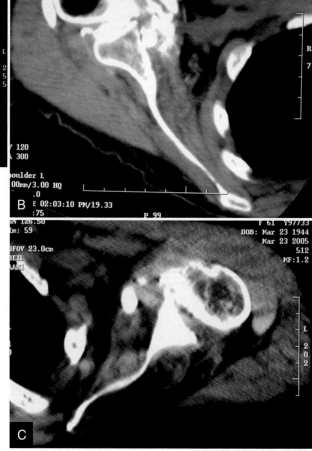

Figure 7-25 Fatty infiltration of the infraspinatus on computed tomography using a three-tiered modification of the Goutallier classification.[7] In this system, mild fatty infiltration (Goutallier stage 0 and stage 1) is defined by essentially normal muscle without any or with minimal fatty streaks (**A**). Moderate fatty infiltration (Goutallier stage 2) is characterized by marked fatty infiltration, but there is more muscle than fat (**B**). In severe fatty infiltration (Goutallier stage 3 and stage 4), there is at least as much fat as muscle (**C**). The same classification system is used for the subscapularis.

REFERENCES

1. Jobe FW, Jobe C: Painful athletic injuries of the shoulder. Clin Orthop Relat Res 1983;173:117-124.
2. Hertel R, Ballmer FT, Lambert SM, et al: Lag signs in the diagnosis of rotator cuff rupture. J Shoulder Elbow Surg 1996;5:307-313.
3. Gerber C, Vinh TS, Hertel R, Hess CW: Latissimus dorsi transfer for the treatment of massive tears of the rotator cuff: A preliminary report. Clin Orthop Relat Res 1988; 232:51-61.
4. Gerber C, Krushell RJ: Isolated rupture of the tendon of the subscapularis muscle: Clinical features in 16 cases. J Bone Joint Surg Br 1991;73:389-394.
5. Walch G, Badet R, Boulahia A, Khoury A: Morphologic study of the glenoid in primary glenohumeral osteoarthritis. J Arthroplasty 1999;14:756-760.
6. Edwards TB, Boulahia A, Kempf JF, et al: The influence of the rotator cuff on the results of shoulder arthroplasty for primary osteoarthritis: Results of a multicenter study. J Bone Joint Surg Am 2002;84:2240-2248.
7. Goutallier D, Postel JM, Bernageau J, et al: Fatty muscle degeneration in cuff rupture. Clin Orthop Relat Res 1994;304:78-83.

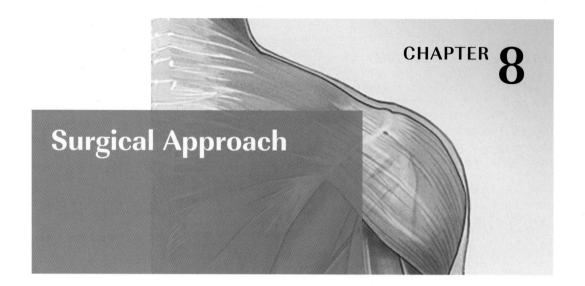

CHAPTER 8

Surgical Approach

For primary unconstrained shoulder arthroplasty we use a deltopectoral approach in all cases. This chapter details this commonly used surgical approach to the glenohumeral joint.

The surgical approach begins with identification of the topographic anatomy (Fig. 8-1). The coracoid process is readily palpable in all but the most obese patients and those who have previously undergone a surgical procedure involving the coracoid process. In thin patients, the deltopectoral interval may be palpable and is useful in guiding orientation of the skin incision. The skin incision, made with a no. 10 scalpel blade, is extended distally and laterally along the anticipated location of the deltopectoral interval from the tip of the coracoid process for 10 to 15 cm, depending on the size of the patient (Fig. 8-2). To minimize hemorrhage, we use a needle tip electrocautery for subcutaneous dissection and for most of the deep dissection throughout the procedure. Medium-size skin rakes are used for retraction during this portion of the approach. The cephalic vein is located to identify the interval between the deltoid and the pectoralis major. In many cases the cephalic vein is covered with a layer of fatty tissue, and identification of this tissue aids in location of the vein (Fig. 8-3). If difficulty is encountered in locating the cephalic vein (congenitally small or absent vein), the deltopectoral interval can be readily detected proximally by identifying a small triangular area devoid of muscle tissue between the proximal portions of the deltoid and pectoralis major muscles (Fig. 8-4). Once located, the cephalic vein is dissected free of the pectoralis major muscle with Metzenbaum scissors. We prefer to retract the cephalic vein laterally with the deltoid because most of the branches of the cephalic vein are based on the deltoid. Medial retraction of the cephalic vein with the pectoralis major disrupts these deltoid branches and introduces unwanted hemorrhage.

After the deltopectoral interval has been identified and developed, Army-Navy retractors are used to maintain the interval. The humeral insertion of the pectoralis major tendon is identified. Dividing the superior centimeter of the pectoralis major tendon enhances exposure of the inferior aspect of the subscapularis, the anterior humeral circumflex vessels, and the axillary nerve (Fig. 8-5). A self-retaining deltopectoral retractor—we prefer a cerebellar-type retractor—is inserted to maintain exposure. Next, the conjoined tendon is identified and traced proximally to its insertion on the coracoid process. Large curved Mayo scissors are used to create a space superior to the coracoid process by placing the scissors just over the top of the coracoid and spreading the blades. Creating this space allows the surgeon to place the tip of a Hohmann-type retractor behind the base of the coracoid process to provide proximal retraction (Fig. 8-6).

The arm is placed in an abducted and externally rotated position, and the apex that is formed by the insertions of the coracoacromial ligament and conjoined tendon to the coracoid process is identified (Fig. 8-7). This apex is developed with the needle tip electrocautery. The lateral aspect of the conjoined tendon is released with the electrocautery, and the conjoined tendon is retracted medially with a narrow Richardson retractor to expose the subscapularis tendon and

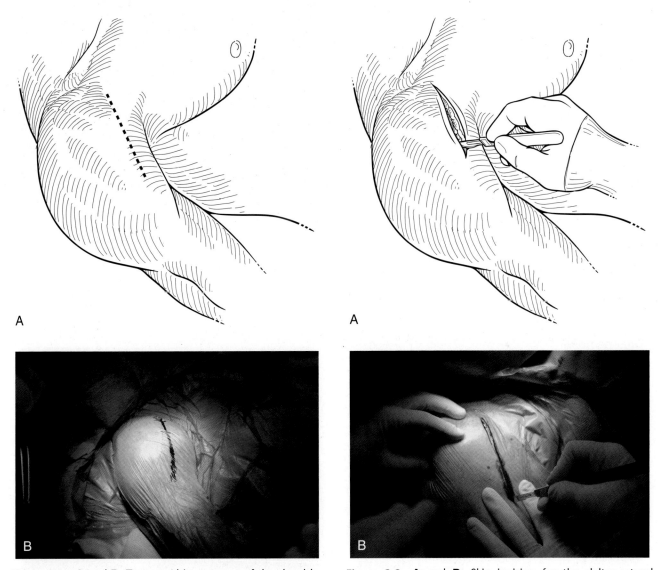

Figure 8-1   **A** and **B,** Topographic anatomy of the shoulder delineated for use in the deltopectoral approach.

Figure 8-2   **A** and **B,** Skin incision for the deltopectoral approach.

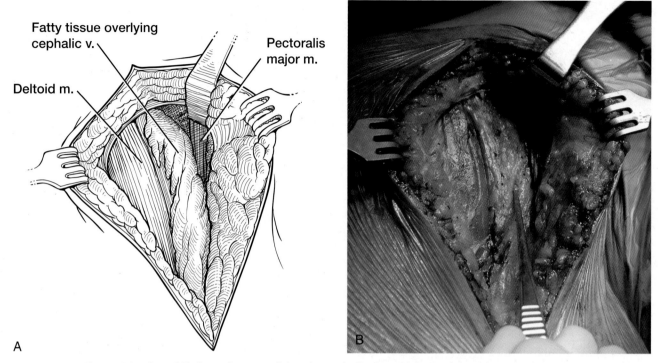

Fatty tissue overlying cephalic v.

Deltoid m.

Pectoralis major m.

A

B

Figure 8-3   **A** and **B,** Fatty tissue overlying the cephalic vein aids in its detection and subsequent identification of the deltopectoral interval.

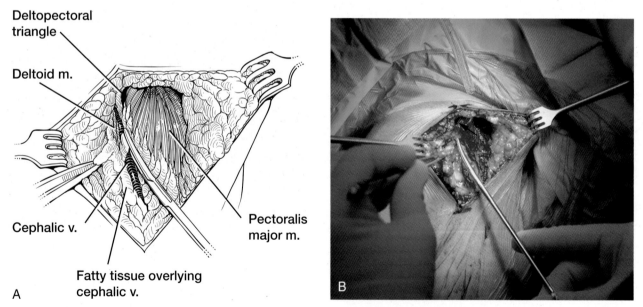

Deltopectoral triangle

Deltoid m.

Cephalic v.

Pectoralis major m.

Fatty tissue overlying cephalic v.

A

B

Figure 8-4   **A** and **B,** Proximal deltopectoral interval. Note the triangular area devoid of muscle tissue (*arrow* in **B**), which aids in identification of this interval.

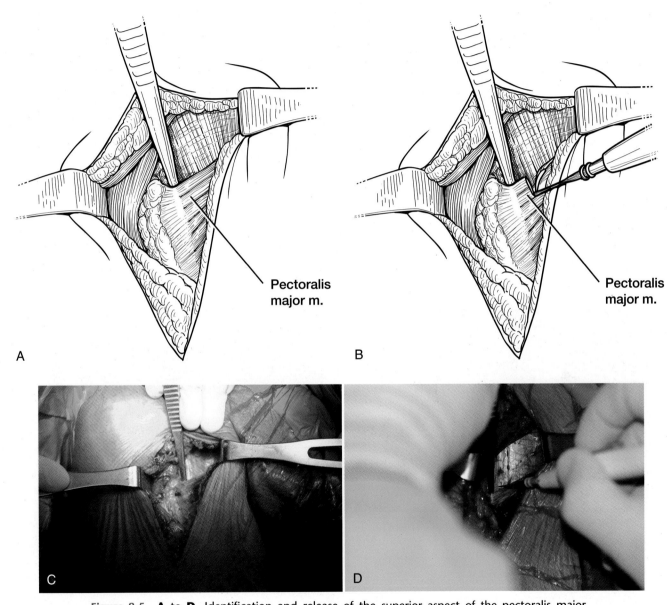

Figure 8-5 **A** to **D,** Identification and release of the superior aspect of the pectoralis major tendon.

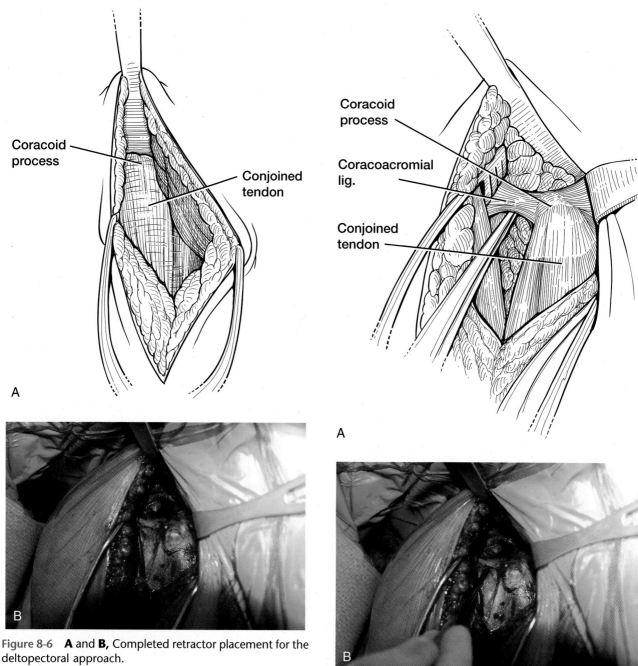

Figure 8-6 **A** and **B,** Completed retractor placement for the deltopectoral approach.

Figure 8-7 **A** and **B,** Identification of the coracoacromial ligament and lateral aspect of the conjoined tendon.

anterior humeral circumflex vessels (the "three sisters") (Fig. 8-8). We prefer to use a narrow Richardson retractor for the conjoined tendon instead of a self-retaining type of retractor because we believe that it minimizes the possibility of prolonged compression and damage to the musculocutaneous nerve.

With the arm externally rotated, the anterior humeral circumflex vessels are suture-ligated at the inferior border of the subscapularis with no. 0 dyed

absorbable braided suture. The proper site of ligation approximates the location of the anatomic neck of the humerus, with the vessels being ligated on each side of the anatomic neck. The suture limbs are cut approximately 15 mm long. This, combined with the dyed suture, allows easier identification of the ligation

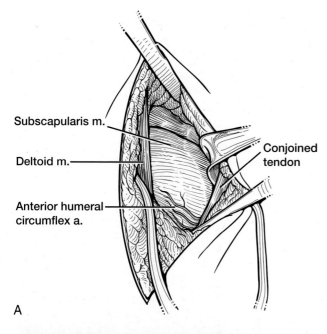

Subscapularis m.

Deltoid m.

Anterior humeral
circumflex a.

Conjoined
tendon

A

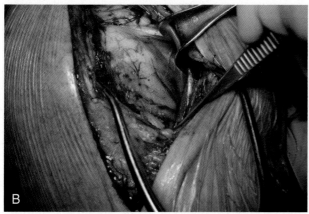

B

Figure 8-8   **A** and **B**, Medial retraction of the conjoined tendon allows visualization of the subscapularis muscle and anterior humeral circumflex vessels.

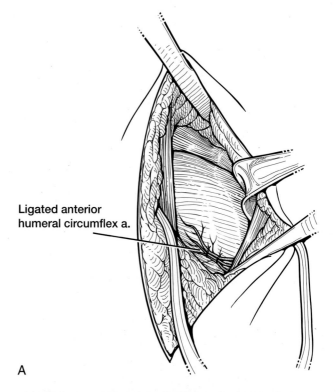

Ligated anterior
humeral circumflex a.

A

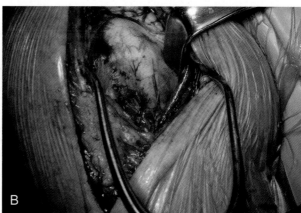

B

Figure 8-9   **A** and **B**, Ligation of the anterior humeral circumflex vessels on each side of the anatomic neck of the humerus. The suture is of the dyed variety and the suture limbs are cut long to allow easier identification of this site during subsequent subscapularis tenotomy.

site during subsequent subscapularis tenotomy (Fig. 8-9).

The axillary nerve is next identified by direct visualization. The narrow Richardson retractor is moved slightly inferiorly along the conjoined tendon to just below the location of the anterior humeral circumflex vessels. The arm is flexed forward in neutral rotation, and blunt dissection is undertaken by spreading the tips of Metzenbaum scissors in the axillary fat inferior and deep to the humeral circumflex vessels. Identification of the axillary nerve ensures its protection throughout the procedure (Fig. 8-10). We identify the axillary nerve routinely. In primary surgery this vital

nerve is almost always in its normal location, but in revision surgery this is rarely the case. The experience gained by dissecting the nerve in primary surgery pays great dividends when the surgeon must find the nerve in the scar tissue associated with revision operations. Table 8-1 lists the steps in the deltopectoral approach for easy reference.

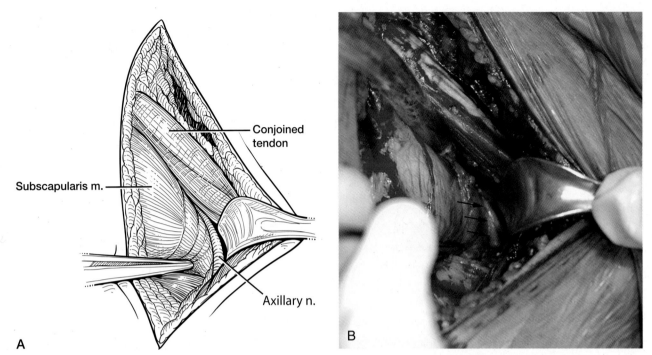

Figure 8-10 **A** and **B,** Identification of the axillary nerve (*arrows* in **B**) through direct visualization.

Table 8-1   STEPS IN THE DELTOPECTORAL APPROACH

Step	Procedure
1	Palpate the coracoid process
2	Perform skin incision of the tip of the coracoid process 15 cm along the deltopectoral interval
3	Perform subcutaneous dissection with needle tip electrocautery
4	Dissect and retract the cephalic vein laterally with the deltoid
5	Identify the pectoralis major tendon insertion on the humerus and divide the superior 1 cm
6	Apply self-retaining retractor to the deltopectoral interval
7	Identify the conjoined tendon and trace it to the coracoid process
8	Place a Hohmann retractor superior to the coracoid process
9	Abduct and externally rotate the arm
10	Identify the lateral aspect of the conjoined tendon
11	Release the lateral aspect of the conjoined tendon
12	Retract the conjoined tendon medially with a narrow Richardson retractor
13	Expose the subscapularis and anterior humeral circumflex vessels
14	Suture-ligate the anterior humeral circumflex vessels with dyed no. 0 braided suture
15	Move the Richardson retractor slightly inferiorly along the conjoined tendon
16	Flex the arm to neutral
17	Identify the axillary nerve in fat inferior and deep to the circumflex vessels

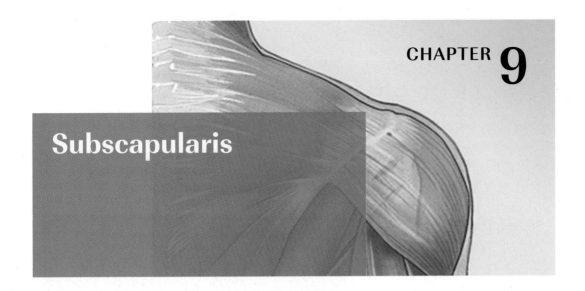

CHAPTER **9**

Subscapularis

After the deltopectoral surgical approach is completed, the next step in performing unconstrained shoulder arthroplasty is management of the subscapularis musculotendinous unit. Various techniques for obtaining anterior access to the glenohumeral joint during shoulder arthroplasty have been described, including complete and partial subscapularis tenotomy, lesser tuberosity osteotomy, and access to the joint solely through the rotator interval. In many patients in whom shoulder arthroplasty is performed the subscapularis lacks normal excursion, thereby creating loss of external rotation. In such cases, surgical techniques must address this soft tissue contracture to allow sufficient postoperative external rotation and minimize the incidence of postoperative dehiscence of the subscapularis. This chapter details our preferred technique for handling the subscapularis, including accessing the glenohumeral joint and addressing loss of external rotation caused by subscapularis contracture.

TECHNIQUE FOR HANDLING THE SUBSCAPULARIS

After the conjoined tendon is retracted medially with a narrow Richardson retractor, the subscapularis is readily visualized. In some cases a hypertrophic subscapularis bursa may be present, and a bursectomy is necessary to allow adequate visualization of the subscapularis tendon. To minimize hemorrhage, we perform bursectomy with the needle tip electrocautery. Once the subscapularis tendon is adequately visualized, two stay sutures of no. 1 nonabsorbable braided suture are double-passed through the tendon approximately 15 mm lateral to the musculotendinous junc-

tion, one in the superior half and one in the inferior half of the tendon (Fig. 9-1).

The glenohumeral joint is opened initially through the rotator interval. The tips of large curved Mayo scissors are passed tangential and just superior to the subscapularis tendon and used to puncture the rotator interval tissue for access to the glenohumeral joint. Once the glenohumeral joint is entered, the scissors are spread to enlarge the arthrotomy (Fig. 9-2). Usually after the Mayo scissors are spread, synovial fluid egresses from the joint.

The next step involves elevation of the subscapularis from its humeral insertion to allow further access to the glenohumeral joint. We prefer performing a complete subscapularis tenotomy because it allows unhindered access to the glenohumeral joint and sufficient release of subscapularis contracture. Additionally, tenotomy does not risk disruption of the existing proximal humeral osseous anatomy, as may occur with lesser tuberosity osteotomy. The location of the tenotomy is critical to allow adequate repair after insertion of the prosthesis is completed. We perform the tenotomy along the anatomic neck of the humerus while leaving a small amount of tendon on the lesser tuberosity to use in later subscapularis closure. The shoulder is placed in neutral to slight external rotation during this portion of the procedure. To identify the anatomic neck of the humerus, a no. 10 scalpel blade on a long handle is used to further open the rotator interval from the initial arthrotomy site extending laterally along the superior border of the subscapularis tendon (Fig. 9-3). Once the anatomic neck of the humerus is identified by observing the lateral extent of the articular surface, the scalpel blade is directed inferiorly to transect the superior two thirds of the subscapularis tendon along

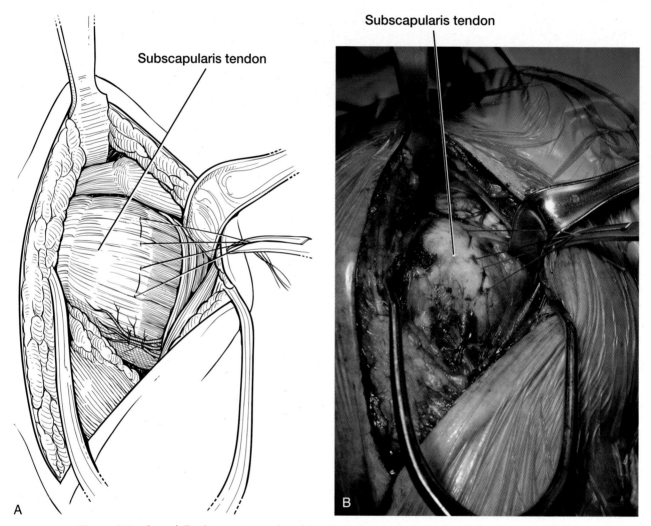

Figure 9-1 A and **B,** Stay sutures placed in the subscapularis tendon before subscapularis tenotomy.

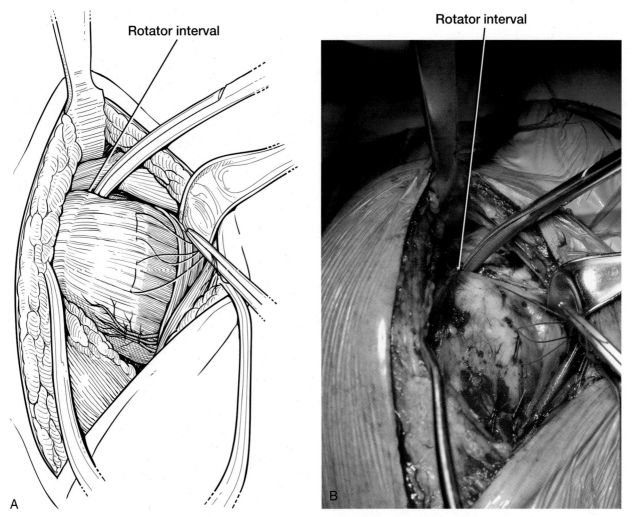

Figure 9-2 **A** and **B,** Arthrotomy of the glenohumeral joint through the rotator interval with large Mayo scissors.

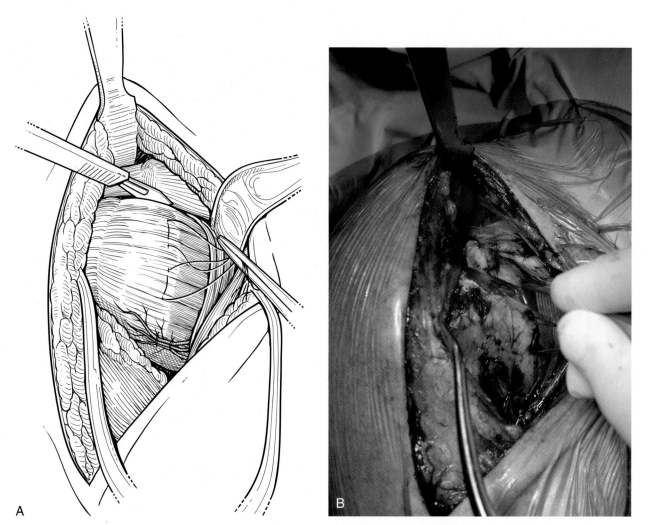

A

B

Figure 9-3 **A** and **B,** Extension of the rotator interval arthrotomy laterally to the anatomic neck in preparation for subscapularis tenotomy.

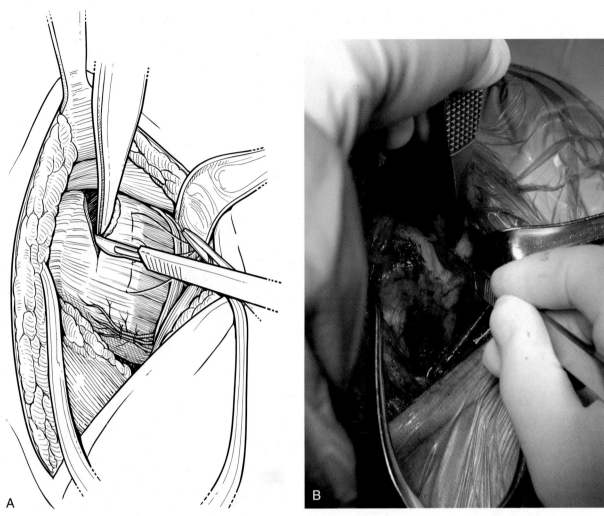

Figure 9-4 Performance of subscapularis tenotomy. **A** and **B,** The superior two thirds of the tendon is transected with the scalpel.

Continued

the anatomic neck of the humerus (Fig. 9-4A). At the inferior third of the subscapularis, we switch to the needle tip electrocautery and complete the tenotomy. The needle tip passes between the previously placed anterior humeral circumflex ligation sutures and cauterizes these vessels (Fig. 9-4B). As the subscapularis tenotomy is completed, the shoulder is progressively externally rotated to allow visualization of the inferior humeral capsular attachment (Fig. 9-4C and D). This capsule is released from the humerus with the needle tip electrocautery while keeping the electrocautery in contact with the humerus (Fig. 9-5).

A humeral head retractor (we prefer the Trillat type of retractor) is placed in the glenohumeral joint and the humeral head is retracted posteriorly. To facilitate insertion of this retractor, the shoulder is initially externally rotated and moved into internal rotation as the retractor is pushed posteriorly between the humeral

head and the glenoid. With the humeral head retracted posteriorly and traction applied to stay sutures in the subscapularis tendon, the glenohumeral ligaments are readily visualized (Fig. 9-6). To increase subscapularis excursion, circumferential release of the subscapularis tendon is performed. The superior glenohumeral ligament is first released with large curved Mayo scissors along the superior aspect of the subscapularis tendon (Fig. 9-7). The middle glenohumeral ligament, which may be absent in up to a third of patients, is released parallel to the anterior glenoid rim with large curved Mayo scissors (Fig. 9-8). Anteriorly and inferiorly the tissue plane between the capsuloligamentous structures and the primarily muscular inferior portion of the subscapularis is identified and established with large curved Mayo scissors. Once this plane is established, the inferior glenohumeral ligament is divided

Text continued on p. 90

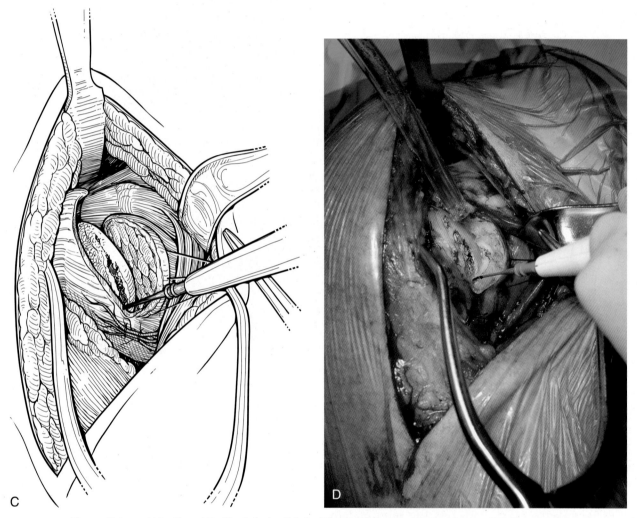

C

D

Figure 9-4, cont'd   **C** and **D,** The inferior third of the tendon is transected by passing the needle tip electrocautery between the ligation sutures previously placed around the anterior humeral circumflex vessels during the surgical approach.

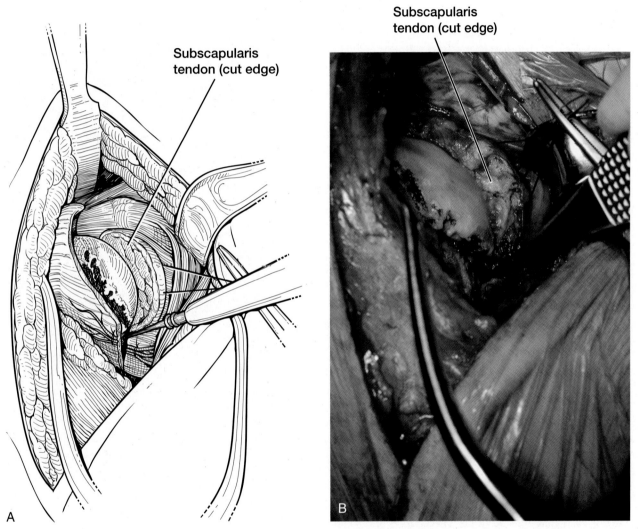

Subscapularis tendon (cut edge)

Subscapularis tendon (cut edge)

A

B

Figure 9-5 A and **B,** Release of the medial joint capsule from the humerus with the needle tip electrocautery.

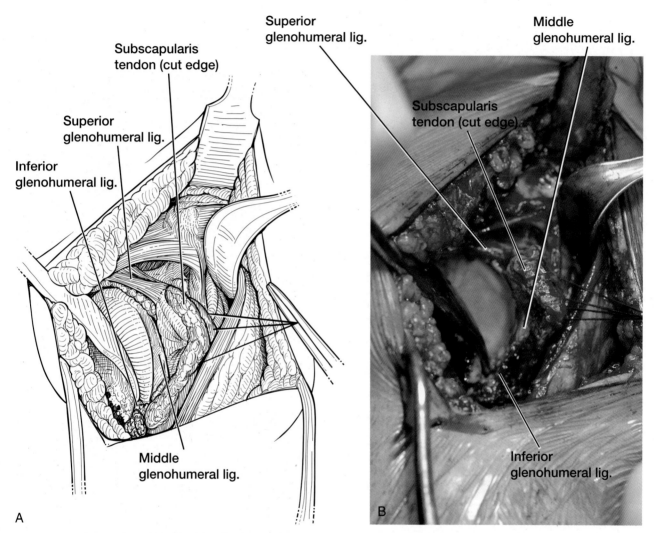

Figure 9-6 **A** and **B,** Visualization of the superior, middle, and inferior glenohumeral ligaments after subscapularis tenotomy.

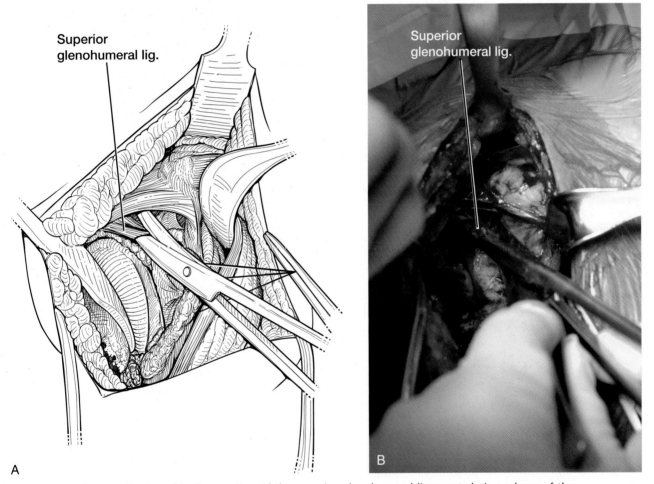

Superior
glenohumeral lig.

Superior
glenohumeral lig.

A

B

Figure 9-7 **A** and **B,** Transection of the superior glenohumeral ligament during release of the
subscapularis tendon.

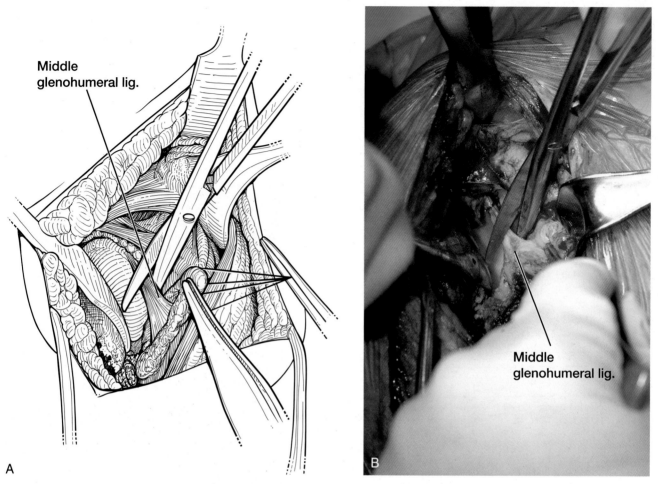

Middle
glenohumeral lig.

Middle
glenohumeral lig.

A

B

Figure 9-8 **A** and **B,** Transection of the middle glenohumeral ligament during release of the subscapularis tendon.

with the scissors. Risk of injury to the axillary nerve is avoided because the muscular portion of the subscapularis isolates it from the path of the scissors (Fig. 9-9). After release of the glenohumeral ligaments, the intra-articularly located subscapularis recess is readily accessible. This recess should be routinely inspected for loose bodies. We remove all loose bodies (Fig. 9-10). In most cases these loose bodies are osseous and may be anticipated by identification

on preoperative imaging studies. Finally, blunt dissection with a Cobb elevator is used to release any adhesions that remain anterior to the subscapularis (Fig. 9-11). After release of the subscapularis, which effectively lengthens the contracted tendon, increased excursion should be possible. A sponge is used to tuck the subscapularis into the subscapularis fossa, and it is held with a small glenoid rim retractor (Fig. 9-12).

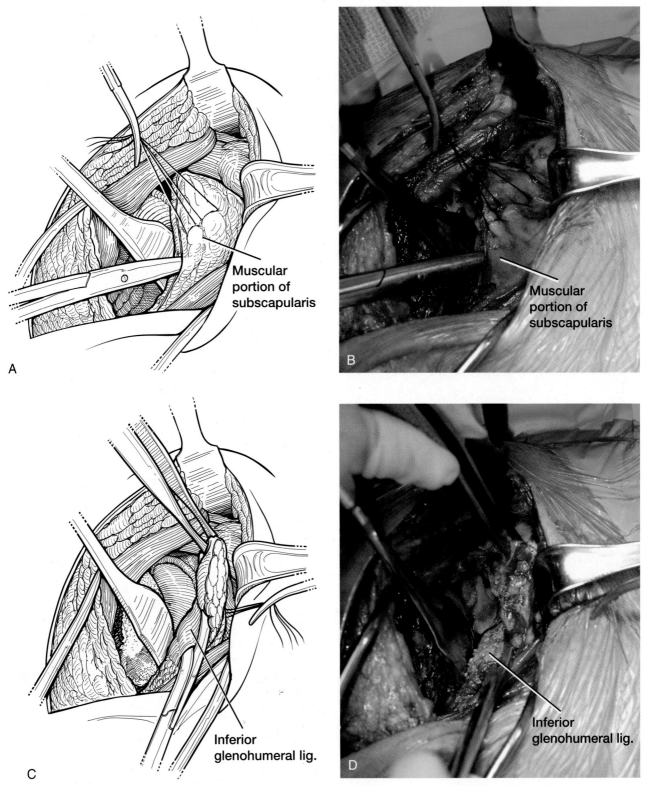

Figure 9-9 A to D, Transection of the inferior glenohumeral ligament during release of the subscapularis. The muscular portion of the subscapularis inferiorly protects the axillary nerve during release.

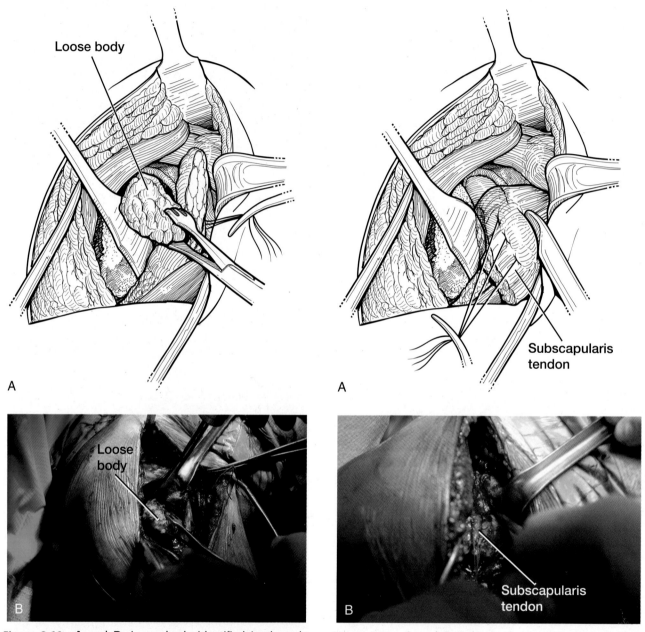

Figure 9-10   **A** and **B,** Loose body identified in the subscapularis recess after release of the glenohumeral ligaments.

Figure 9-11   **A** and **B,** Release of extra-articular adhesions anterior to the subscapularis with a Cobb elevator.

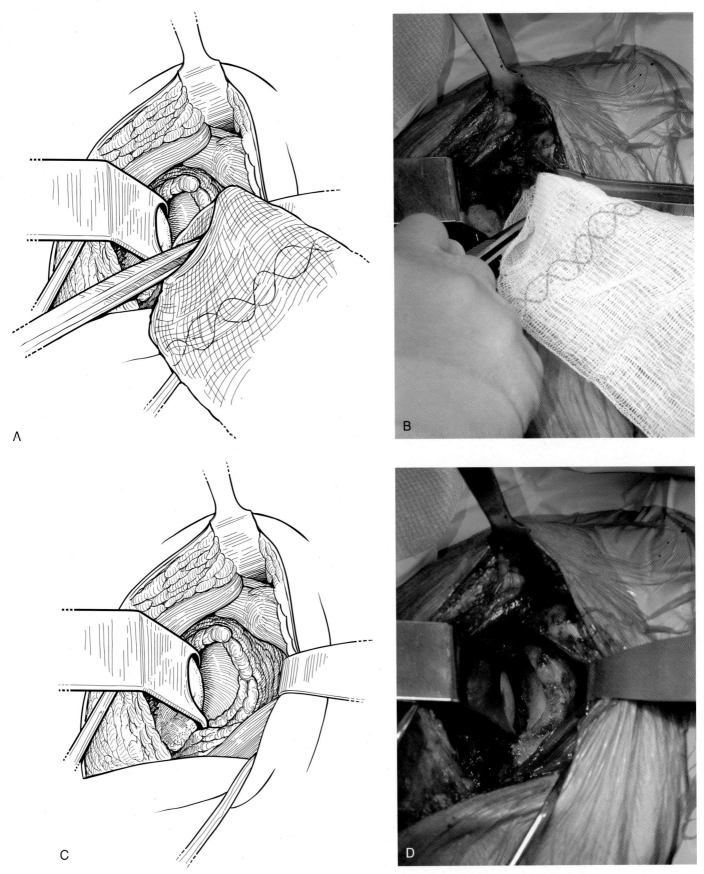

A

B

C

D

Figure 9-12   A sponge is used to tuck the subscapularis into the subscapularis fossa (**A** and **B**), and it is held with a small glenoid rim retractor (**C** and **D**).

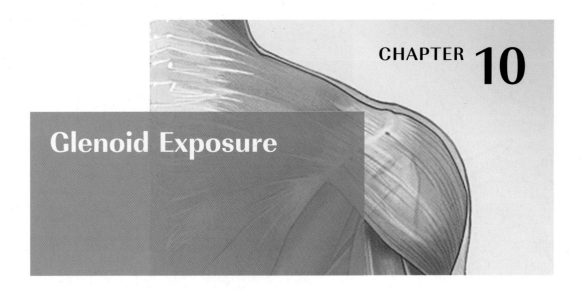

CHAPTER 10

Glenoid Exposure

Whenever we question surgeons who routinely perform hemiarthroplasty instead of total shoulder arthroplasty for conditions such as primary osteoarthritis about why they chose not to resurface the glenoid, by far the most common response is that they encounter problems with glenoid exposure. When questioned further, it is evident that most of these surgeons simply lack the information necessary to correctly and reliably provide visualization of the osseous glenoid. Glenoid exposure can be simplified by following a sequence of surgical steps. This chapter outlines our systematic technique of capsular release that provides sufficient visualization for glenoid resurfacing.

TECHNIQUE FOR GLENOID EXPOSURE

Anterior Release

After the subscapularis is retracted medially with a sponge and small glenoid rim retractor, attention is turned to glenoid exposure. A needle tip electrocautery is used to excise any remaining labrum beginning at the base of the coracoid process and extending inferiorly to the 5 o'clock position in a right shoulder (7 o'clock in a left shoulder). This allows identification of the osseous anterior margin of the glenoid (Fig. 10-1).

Inferior Release

In nearly all cases, implantation of a glenoid component requires release of the inferior capsule to obtain adequate exposure. The tip of the electrocautery is used to release the inferior capsule directly off the rim of the glenoid bone (Fig. 10-2). To avoid damaging the axillary nerve, the tip of the electrocautery must be kept in contact with glenoid bone. This release is extended sufficiently medially toward the axillary border of the scapula to completely transect the capsule and expose the muscular fibers of the triceps inserting on the inferior osseous glenoid. Visualization of the muscular fibers of the triceps or the axillary border of the scapula indicates that dissection of the capsule is sufficient.

Posterior Release

The amount of posterior subluxation present on preoperative secondary imaging studies (computed tomography, magnetic resonance imaging) determines the posterior extent of release. In shoulders without posterior subluxation, the release continues posteriorly to the 8 o'clock position for right shoulders (4 o'clock position for left shoulders). In shoulders that have preexisting posterior subluxation, either with or

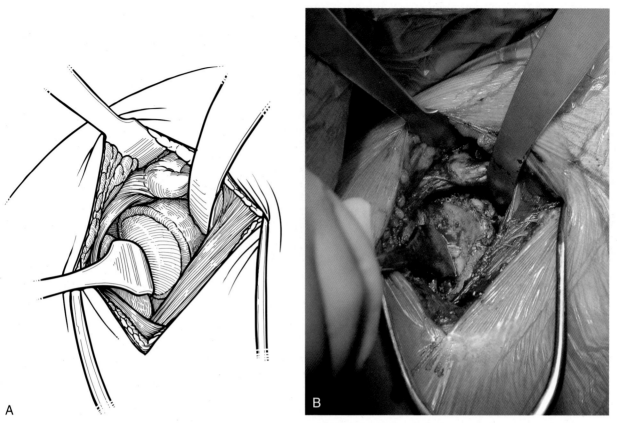

Figure 10-1   **A** and **B,** Identification of the anterior osseous margin of the glenoid after excision of the anterior glenoid labrum.

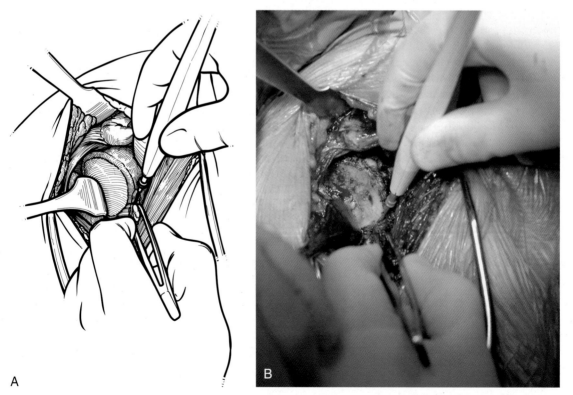

Figure 10-2   **A** and **B,** Release the inferior capsule directly off the rim of the glenoid with the electrocautery.

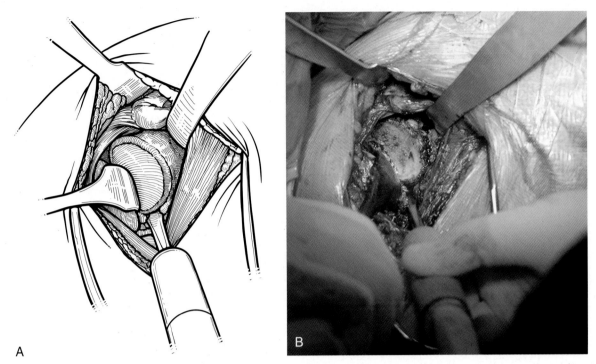

Figure 10-3 **A** and **B,** A Cobb elevator is used to check the adequacy of the inferior capsular release.

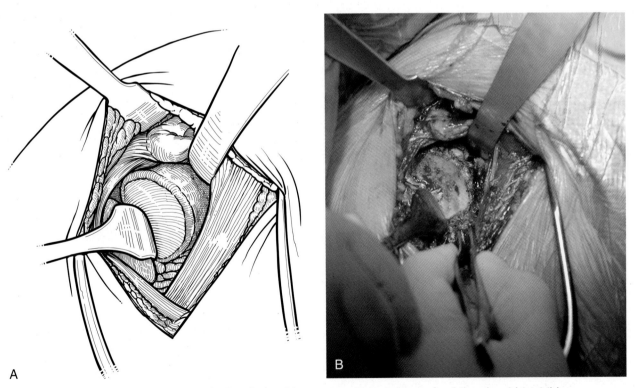

Figure 10-4 **A** and **B,** Completed glenoid exposure. Note how much of the glenoid is visible even before humeral head resection.

without posterior glenoid erosion, the release continues initially to only the 6 o'clock position. These patients often have a distended posterior capsule, so to avoid further compromising these posterior structures, no more release is performed than is absolutely necessary. If release to only the 6 o'clock position proves inadequate later during glenoid reaming, the release can be extended at that time. A Cobb elevator can be used to check the release for completeness (Fig. 10-3). Figure 10-4 shows the completed release.

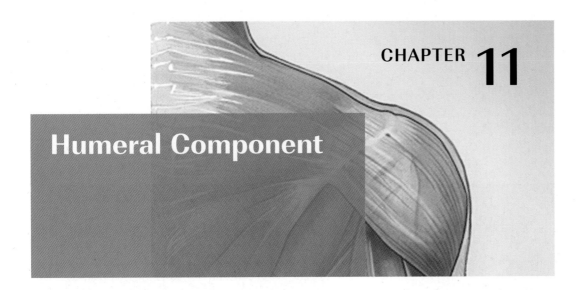

CHAPTER 11

Humeral Component

For unconstrained shoulder arthroplasty, both cemented and uncemented humeral stemmed components are available (Figs. 11-1 and 11-2). The incidence of aseptic loosening of cemented humeral stems is less than 2%.[1] Similarly, the incidence of aseptic loosening of uncemented textured humeral stems is negligible.[2] Implantation of smooth, polished humeral components without cement has led to a 55% incidence of humeral loosening and should be avoided.[1] In most cases of unconstrained shoulder arthroplasty, the choice of cemented or uncemented humeral stems is based on surgeon preference. In our practice we prefer the use of uncemented humeral stems in most cases. Use of uncemented humeral stems eliminates the time required for cement preparation and insertion. Our indication for use of a cemented humeral stem is pre-existing deformity of the proximal humerus or severe proximal humeral osteopenia precluding initial fixation of an uncemented humeral stem (Fig. 11-3). Many different prosthetic systems are available for unconstrained shoulder arthroplasty, and it is beyond the scope of this textbook to describe the specific techniques used for each of these systems. This chapter describes the technique for preparation of the proximal humerus with our preferred prosthetic system. Most of the steps are applicable regardless of the system used.

TECHNIQUE FOR INSERTION OF AN UNCEMENTED HUMERAL COMPONENT

Once the inferior capsule is released from the neck of the glenoid as described in Chapter 10, humeral preparation begins. The humeral head retractor is removed, and the humeral head is dislocated by externally rotating and extending the arm (Fig. 11-4). A Hohmann retractor positioned superior to the coracoid process is moved to the margin of the bare area of the humeral head articular surface (junction of the supraspinatus and infraspinatus), and a modified Hohmann retractor (see Chapter 3) is placed inferiorly and medially at the surgical neck of the humerus. This completes the proximal humeral exposure (Fig. 11-5). The presence and extent of humeral head osteophytes vary with the underlying diagnosis. Whereas conditions such as primary osteoarthritis typically have large osteophytes, other conditions such as rheumatoid arthritis have a paucity of osteophytes. The anteroposterior radiograph is helpful in determining the presence and extent of humeral osteophytes. To identify the true anatomic neck of the humerus, the osteophytes are removed with a $^1/_2$-inch straight osteotome (Fig. 11-6). Typically, a layer of adipose tissue is present between the osteophytes and the native humerus and aids in identification of the normal margin of the humeral head articular surface (Fig. 11-7). The insertion of the infraspinatus tendon should be readily visible on the posterior aspect of the humerus (Fig. 11-8). It is critical to visualize the infraspinatus to prevent damage to the posterior rotator cuff during humeral head resection. Additionally, when using a prosthesis with an anatomic design, the location of the posterior rotator cuff (infraspinatus) defines humeral version (which varies from 7 degrees of anteversion to 48 degrees of retroversion) and, consequently, version of the humeral head cut.[3] After identification of the insertion of the

Text continued on p. 104

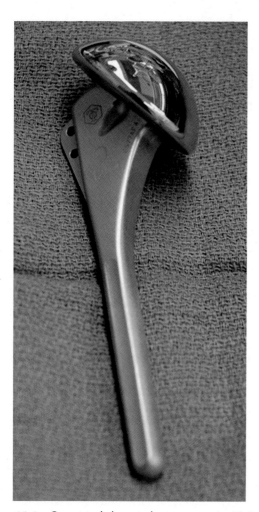

Figure 11-1 Cemented humeral component. Note the smooth, polished stem design.

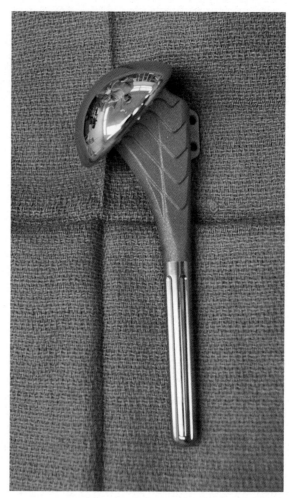

Figure 11-2 Uncemented humeral component. Note the textured proximal finish with the fluted distal stem designed to resist motion at the prosthesis-bone interface.

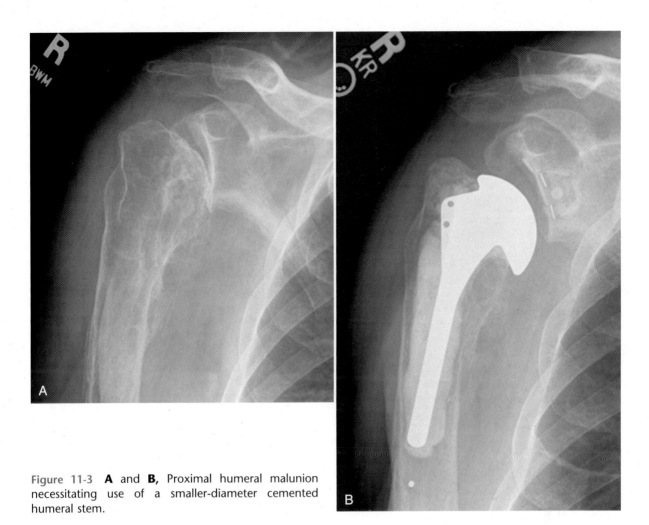

Figure 11-3 A and **B,** Proximal humeral malunion necessitating use of a smaller-diameter cemented humeral stem.

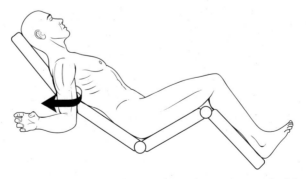

Figure 11-4 Maneuver (external rotation and extension) for dislocation of the humeral head.

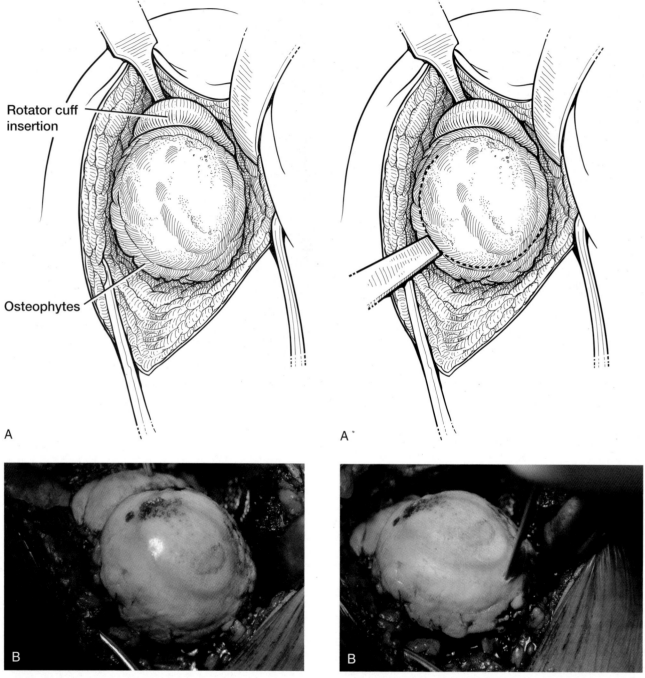

Rotator cuff
insertion

Osteophytes

A

A

B

B

Figure 11-5 **A** and **B,** The dislocated proximal humerus reveals peripheral osteophytes.

Figure 11-6 **A** and **B,** Peripheral humeral osteophytes are removed with an osteotome to expose the anatomic neck of the humerus.

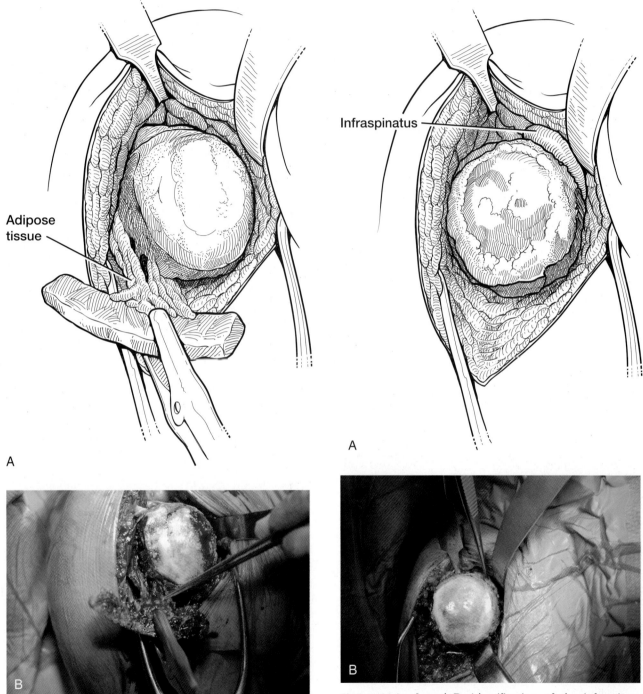

Figure 11-7 **A** and **B,** Layer of adipose tissue interposed between the osteophytes and the native humerus.

Figure 11-8 **A** and **B,** Identification of the infraspinatus insertion on the greater tuberosity at the posterior aspect of the humerus.

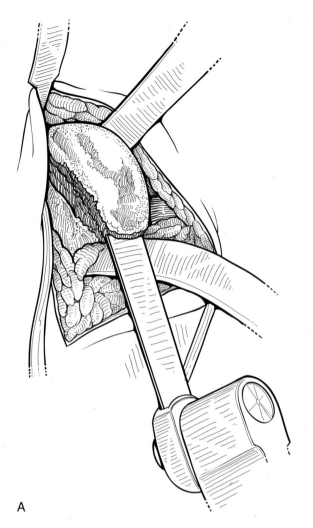

A

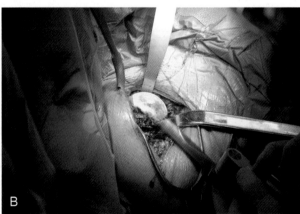

B

Figure 11-9 **A** and **B,** Resection of the humeral head with an oscillating saw.

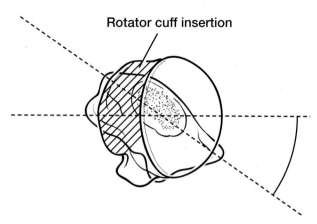

Figure 11-10 Depiction of the relationship between the insertion of the posterior rotator cuff (infraspinatus) and humeral version.

during humeral head resection. Proper head resection at the anatomic neck correctly replicates humeral version. Figure 11-10 depicts the relationship between humeral version and insertion of the rotator cuff.

We use an adaptable anatomic prosthetic system (Aequalis Prosthetic System, Tornier, Inc., Stafford, TX) with the goal of reproducing the normal anatomy of each patient. This system permits specification of humeral stem diameter, humeral head diameter, anatomic neck inclination, and humeral head offset. With this system the humeral canal is identified and entered with an awl; the entry point is typically on the anterior and lateral aspect of the cut surface because of the normal posterior and medial offset of the humeral head with respect to the humeral diaphysis (Fig. 11-11). Progressive diaphyseal reaming is performed with manual instrumentation to reach the inner humeral cortex. The preoperative anteroposterior radiograph is helpful to estimate intramedullary canal diameter (Fig. 11-12). It is not critical that the diaphyseal fit be excessively "tight." We prefer to use a smaller diaphyseal reamer rather than risk humeral fracture. The neck inclination guide is used to select the appropriate inclination of the prosthesis, which varies between 125 and 140 degrees in 5-degree increments (Fig. 11-13). If the neck inclination angle is not divisible by 5, we select the smaller angle; that is, we would select a 130-degree component if the actual measurement were 133 degrees. The proximal humerus seems to be able to better adapt to a smaller neck inclination angle than to one that is too large, hence our reason for selecting the prosthesis with the smaller inclination angle. Progressive metaphyseal broaching is performed to match the size of the largest reamer used (Fig. 11-14) while taking care to keep the broaches perpendicular to the cut surface of the humerus for maintenance of correct humeral version. The humeral inclination angle is

infraspinatus, the humeral head is removed at the anatomic neck of the humerus with an oscillating saw (Fig. 11-9). We believe it acceptable to leave the bare area of the humeral head because this allows a margin of error for protection of the posterior rotator cuff

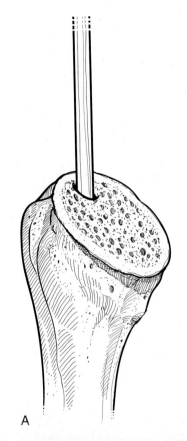

A

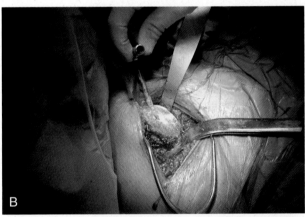

B

Figure 11-11 A and **B,** An awl is used to locate and open the humeral canal. The entry point is generally located on the anterior and lateral aspect of the cut surface because of the normal posterior and medial offset of the humeral head with respect to the humeral diaphysis.

marked on the broach to help the surgeon determine the appropriate depth to advance it (Fig. 11-15). Once reaming and broaching are complete, a trial stem is inserted (Fig. 11-16). The trial stem is assembled before insertion by combining a metaphyseal-diaphyseal portion that matches the largest size broach used and a humeral neck portion that matches the neck inclina-

tion angle selected (Fig. 11-17). A trial prosthetic humeral head is selected to match the size of the resected humeral head (Fig. 11-18). Most humeral heads are slightly elliptical; if this is the case, the smaller diameter is selected. Additionally, if the resected humeral head is between the sizes available in the prosthetic system, the smaller size is initially selected to avoid "overstuffing" the glenohumeral joint. The trial head is then placed on the trial stem. The Aequalis system incorporates variable medial and posterior head offset to allow the surgeon to position the head at one of eight indexed positions. The position that provides the best coverage of the cut humeral surface is selected (Fig. 11-19). Care is taken to avoid overhang of the prosthetic head anteriorly, superiorly, and posteriorly to prevent impingement of the rotator cuff. Inferior overhang, though not ideal, is acceptable. If a large amount of overhang is observed at any index, the selected head is probably too large. In areas in which the prosthetic head does not quite cover the cut humeral surface, a rongeur can be used to trim the cut surface and create a better fit. The entire humeral trial component is then removed. If a glenoid component is to be inserted, the cut humeral surface is covered with a humeral cut protector to prevent deformation of the humeral cut surface during glenoid preparation and implantation (Fig. 11-20). Care is taken to note the humeral head offset index before disassembling the trial humeral component so that the final humeral implant may be properly assembled. Except in cases in which we have selected the smallest humeral stem, we use a cut protector (assembled similar to the trial humeral implant except that the neck portion is replaced with a flat surface matching the selected inclination angle) with a metaphyseal-diaphyseal portion 1 size smaller than what has been selected for the trial stem to allow easier removal later in the procedure (Fig. 11-21). In cases in which the smallest humeral stem has been selected, the same size cut protector is used.

After the cut protector has been inserted, tenotomy or tenodesis of the biceps tendon is performed (as described in Chapter 5), the glenoid is addressed (as described in Chapter 12), and soft tissue balancing is completed (as described in Chapter 13) in cases of total shoulder arthroplasty. While the glenoid cement is curing, the final humeral implant is assembled on the back table by an assistant (Fig. 11-22). Before insertion of the final humeral implant, three no. 2 nonabsorbable braided sutures are placed first through the humeral stump of the subscapularis tendon, into the lesser tuberosity, and out through the intramedullary canal of the humerus to be used in later reattachment

Text continued on p. 112

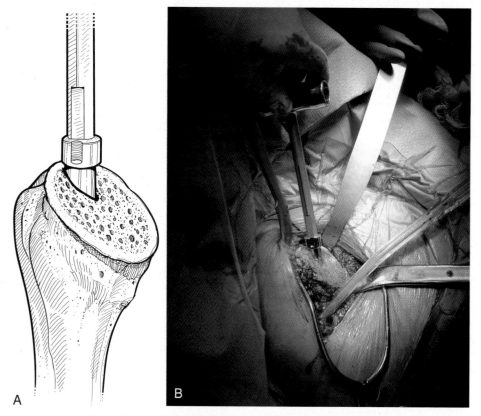

Figure 11-12 **A** and **B,** Reaming of the humeral diaphysis.

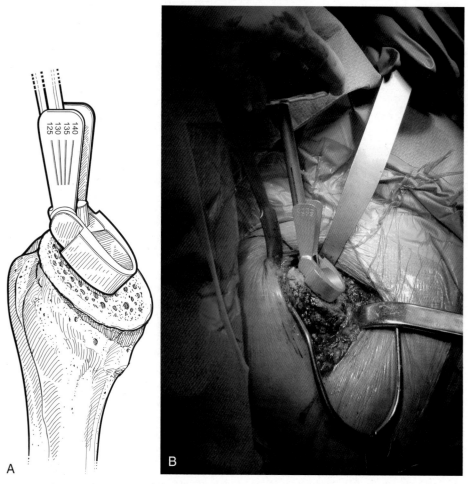

Figure 11-13 **A** and **B,** Selection of the humeral neck inclination angle.

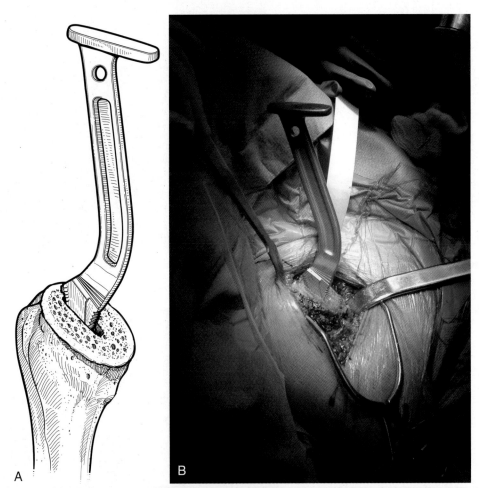

A

B

Figure 11-14 **A** and **B,** Progressive metaphyseal broaching is performed.

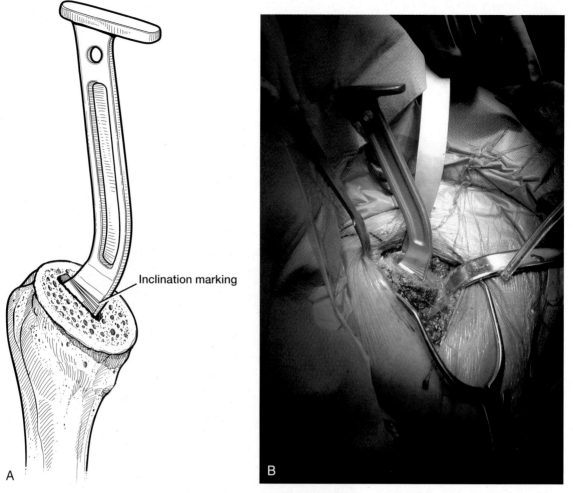

Figure 11-15   **A** and **B,** Markings along the neck of the broach identify the different humeral neck inclination angles available.

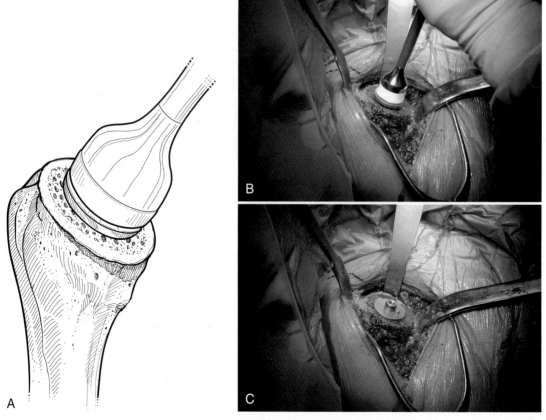

Figure 11-16   **A** to **C,** Placement of the trial stem.

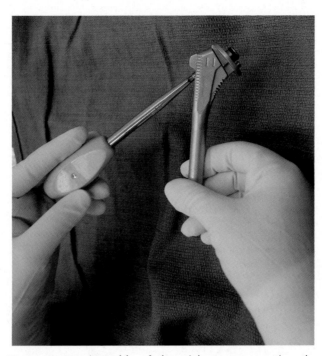

Figure 11-17 Assembly of the trial stem connecting the metaphyseal-diaphyseal portion with the humeral neck portion.

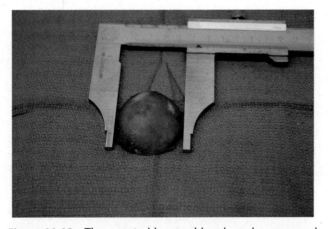

Figure 11-18 The resected humeral head can be measured with calipers or compared in size to the trial humeral heads available.

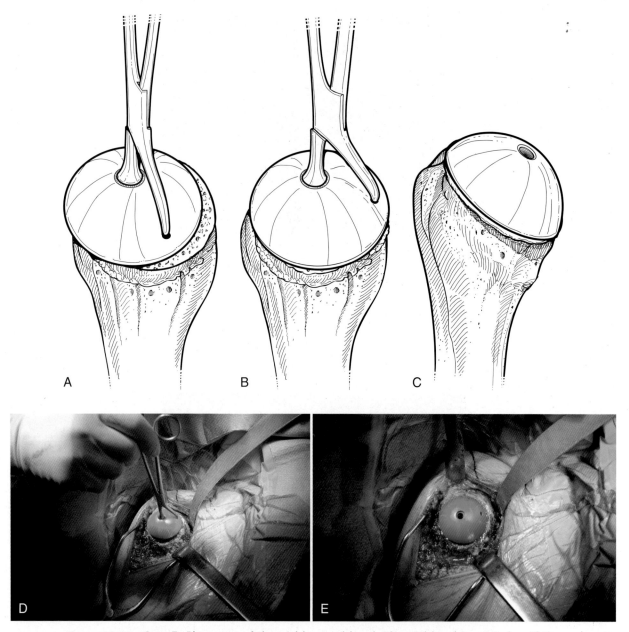

Figure 11-19 **A** to **E**, Placement of the trial humeral head. The trial head is rotated until the indexed position providing the best coverage of the cut humeral surface is discovered.

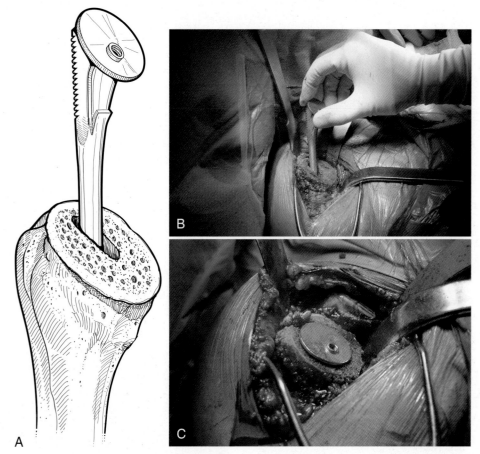

Figure 11-20 **A** to **C,** A humeral cut protector is placed after removal of the trial humeral component and before glenoid preparation.

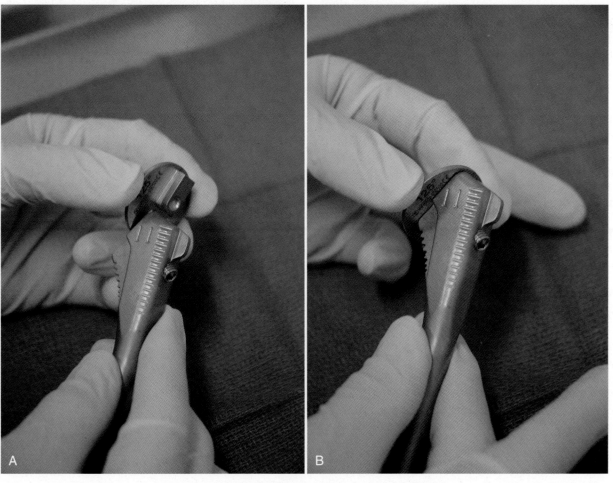

Figure 11-21 **A** and **B,** Assembly of the cut protector.

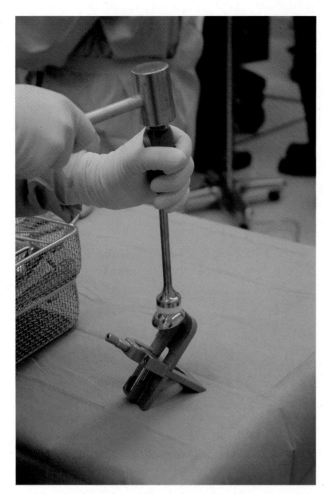

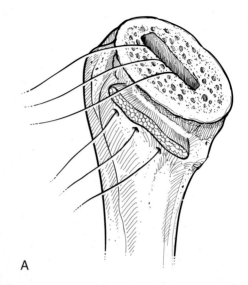

Figure 11-22 Assembly of the humeral implant. The humeral head is impacted onto the humeral stem at the selected posterior medial offset index.

of the subscapularis (Fig. 11-23). These sutures are tagged with three different types of hemostats to identify the sutures as superior, middle, and inferior (we use a curved Kelly hemostat superiorly, a mosquito hemostat on the middle suture, and a regular hemostat inferiorly). The humeral implant is then impacted into place while making sure to avoid inadvertent rotation of the component during insertion (Fig. 11-24).

TECHNIQUE FOR INSERTION OF A CEMENTED HUMERAL COMPONENT

The technique for insertion of a cemented humeral stem is not too dissimilar from the technique described for insertion of an uncemented humeral stem. The main differences are in the instrumentation used to prepare the proximal humerus to receive the humeral implant.

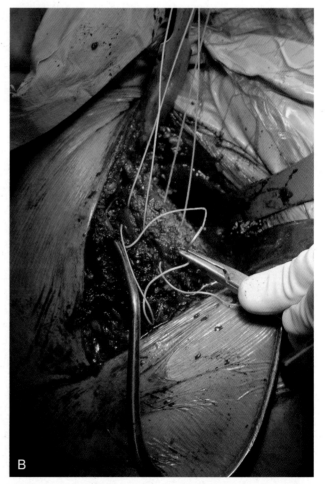

Figure 11-23 A and **B,** Placement of transosseous sutures for later reattachment of the subscapularis.

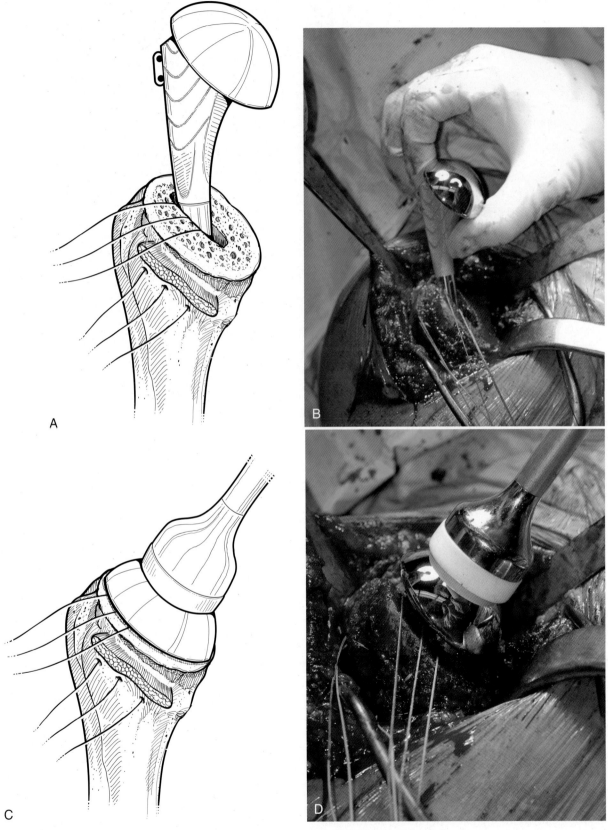

Figure 11-24   **A** to **D,** Insertion of the humeral implant.

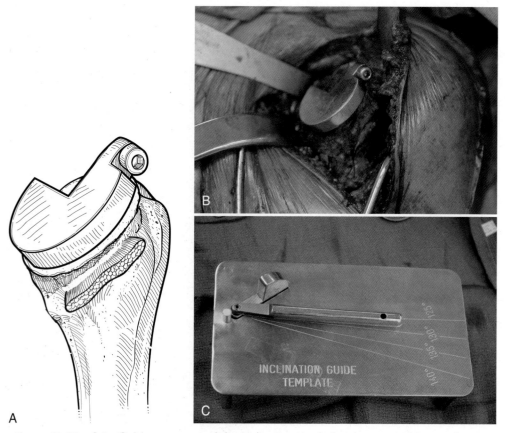

Figure 11-25   A to **C,** Measurement of the inclination angle for a cemented humeral stem.

Humeral exposure and the osteotomy are performed the same as for an uncemented humeral stem. The humeral canal is entered and the diaphysis reamed just as for an uncemented humeral stem. After the final diaphyseal reamer is selected and used, a specialized instrument corresponding in size to the diameter of the last diaphyseal reamer used is introduced to measure the humeral cut inclination angle. This instrument consists of a stem and a flat surface that sits on the cut humeral surface connected by an adjustable hinge. With the flat surface sitting on the cut humeral surface, the hinge is tightened. The instrument is removed and placed in a measurement device that yields the neck inclination angle (Fig. 11-25). Metaphyseal broaching is performed by advancing broaches similar to those used for an uncemented stem to the line demarcating the selected inclination angle. Insertion of the trial stem and selection of the trial humeral head and its posterior medial offset index are identical to that for an uncemented humeral stem, as are trial removal and insertion of a cut protector. Preparation

of the glenoid and soft tissue balancing are carried out as described in Chapters 12 and 13.

Before insertion of the humeral stem, a cement restrictor is placed 1 cm distal to the distal-most extent of the stem with an insertion device (Fig. 11-26). Sutures for reattachment of the subscapularis are placed as described earlier. The humeral canal is irrigated with sterile saline and dried with suction and gauze sponges. Bone cement (we prefer to use DePuy 2 [DePuy, Inc., Warsaw, IN] because of its accelerated curing time of less than 8 minutes) is introduced with a catheter tip syringe (Fig. 11-27). The canal is filled with cement and the assembled humeral stem is seated with an impactor (Fig. 11-28). It is not necessary to pressurize the cement. Excess cement is removed with a Freer elevator. It is not necessary to allow the cement to cure before reducing the glenohumeral joint unless the humeral metaphysis is compromised (tuberosity fracture), in which case the cement should be allowed to cure before reduction of the glenohumeral joint.

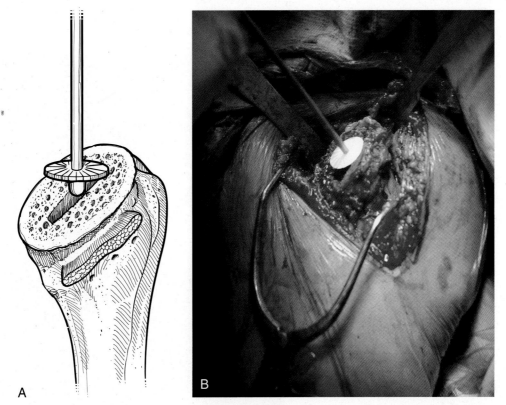

Figure 11-26 **A** and **B,** Insertion of a cement restrictor before insertion of a cemented humeral stem. The cement restrictor allows 1 cm of cement distal to the tip of the humeral stem.

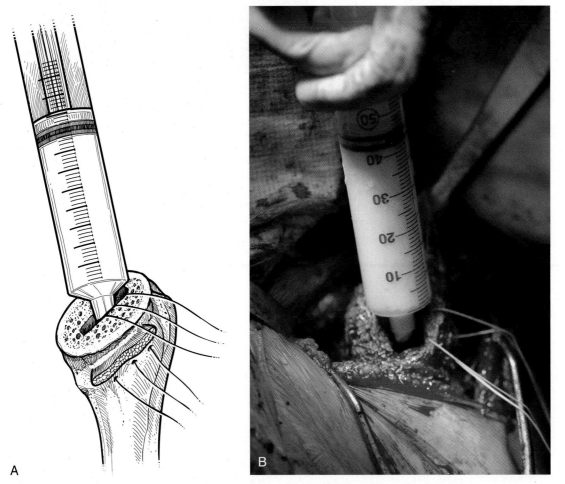

Figure 11-27 **A** and **B,** Cement is inserted into the humeral canal with a catheter tip syringe.

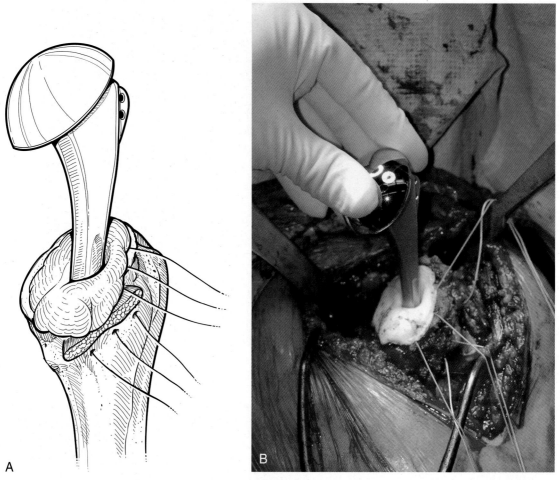

Figure 11-28 **A** and **B,** Insertion of a cemented humeral stem.

REFERENCES

1. Trojani C, Boileau P, Coste JS, Walch G: Aseptic loosening in Aequalis shoulder arthroplasty. In Walch G, Boileau P, Molé D (eds): 2000 Prosthèses d'Epaule . . . Recul de 2 à 10 Ans. Paris, Sauramps Medical, 2001, pp 437-441.
2. Matsen FA III, Iannotti JP, Rockwood CA Jr: Humeral fixation by press-fitting of a tapered metaphyseal stem: A prospective radiographic study. J Bone Joint Surg Am 2003;85:304-308.
3. Boileau P, Walch G: Anatomical study of the proximal humerus: Surgical technique consideration and prosthetic design rationale. In Walch G, Boileau P (eds): Shoulder Arthroplasty. Berlin, Springer, 1999, pp 69-82.

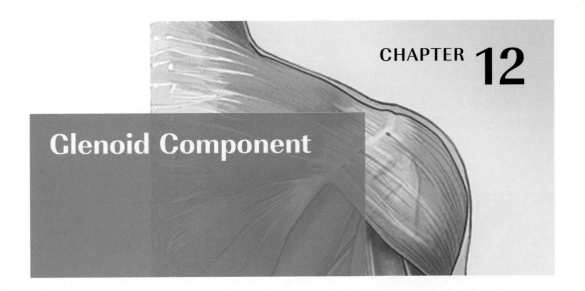

CHAPTER 12

Glenoid Component

Historically, the glenoid component has been the "weak link" of shoulder replacement. In addition to being the most difficult part of the surgical procedure, the glenoid component is the most likely site of component failure, which has led many surgeons to avoid glenoid resurfacing in nearly all cases. Fortunately, glenoid component materials and designs have improved greatly, as have techniques for implantation of glenoid components. Problems with the glenoid component are becoming less common, perhaps leading more surgeons to consider glenoid resurfacing in more cases. As detailed in Chapter 6, we prefer to implant a glenoid component in most nonfracture indications for unconstrained shoulder arthroplasty because of results superior to those of hemiarthroplasty in most diagnoses. The main contraindication to glenoid resurfacing in patients with a competent rotator cuff is insufficient glenoid bone to support implantation of a glenoid component. Such cases are readily identifiable with preoperative imaging studies (Fig. 12-1).

The steps involved in implantation of the glenoid component include obtaining glenoid exposure (detailed in Chapter 10), reaming the glenoid surface, selecting the size of glenoid component to be implanted, selecting the type of glenoid component to be implanted, preparing the native glenoid bone for implantation of the glenoid component, and final implantation of the glenoid component. Each facet of this process is detailed in this chapter.

REAMING THE GLENOID SURFACE

Reaming the glenoid surface serves two purposes: first, it provides a congruent surface that matches the appos-

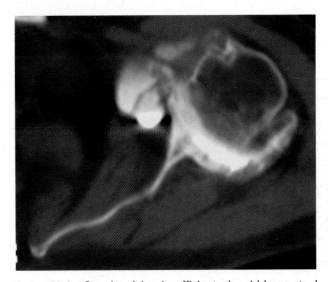

Figure 12-1 Case involving insufficient glenoid bone stock to allow implantation of a glenoid component.

ing surface of the implant by removing any remaining cartilage and smoothing the osseous surface, and second, it corrects any deformity caused by bony wear, as identified on preoperative imaging (Fig. 12-2). If no deformity is present, "light" reaming is performed. In patients with posterior glenoid wear, however, the anterior portion of the glenoid should be preferentially reamed to correct the deformity.

After humeral preparation and insertion of the humeral cut protector (Chapter 11), the humeral head retractor is replaced to retract the proximal humerus posteriorly and expose the glenoid (Fig. 12-3). It is helpful to mark the center point of the glenoid with an electrocautery. It is also important to realize that with severe deformity or biconcavity, the center point will change (the new center point is posterior to the original center point after "reaming away" a portion of the anterior glenoid) by preferentially reaming the anterior glenoid, and this should be considered when identifying the center point. A guide with a stop is

used when drilling a pilot hole through the center point of the glenoid (Fig. 12-4). The tip of a reamer of the appropriate glenoid size (see the next section) is introduced into the pilot hole (Fig. 12-5). Introduction of the reamer is usually the most difficult part of glenoid resurfacing. A few techniques are helpful when performing this portion of the procedure in exceptionally stiff shoulders. We first confirm with the anesthesiologist that the patient is adequately relaxed with paralytic agents. We then determine which posterior glenoid retractor yields the best exposure. We start with the Trillat humeral head retractor. If this proves inadequate, we will also try a Fukada humeral head retractor, a large glenoid rim retractor, or one or more Hohmann retractors (these retractors are shown in Chapter 3). Many times it is necessary for the assistant retracting the humeral head to perform a maneuver with the humeral head retractor to facilitate insertion of the reamer. This is done by first forcefully retracting posteriorly and then relaxing the retractor to allow clearance of the posterior aspect of the reamer. The retractor can be left in place in a relaxed position during the actual reaming. This technique is illustrated in Figure 12-6. Rarely, despite the use of these techniques for exposure of the glenoid and insertion of the reamer, it may not be possible to insert the reamer tip into the pilot hole. In this scenario we remove the humeral head retractor completely and insert a laminar

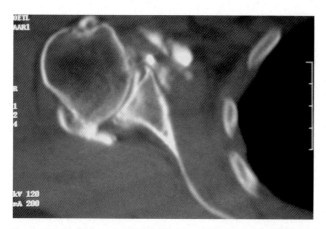

Figure 12-2 Example of identification of a biconcave glenoid deformity identified on preoperative imaging studies. This deformity should be corrected by eccentric reaming during the surgical procedure.

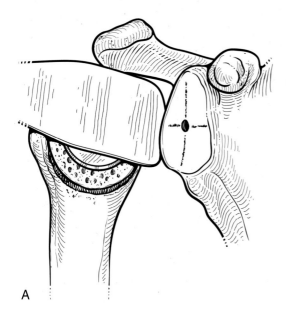

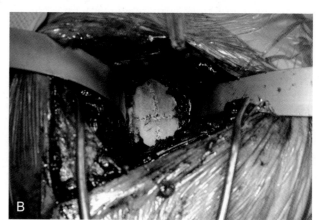

Figure 12-3 Glenoid exposure. The center point of the glenoid has been marked with the electrocautery.

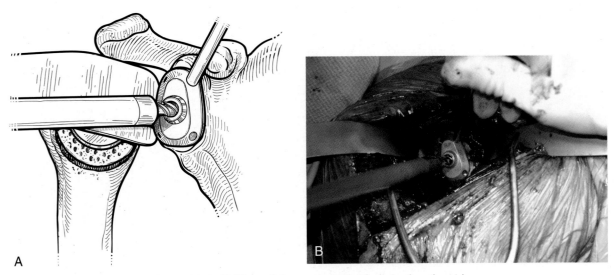

Figure 12-4   Drilling of the central pilot hole in the glenoid.

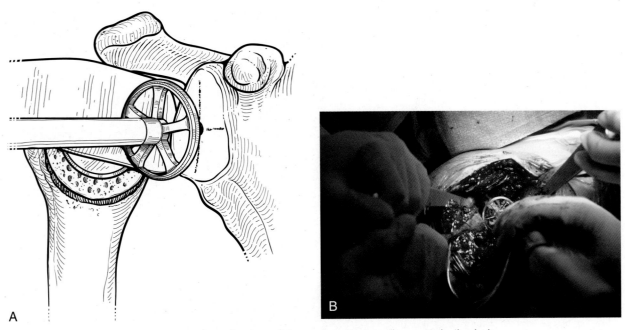

Figure 12-5   Introduction of the reamer tip into the central pilot hole.

spreader between the glenoid and humerus. One limb of the laminar spreader is placed at the most superior aspect of the glenoid surface, and the other limb is placed on the cut surface of the proximal humerus. The laminar spreader is opened to distract the gleno-humeral joint and retract the humerus laterally. This technique allows insertion of the glenoid reamer by eliminating obstruction of the reamer by the posterior

humeral head retractor (Fig. 12-7). By using these techniques sequentially, we have yet to perform a shoulder arthroplasty in which we were unable to resurface the glenoid because of inadequate exposure.

After the tip of the reamer is inserted into the pilot hole, the cutting surface of the reamer is slightly distracted away from the glenoid surface as the reamer is started. This helps avoid glenoid fracture by

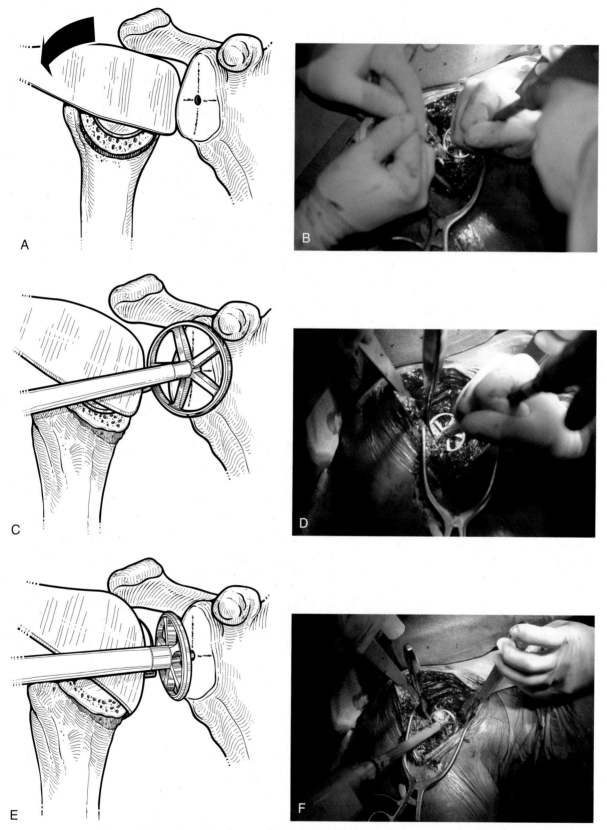

Figure 12-6   A to **F,** Maneuver for insertion of the reamer in a stiff shoulder.

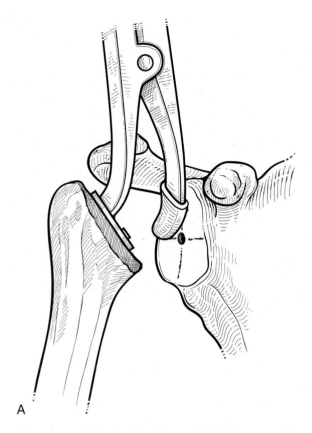

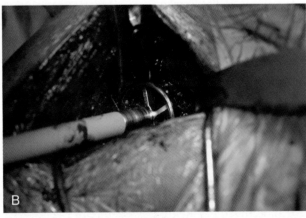

Figure 12-7 Technique for using a laminar spreader to facilitate insertion of the glenoid reamer in an excessively stiff shoulder.

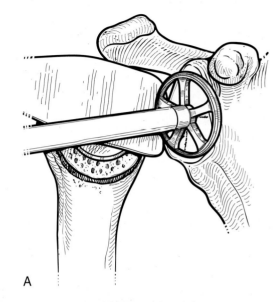

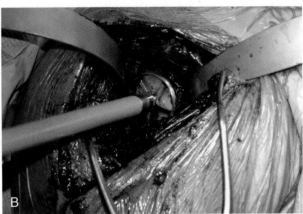

Figure 12-8 Reaming of the glenoid surface.

preventing the reamer from suddenly engaging any prominent areas on the glenoid. The reamer is advanced medially to engage the glenoid bone (Fig. 12-8). In patients with a concentric glenoid (identified on preoperative computed tomography or magnetic resonance imaging; Chapter 7), reaming is performed only until a surface matching the radius of curvature of the reamer (same radius of curvature as on the back side of the glenoid component) is obtained. Any remaining glenoid cartilage should be removed; however, it is unnecessary to ream past the subchondral bone to cancellous bone.

Cases of asymmetric glenoid wear represent a challenging problem. This wear is almost always posterior in primary osteoarthritis and creates a biconcave glenoid with the humeral head articulating with the posterior concavity (Fig. 12-9). This biconcavity may not be grossly apparent during surgical visualization, hence the need for adequate preoperative imaging studies (Chapter 7). In addition to providing a concentric surface for the glenoid component, an additional goal of reaming in this scenario is to eliminate the biconcave glenoid morphology and restore the glenoid to a single-concavity morphology with appropriate version (2 to 8 degrees of retroversion). Preoperative

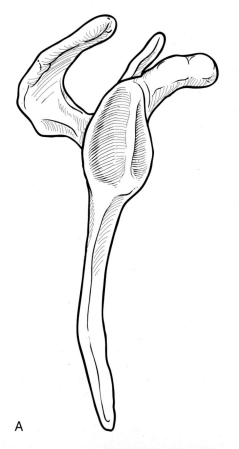

A

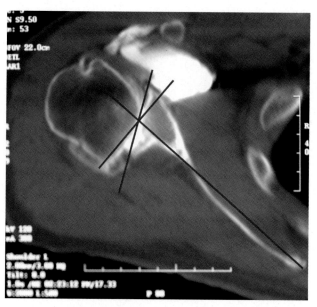

Figure 12-10   Determination of the correction needed in a case of primary osteoarthritis with glenoid biconcavity.

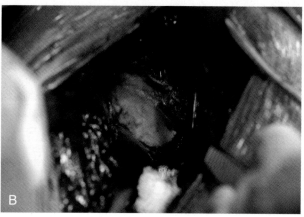

B

Figure 12-9   Glenoid biconcavity in primary osteoarthritis identified on preoperative computed tomography.

planning with computed tomography or magnetic resonance imaging helps determine the amount of correction necessary (Fig. 12-10; see Chapter 7 for more details). When reaming a biconcave glenoid, the anterior glenoid is preferentially reamed until a single concavity is achieved and the glenoid surface has been reoriented into correct version. As reaming progresses, the reamer should be periodically removed and the glenoid surface checked. A ridge on the glenoid surface

demarcating the two concavities of the glenoid surface should move progressively posteriorly until it is no longer visible (Fig. 12-11).

SELECTING THE SIZE OF THE GLENOID COMPONENT

Selection of glenoid component size is based on coverage of the glenoid surface and, more importantly, on glenohumeral component mismatch. Glenohumeral prosthetic mismatch is defined as the difference in radius of curvature between the humeral head and glenoid components. Mismatch of at least 5.5 mm has been associated with fewer postoperative radiolucent lines.[1] Mismatch of greater than 10 mm has been shown biomechanically to risk fracture of the polyethylene glenoid component.[2] In the prosthetic system that we use, the preferred mismatch is obtained by combining a given humeral head size with a given glenoid component size (Table 12-1). The size of the humeral head is first selected as described in Chapter 11. The corresponding glenoid size is selected so that glenohumeral prosthetic mismatch is optimized. Occasionally, the native glenoid surface area is larger than the surface of the selected glenoid component. In this case a larger glenoid component is selected to provide better surface coverage and increased glenohumeral prosthetic mismatch. In the rare scenario in which the selected glenoid component is larger than the native glenoid surface, the preferentially selected glenoid

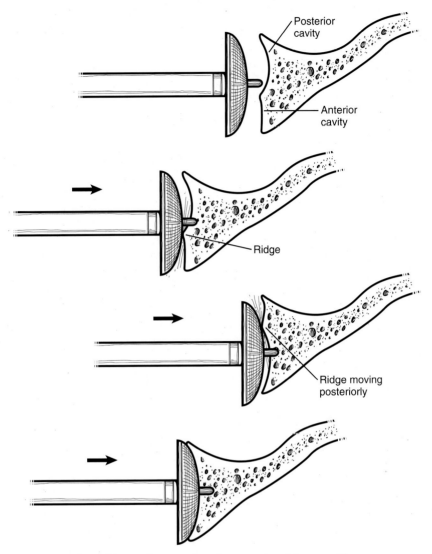

Figure 12-11   The ridge of bone demarcating the two glenoid concavities moves progressively posteriorly during eccentric glenoid reaming.

component is used while some peripheral overhanging of the glenoid component is accepted to respect a mismatch of at least 5.5 mm.

SELECTING THE TYPE OF GLENOID COMPONENT

After the glenoid has been reamed and the size of glenoid component selected, the type of glenoid to be implanted is determined. We use either a keeled component or a pegged component. Both components are all-polyethylene convex-back components inserted with cement (Figs. 12-12 and 12-13). Radiographic studies have shown superior early results with pegged components.[3] Laboratory biomechanical studies have favored fixation of pegged components as well.[4] Clinical outcomes have been equivocal or shown slightly better results with keeled components.[5] In most scenarios, we believe that selection of a keeled or pegged glenoid component is based largely on surgeon preference. In patients with a shallow glenoid vault as determined on preoperative computed tomography or magnetic resonance imaging (type A2 glenoid, see Chapter 7), we prefer a keeled component. If the glenoid vault appears inadequate to place the 15-mm keel of the implant, the tip of the keel can be shortened with a cutting rongeur (Fig. 12-14).

Table 12-1 GLENOHUMERAL PROSTHETIC MISMATCH VALUES AND RECOMMENDATIONS* FOR THE AEQUALIS SHOULDER ARTHROPLASTY SYSTEM†

		Humeral Head Sizes	37 × 13.5	39 × 14	41 × 15	43 × 16	46 × 17	48 × 18	50 × 16	50 × 19	52 × 19	52 × 23	54 × 23	54 × 27
		Radius of Curvature of Humeral Head	19.5	20.6	21.5	22.5	24	25	27.5	26	27.3	26.2	27.35	27
Glenoid Component Sizes	**Radius of Curvature of Glenoid Component**													
Small	27.5		8	6.9	6	5	3.5	2.5	0	1.5	0.2	1.3	0.15	0.5
Medium	28.5		9	7.9	7	6	4.5	3.5	1	2.5	1.2	2.3	1.15	1.5
Large	31		11.5	10.4	9.5	8.5	7	6	3.5	5	3.7	4.8	3.65	4
XL	33		13.5	12.4	11.5	10.5	9	8	5.5	7	5.7	6.8	5.65	6
2XL	33.5		14	12.9	12	11	9.5	8.5	6	7.5	6.2	7.3	6.15	6.5

*Shaded boxes represent recommendations.
†Tornier, Inc., Stafford, TX.

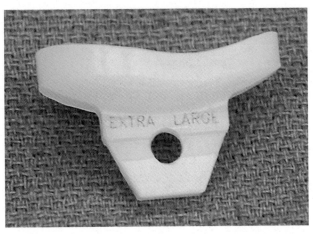

Figure 12-12   Keeled, all-polyethylene convex-back glenoid component.

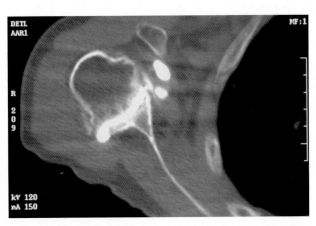

Figure 12-14   Case of A2 glenoid morphology necessitating shortening the length of the glenoid component keel before glenoid resurfacing.

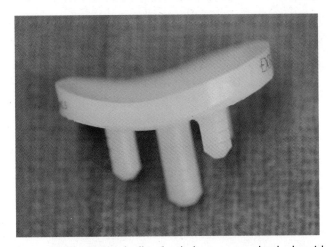

Figure 12-13   Pegged, all-polyethylene convex-back glenoid component.

PREPARING THE GLENOID BONE

The technique used for preparing the native glenoid bone has been shown to influence the radiographic results when a keeled glenoid component has been selected.[6] When implanting a keeled glenoid component we prefer using the bony compaction technique pioneered by Gazielly.[7] Holes are drilled superior and inferior to the original pilot hole with use of a tem-

plate device, and any remaining bony bridge is broken with a rongeur (Fig. 12-15). A keel punch that is the same size as the keel of the glenoid component is impacted into the native glenoid to finish preparation of the keel slot (Fig. 12-16). A trial glenoid component is inserted to ensure full seating of the component (Fig. 12-17). The trial component is removed and the keel slot is irrigated with sterile saline and dried with a sponge, an inexpensive technique shown to be as effective as the use of hemostatic agents and compressed carbon dioxide.[8]

When using a pegged glenoid component, a different template is used to drill the peg holes (Fig. 12-18). The peg holes are then irrigated and dried in the same manner as described for the keel slot.

FINAL IMPLANTATION OF THE GLENOID COMPONENT

The final component is cemented in place with polymethylmethacrylate (we prefer to use DePuy 2 bone cement [DePuy, Inc., Warsaw, IN] because of its accelerated curing time of less than 8 minutes) in the keel slot/peg holes only (Fig. 12-19). An impactor impacts and holds the component in place while the cement cures.

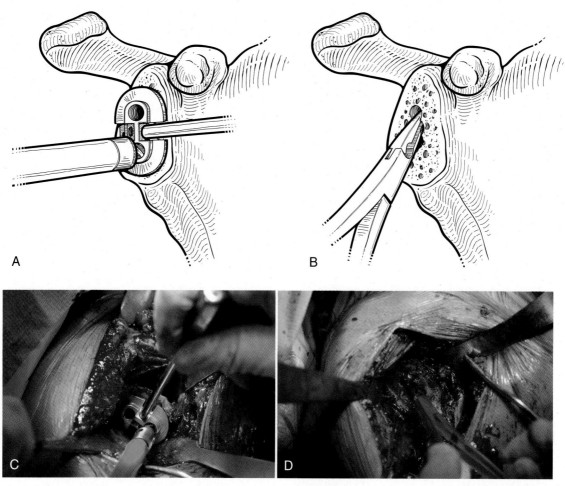

Figure 12-15 **A** to **D,** Creation of the keel slot by first drilling holes superior and inferior to the original pilot hole via a template. The bony bridges between these holes are removed with a small rongeur.

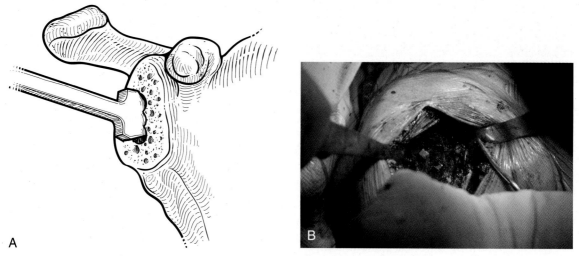

Figure 12-16 **A** and **B,** Compaction of the glenoid vault to complete creation of the keel slot.

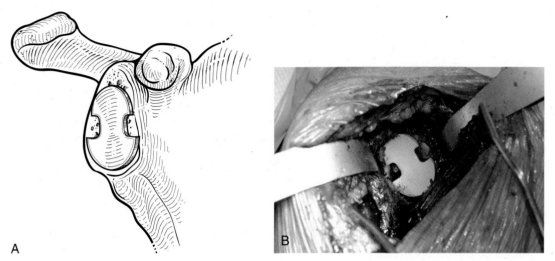

Figure 12-17   A and **B,** Placement of the trial glenoid component to ensure that the component fully seats.

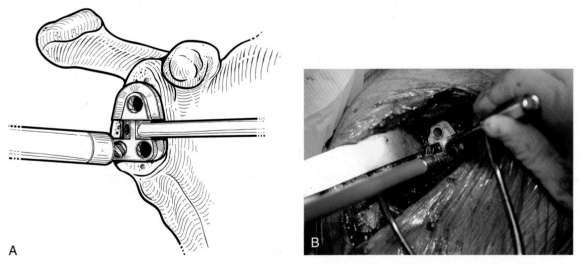

Figure 12-18   A and **B,** Preparation of the glenoid for a pegged glenoid component.

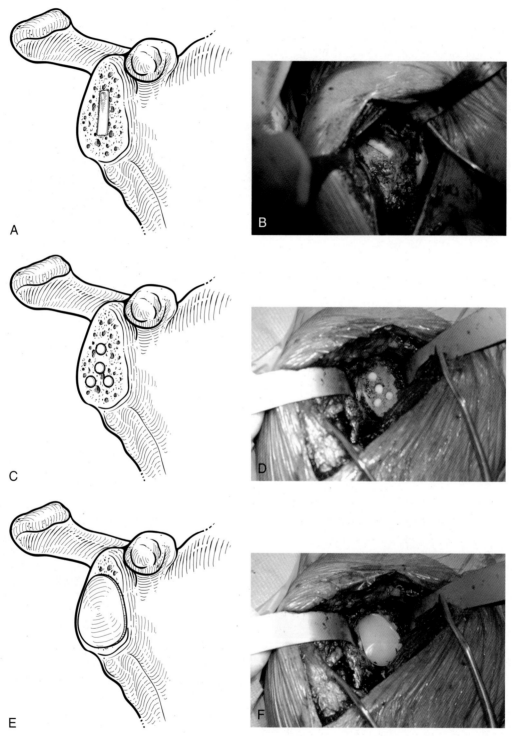

Figure 12-19 **A** to **F,** Cementing the final glenoid component. **A** and **B,** Keeled component. **C** and **D,** Pegged component. **E** and **F,** Final component in place.

REFERENCES

1. Walch G, Edwards TB, Boulahia A, et al: The influence of glenohumeral prosthetic mismatch on glenoid radiolucent lines: Results of a multicentric study. J Bone Joint Surg Am 2002;84:2186-2191.
2. Friedman RJ, An YH, Draughn RA: Glenohumeral congruence in total shoulder arthroplasty. Orthop Trans 1997; 21:17.
3. Gartsman GM, Elkousy HA, Warnock KM, et al: Radiographic comparison of pegged and keeled glenoid components. J Shoulder Elbow Surg 2005;14:252-257.
4. Anglin C, Wyss UP, Nyffeler RW, Gerber C: Loosening performance of cemented glenoid prosthesis design pairs. Clin Biomech 2001;16:144-150.
5. Gazielly D, El-Abiad R: Comparative results of three types of polyethylene cemented glenoid components. In Walch G, Boileau P, Molé D (eds): 2000 Prosthèses d'Epaule . . . Recul de 2 à 10 Ans. Paris, Sauramps Medical, 2001, pp 483-488.
6. Szabo I, Buscayret F, Edwards TB, et al: Radiographic comparison of two different glenoid preparation techniques in total shoulder arthroplasty. Clin Orthop Relat Res 2005;431:104-110.
7. Gazielly DF, Allende C, Pamelin E: Results of cancellous compaction technique for glenoid resurfacing. Paper presented at the 9th International Congress on Surgery of the Shoulder, May 2004, Washington, DC.
8. Edwards TB, Sabonghy EP, Elkousy HA, et al: Glenoid component insertion in total shoulder arthroplasty: Comparison of three techniques for drying the glenoid prior to cementation. J Shoulder Elbow Surg 2007;16(3 Suppl): S107-S110.

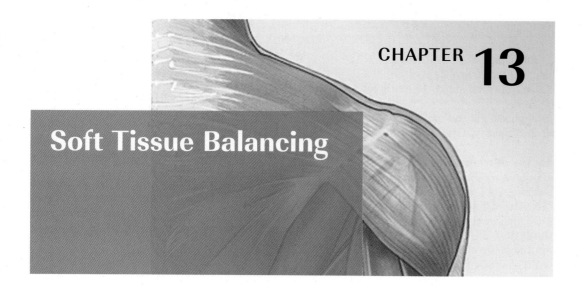

CHAPTER 13

Soft Tissue Balancing

The use of a prosthetic system that adapts to the patient's anatomy decreases the need for soft tissue balancing. In most cases, little additional soft tissue balancing is necessary after the steps of the procedure are followed as described in this textbook. Two notable exceptions exist. The first is in an individual, usually with a diagnosis of primary osteoarthritis or instability arthropathy, who has marked posterior glenoid wear and posterior glenohumeral subluxation on preoperative computed tomography or magnetic resonance imaging. The second is in an individual with an exceptionally tight posterior capsule, most commonly seen in our practice in patients with juvenile-onset inflammatory arthropathy.

EVALUATING THE NEED FOR SOFT TISSUE BALANCING

In patients with posterior glenoid wear (type B2 glenoid morphology; see Chapter 7), the sequence of surgical steps is altered. After the glenoid component is implanted, we insert the trial humeral prosthesis instead of the final humeral implant. This is helpful in judging prosthetic stability. After the trial humeral component is reinserted, the glenohumeral joint is reduced. With the arm externally rotated 30 degrees, force is applied in a posterior direction to the proximal humerus. There are two keys that allow the surgeon to determine whether the soft tissues are properly balanced. First, the prosthetic humeral head should sub-

luxate posteriorly approximately 30% to 50% of its diameter and spontaneously reduce on release of the posteriorly directed force. If spontaneous reduction does not occur, posterior capsulorrhaphy may be necessary. Second, if posterior translation of at least 30% of the diameter of the humeral head is not possible, posterior capsular release may be necessary.

PERFORMING A POSTERIOR CAPSULORRHAPHY

In many patients with posterior glenoid wear and posterior humeral head subluxation, the posterior capsule has become distended and ineffective in maintaining posterior glenohumeral stability, even after the osseous glenoid deformity has been corrected by reaming (Fig. 13-1). In such cases, posterior capsulorrhaphy serves to tighten the posterior capsule and prevent posterior instability. To perform this procedure, the trial humeral implant is removed and a laminar spreader with protective rubber sleeves on the tips is placed between the humerus and glenoid to expose the posterior capsule (Fig. 13-2). Three no. 1 braided absorbable sutures (one superior, one in the middle, and one inferior) are passed through the posterior capsule in a mediolateral direction to imbricate the posterior capsule (Fig. 13-3). The laminar spreader is removed and the sutures tied sequentially. The excess suture limbs are cut from the superior and middle capsulorrhaphy sutures, but the inferior suture is left uncut (Fig. 13-4). The sutures for

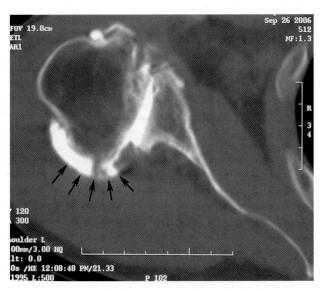

Figure 13-1 Computed tomography showing posterior glenoid wear. The posterior glenoid capsule has been enhanced to show its marked distention (*arrows*).

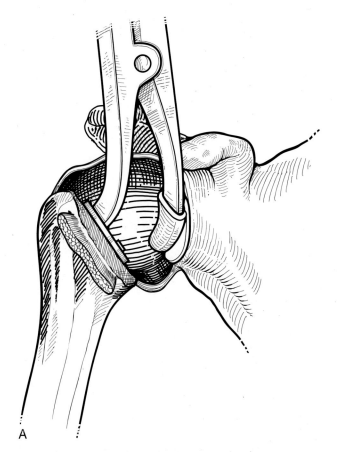

subscapularis repair and the final humeral implant are placed (see Chapter 11) after posterior capsulorrhaphy, and stability is re-evaluated. Stability is usually greatly improved after posterior capsulorrhaphy. In the rare circumstance in which the glenohumeral joint remains dislocated on stability testing after posterior capsulorrhaphy is performed, the excess inferior suture limbs can be brought through the glenohumeral joint and rotator interval and sutured to the coracoacromial ligament just lateral to its insertion on the coracoid. This helps avoid posterior instability in the early postoperative phase (Fig. 13-5). Because these sutures are absorbable, no long-term consequence of passing the sutures through the glenohumeral joint have been observed when they have been necessary.

PERFORMING A POSTERIOR CAPSULAR RELEASE

Rarely, posterior translation of at least 30% of the diameter of the humeral head will be impossible during stability testing. We have observed this scenario most commonly in patients with inflammatory arthropathy as the underlying condition for which they are undergoing shoulder arthroplasty. When this occurs, we perform a posterior capsular release in which the final humeral implant is left in place and a laminar spreader with protective rubber sleeves on the tips is placed between the humeral and glenoid components to

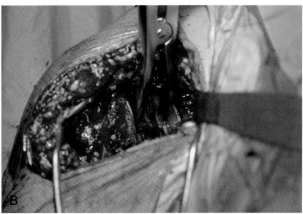

Figure 13-2 **A** and **B,** Laminar spreader placed between the humerus and glenoid to expose the posterior capsule.

expose the posterior capsule (Fig. 13-6). The posterior capsule is then released under direct visualization just adjacent to the glenoid component with a no. 10 scalpel blade on a long handle from the 12 o'clock to the 6 o'clock position (Fig. 13-7). After posterior capsular release, stability is re-evaluated. In the rare scenario in which the posterior capsule remains too tight after posterior capsular release, consideration is given to decreasing the size of the prosthetic head.

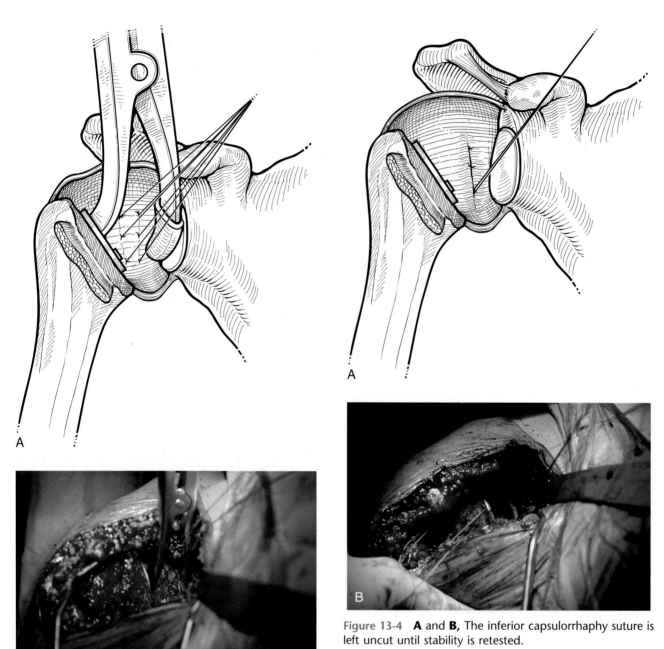

Figure 13-3 A and **B,** Imbrication sutures placed in the posterior capsule.

Figure 13-4 A and **B,** The inferior capsulorrhaphy suture is left uncut until stability is retested.

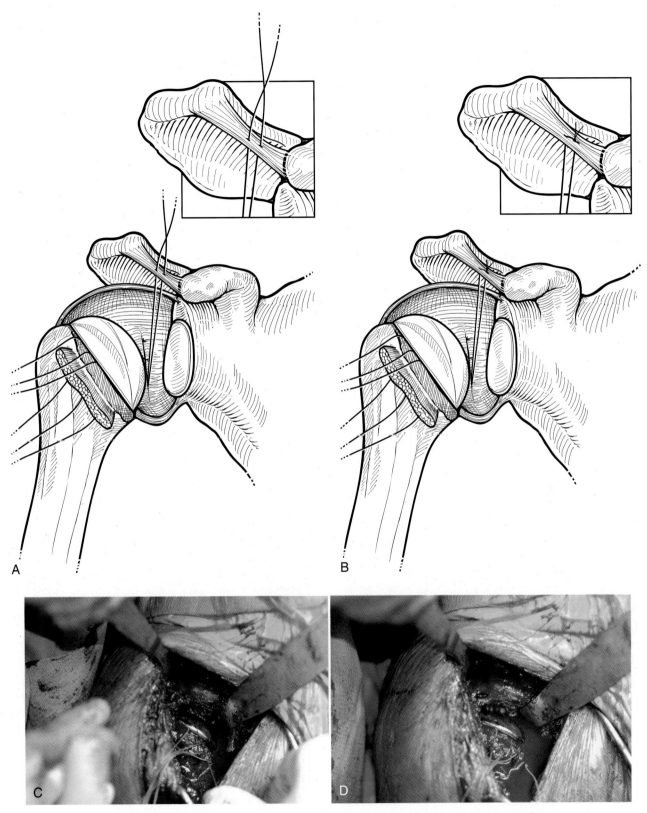

Figure 13-5 **A** to **D,** Suturing the inferior capsulorrhaphy suture to the coracoacromial ligament in cases of residual posterior instability after posterior capsulorrhaphy.

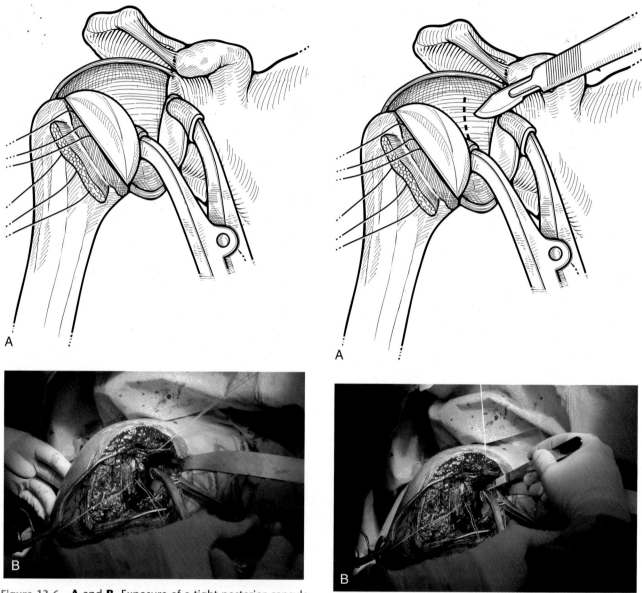

Figure 13-6 **A** and **B**, Exposure of a tight posterior capsule with the laminar spreader.

Figure 13-7 **A** and **B**, Release of a tight posterior capsule with a scalpel.

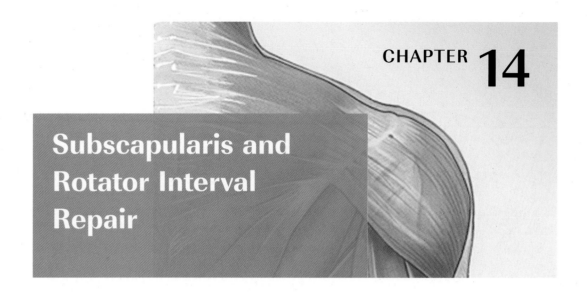

CHAPTER 14

Subscapularis and Rotator Interval Repair

Failure of subscapularis repair occurs in 2% of patients after shoulder arthroplasty for primary osteoarthritis.[1] Prognostic factors for the development of symptoms after subscapularis failure are unclear. Many patients will be asymptomatic after failure of subscapularis repair, with subscapularis weakness detected only on postoperative examination. However, symptoms of weakness or anterior instability (or both) will develop in some patients. Additionally, even in patients who are asymptomatic, concern exists over subscapularis failure's causing eccentric anterior loading and subsequent loosening of the glenoid component. For these reasons every effort should be made to perform a secure subscapularis repair. We prefer a repair that incorporates both transosseous and transtendinous components. In addition to subscapularis repair, we also routinely close the rotator interval to further decrease the risk for postoperative glenohumeral instability.

TECHNIQUE FOR REPAIR OF THE SUBSCAPULARIS AND ROTATOR INTERVAL

After completing soft tissue balancing, final preparations are made for implantation of the humeral component and subsequent subscapularis repair. Three no. 2 nonabsorbable braided sutures are placed through the lesser tuberosity and the humeral stump of the subscapularis tendon, as detailed in Chapter 11, to be used for reattachment of the subscapularis (Fig. 14-1). These sutures are placed just before insertion of the final humeral implant. The final humeral implant is

then impacted into place and its stability checked (Chapters 11 and 13).

The small anterior glenoid rim retractor is removed and replaced with a narrow Richardson retractor, which is used to retract the conjoined tendon medially. The previously placed sponge is visualized and removed from the subscapularis fossa with a Kocher clamp (Fig. 14-2). Removal of this sponge reveals the stay sutures placed in the subscapularis tendon during the surgical approach. The Kocher clamp is placed on these stay sutures to obtain control of the subscapularis (Fig. 14-3). The limb of the superior suture exiting the medullary canal is passed from deep to superficial through the superior portion of the subscapularis tendon not more than 1 cm medial to its terminus. The same limb is then passed through the humeral stump of the subscapularis and back through the superior portion of the subscapularis tendon, as before (Fig. 14-4). This suture is tied with a square surgeon's knot using five throws. The subscapularis stay sutures are removed, and the suture passing and tying procedure is repeated for the middle suture and then the inferior suture. This technique yields a transosseous and transtendinous repair (Fig. 14-5). No effort is made to imbricate the subscapularis or to medialize its insertion; the repair should be as anatomic as possible.

The rotator interval is closed with a single figure-of-eight stitch with the residual no. 2 braided nonabsorbable suture from the subscapularis repair (Fig. 14-6). The repaired tissue should consist of the rotator interval capsule. Direct suturing of the subscapularis tendon to the supraspinatus tendon should be avoided because this could substantially limit external rotation postoperatively. Additionally, care is required to avoid imbricating the rotator interval, which could also lead to

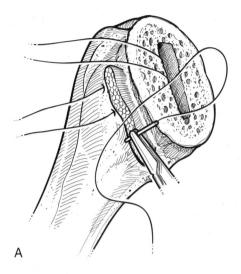

A

Figure 14-1   **A** to **C,** Placement of transosseous sutures for later subscapularis repair.

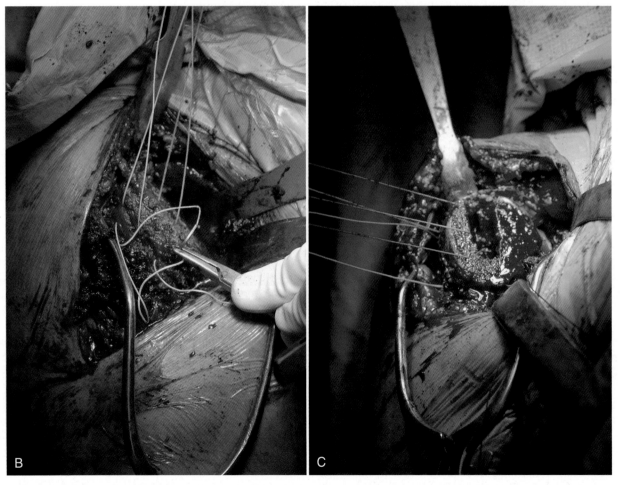

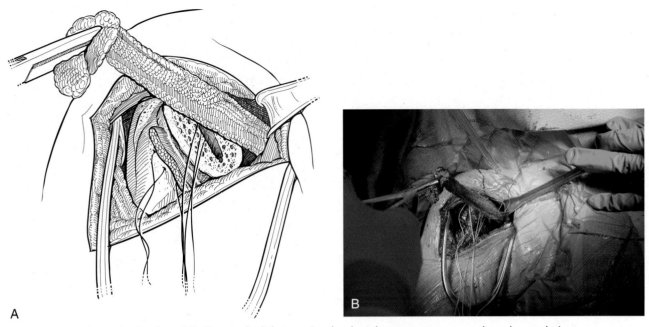

Figure 14-2   **A** and **B,** Removal of the previously placed sponge to expose the subscapularis.

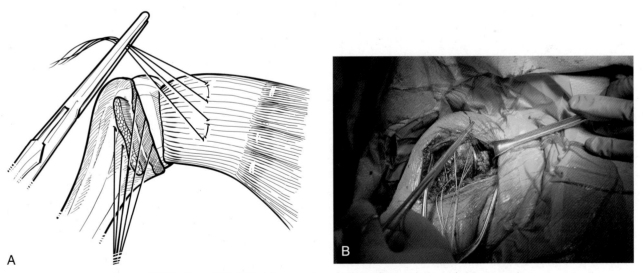

Figure 14-3   **A** and **B,** Obtaining control of the subscapularis with stay sutures.

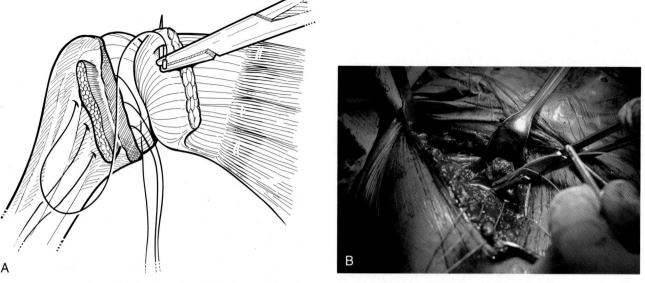

Figure 14-4 **A** and **B,** Technique of passing suture through the subscapularis during repair.

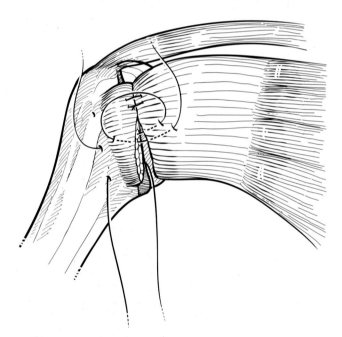

Figure 14-5 This repair technique yields a transosseous and transtendinous repair.

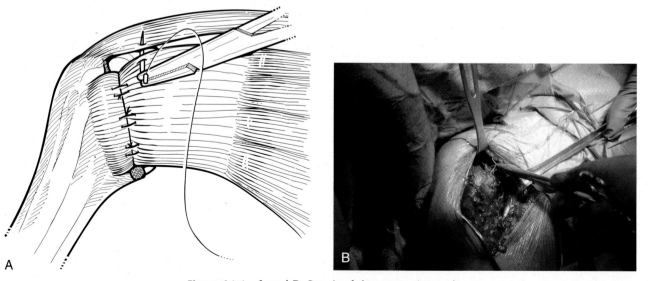

Figure 14-6 **A** and **B,** Repair of the rotator interval.

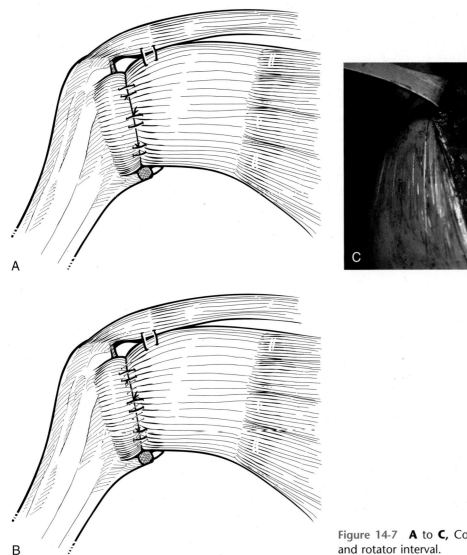

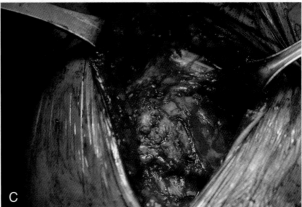

Figure 14-7 **A** to **C,** Completed repair of the subscapularis and rotator interval.

postoperative limitation of external rotation. The rotator interval and subscapularis repair are then reinforced with a no. 1 braided absorbable suture in a running nonlocking technique. The final repair is shown in Figure 14-7. After the subscapularis and rotator interval are closed, passive external rotation with the arm at the patient's side is documented to assist in directing postoperative rehabilitation (Fig. 14-8). Ideally, we like to observe at least 30 degrees of external rotation with the arm at the side after repair

of the subscapularis and rotator interval. If unable to obtain this, we remove the rotator interval suture. If external rotation remains less than 30 degrees (as may be the case in patients with severe preoperative stiffness), we accept whatever external rotation is obtained after removal of the rotator interval suture. We do not recommend heroic attempts such as Z-plasty tendon lengthening of the subscapularis to obtain more external rotation because such attempts can seriously compromise the integrity of the subscapularis tendon.

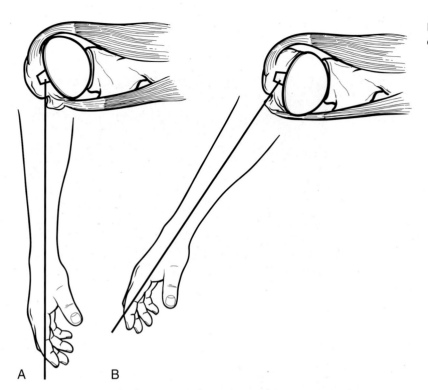

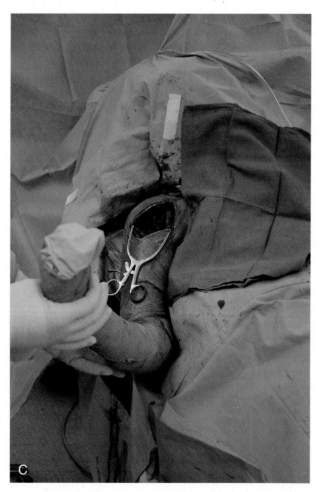

Figure 14-8 **A** to **C**, Assessment of passive external rotation after subscapularis repair.

REFERENCE

1. Lafosse L, Kempf JF: Omarthrose primitive: Resultats cliniques et radiologiques. In Walch G, Boileau P, Molé D (eds): 2000 Prosthèses d'Epaule . . . Recul de 2 à 10 Ans. Paris, Sauramps Medical, 2001, pp 73-85.

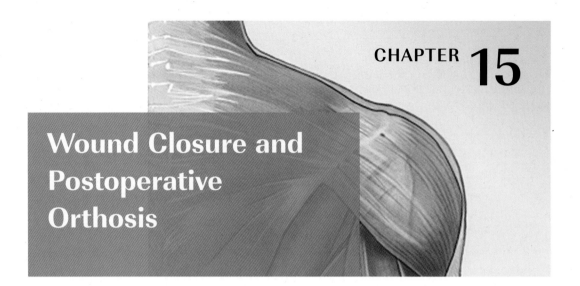

Wound Closure and Postoperative Orthosis

The final steps of the operative procedure are wound closure and placement of the postoperative orthosis. These steps are relatively elementary but no less important than other aspects of the procedure.

TECHNIQUE FOR WOUND CLOSURE

After closure of the subscapularis and rotator interval, the wound is irrigated with 800 mL of antibiotic-impregnated sterile saline (50,000 units bacitracin per liter sterile normal saline) via a bulb syringe. The wound is checked to ensure that adequate hemostasis has been achieved. The electrocautery is used as necessary to minimize any residual hemorrhage. No drain is used because it has been shown to be unnecessary during unconstrained shoulder arthroplasty.[1] We do not close the deltopectoral interval but initiate our closure with the overlying fascial layer. This layer is reapproximated with no. 0 braided absorbable suture via an interrupted figure-of-eight technique (Fig. 15-1). The subcutaneous fascia is reapproximated with 2-0 braided absorbable suture via an interrupted figure-of-eight technique (Fig. 15-2). The skin is reapproximated with 3-0 undyed absorbable monofilament suture in a subcuticular running closure (Fig. 15-3).

The occlusive draping is removed adjacent to the incision, and the skin is cleansed of blood with a saline-soaked sponge and then dried. Half-inch Steri-Strips are placed over the incision (Fig. 15-4). Sterile gauze is placed over the incision and a sterile absorbent pad is placed over the gauze (Fig. 15-5). The dressing is secured with 3-inch foam tape (Fig. 15-6). The remaining surgical drapes are then removed.

The dressing is maintained in place until postoperative day 3, at which time it is removed and not replaced. After removal of the dressing, the patient is allowed to shower, but submerging the incision in a bathtub is prohibited until 2 weeks postoperatively. The patient removes the Steri-Strips progressively as they lose their adhesion to the skin.

POSTOPERATIVE ORTHOSIS

The postoperative orthosis is placed in the operating room immediately after the dressing is applied. The type of orthosis used is determined by the procedures performed. We use two types of postoperative orthoses. For unconstrained shoulder arthroplasty without an associated posterior capsulorrhaphy, we use a simple sling (Fig. 15-7). This is used for the patient's comfort and protection and is discontinued whenever the patient decides that it is no longer required, usually between 2 and 4 weeks postoperatively. We ask patients to avoid externally rotating beyond neutral for 4 weeks (6 weeks for inflammatory arthropathy) and to avoid pushing or pulling their body weight with the operated extremity for 8 weeks to protect the subscapularis repair.

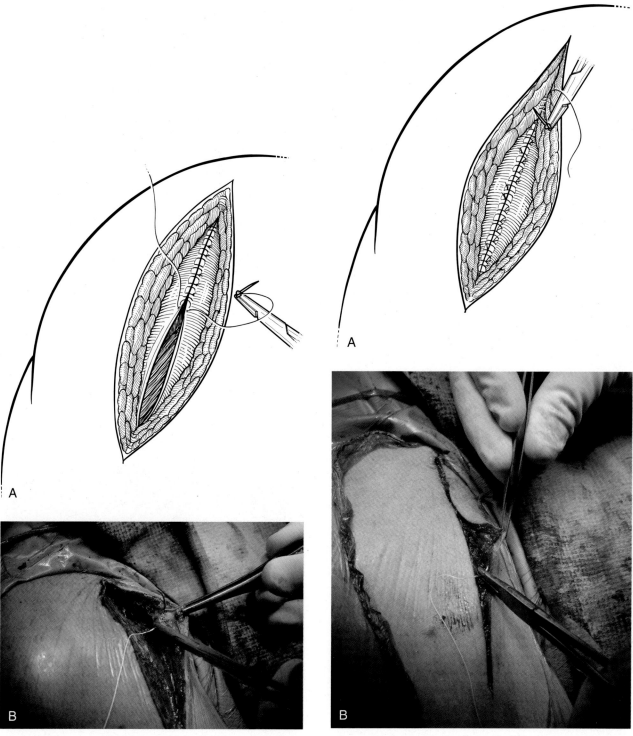

Figure 15-1   **A** and **B,** Closure of the deep fascial layer.

Figure 15-2   **A** and **B,** Closure of the subcutaneous fascia.

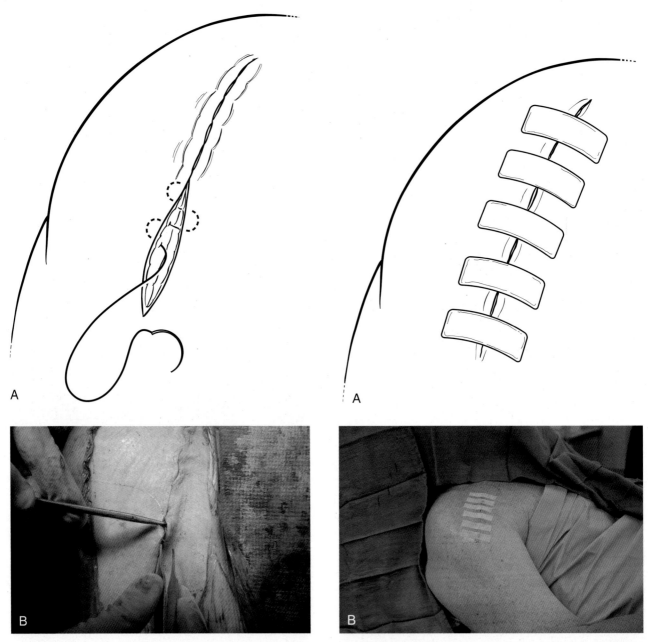

Figure 15-3   **A** and **B,** Subcuticular skin closure.

Figure 15-4   **A** and **B,** Steri-Strips covering the incision.

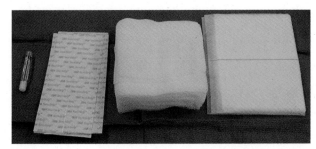

Figure 15-5 Sterile dressings used after shoulder arthroplasty.

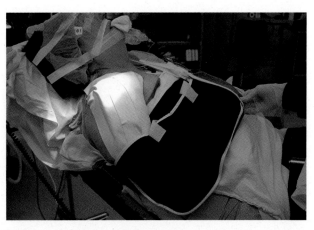

Figure 15-7 Simple sling used in most cases of unconstrained shoulder arthroplasty.

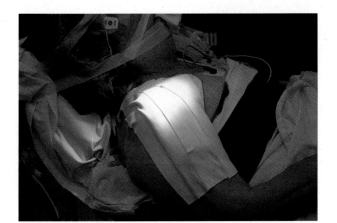

Figure 15-6 Completed postoperative dressing.

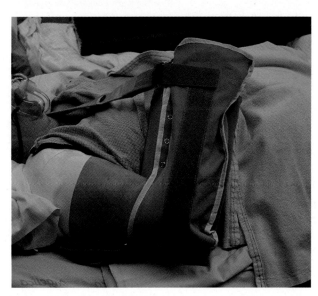

Figure 15-8 Application of a neutral rotation sling in patients who have undergone an associated posterior capsulorrhaphy.

In patients who have undergone an associated posterior capsulorrhaphy, we use a neutral-rotation sling (Fig. 15-8). This sling is maintained for 4 weeks to protect the posterior capsulorrhaphy. Patients are allowed to remove the sling only for hygiene and rehabilitative exercises. Additionally, patients who have undergone posterior capsulorrhaphy are cautioned against cross-body adduction and internal rotation behind the back for the first 4 postoperative weeks.

REFERENCE

1. Gartsman GM, Milne JC, Russell JA: Closed wound drainage in shoulder surgery. J Shoulder Elbow Surg 1997;6: 288-290.

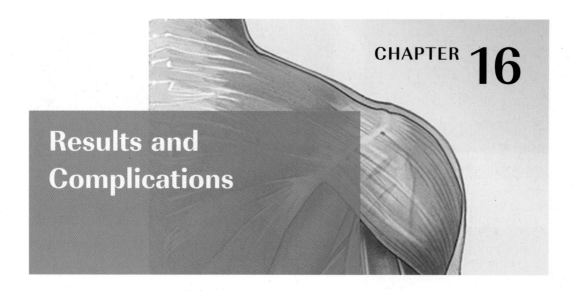

CHAPTER 16

Results and Complications

The results of unconstrained shoulder arthroplasty have been reported by multiple investigators. The results vary predominantly according to the underlying indication for which the arthroplasty has been performed. To our knowledge, the largest reported database of results of unconstrained shoulder arthroplasty was presented in Nice, France, in 2001.[1] Because of the large number of patients enrolled, this multicenter study has allowed meaningful conclusions to be made about the outcomes and complications of unconstrained shoulder arthroplasty. Our results have largely mirrored those reported in the Nice study. This chapter reports the results of unconstrained shoulder arthroplasty for the treatment of nonfracture conditions by drawing from information in the Nice database and our arthroplasty database that was prospectively established in 2003. Additionally, the most frequent complications and their treatment are outlined.

RESULTS

The results of unconstrained shoulder arthroplasty vary mainly with the cause for which the arthroplasty is performed. The best results are obtained in the treatment of primary osteoarthritis and osteonecrosis, whereas results are least satisfactory for post-traumatic arthritis and rotator cuff tear arthropathy. Tables 16-1 and 16-2 detail the results of unconstrained shoulder arthroplasty for the most common indications for which it is performed.[2-8] These tables express the results in terms of active mobility; patient satisfaction; the Constant score, a shoulder-specific outcomes device incorporating pain, mobility, activity,

and strength; and the age- and gender-adjusted Constant score.[9,10]

INTRAOPERATIVE COMPLICATIONS

Intraoperative complications are uncommon during shoulder arthroplasty and may be divided into complications involving the humerus, glenoid, musculotendinous soft tissues (rotator cuff), and neurovascular structures.

Humerus

Intraoperative complications involving the humerus are rare. The most common humeral complication is iatrogenic fracture, which usually results from performing an overly aggressive dislocation maneuver without previous adequate soft tissue release. Patients with osteopenia (i.e., inflammatory arthropathy patients) and those with severe preoperative stiffness (i.e., post-traumatic arthritis) are at most risk for this complication. These fractures may occur at the humeral diaphysis or proximally and involve the tuberosities. Fractures involving the humeral diaphysis should be reduced and a long-stem humeral implant placed. Allograft struts and cerclage cables may be added in patients with severe osteopenia (Fig. 16-1).

Intraoperative fractures involving the greater or lesser tuberosities (or both) are usually nondisplaced. Many of these fractures are stable or become stable once the humeral implant is placed (Fig. 16-2). If a tuberosity fracture is not satisfactorily stable, suture fixation of the tuberosity is performed and the

Table 16-1 RESULTS OF UNCONSTRAINED SHOULDER ARTHROPLASTY ACCORDING TO UNDERLYING CAUSE IN THE NICE MULTICENTER STUDY

Etiology	Absolute Constant Score (Points)		Adjusted Constant Score (%)		Active Forward Flexion (Degrees)		Active External Rotation (Degrees)		Excellent/Good Subjective Results (%)
	Preoperative	Postoperative	Preoperative	Postoperative	Preoperative	Postoperative	Preoperative	Postoperative	
Primary osteoarthritis (n = 689)[2]	32	71	43	96	92	142	8	41	93
Rheumatoid arthritis (n = 172)[3]	26	56	34	73	79	120	15	39	90
Osteonecrosis (n = 80)[4]	30	70	37	88	89	142	15	41	90
Post-traumatic arthritis (n = 203)[5]	27	57	NA*	NA	80	112	2	30	81
Fixed dislocation (n = 11)[6]	21	46	28	60	49	90	13	26	73
Cuff tear arthropathy (n = 66)[7]	25	46	NA	NA	76	96	10	22	NA
Instability arthropathy (n = 55)[8]	301	66	38	80	82	139	4	39	94

*Not available. These data were not reported in the referenced article/chapter.

From Walch G, Boileau P, Molé D (eds): 2000 Prosthèses d'Epaule . . . Recul de 2 à 10 Ans. Paris, Sauramps Medical, 2001, pp 11-20.

Table 16-2   RESULTS OF UNCONSTRAINED SHOULDER ARTHROPLASTY ACCORDING TO UNDERLYING CAUSE IN THE AUTHORS' PROSPECTIVE DATABASE FROM 2003 TO 2006

Etiology	Absolute Constant Score (Points)		Adjusted Constant Score (%)		Active Forward Flexion (Degrees)		Active External Rotation (Degrees)		Excellent/ Good Subjective Results (%)
	Preoperative	Postoperative	Preoperative	Postoperative	Preoperative	Postoperative	Preoperative	Postoperative	
Primary osteoarthritis (*n* = 159)	33	78	42	97	98	156	17	48	92
Rheumatoid arthritis (*n* = 8)	22	57	37	91	83	128	34	38	75
Osteonecrosis (*n* = 15)	32	62	45	89	98	148	24	40	100
Post-traumatic arthritis (*n* = 14)	22	51	30	72	77	128	13	40	66
Cuff tear arthropathy (*n* = 1)	19	32	27	46	80	80	0	10	100
Instability arthropathy (*n* = 22)	32	80	37	86	97	143	10	35	88

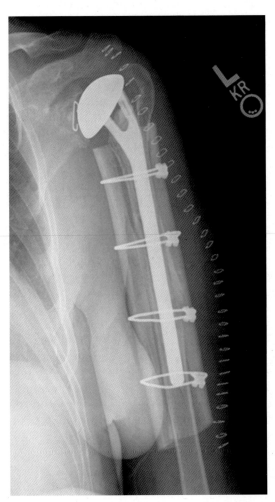

Figure 16-1 Fixation of an intraoperative humeral diaphyseal fracture with a long-stem humeral implant, allograft cortical struts, and cerclage cables.

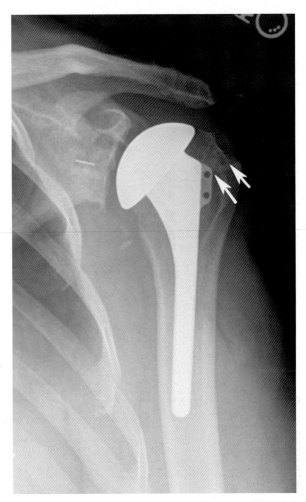

Figure 16-2 Nondisplaced fractures of the greater tuberosity (*arrows*) are usually sufficiently stable after placement of the humeral implant.

postoperative rehabilitation adjusted accordingly to allow healing of the tuberosity.

Glenoid

Intraoperative glenoid fractures are more common than humeral injury. These fractures almost always occur during preparation (reaming) of the glenoid. Patients with osteopenia are most at risk. Fractures may involve only the peripheral glenoid rim or may extend significantly into the articular surface. Adequate capsular release helps minimize the risk of glenoid fracture. Additionally, a motorized reamer (not a drill) should be used to prepare the glenoid surface. The reamer should be started before the surgeon applies force to engage the reamer onto the glenoid face. This avoids having the reamer "catch" an edge of the glenoid, which may cause a fracture.

Fractures that involve only a small portion of the peripheral rim usually require no treatment, and the glenoid component can be inserted as planned. Glenoid fractures that extend into the central portion of the glenoid (keel slot or peg holes) should be bone-grafted with the humeral head, and placement of a glenoid component should be avoided. Placement of a glenoid component in a patient with a fracture involving the central portion of the glenoid can result in early glenoid failure (Fig. 16-3).

Rotator Cuff

With proper glenoid exposure, intraoperative injury to the rotator cuff is rare. The key to avoiding rotator cuff injury during unconstrained shoulder arthroplasty is adequate visualization of the rotator cuff before resection of the humeral head (see Chapter 11). If the

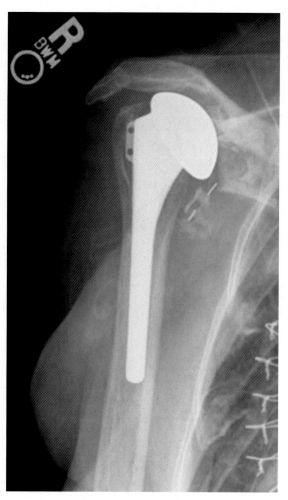

Figure 16-3 Early glenoid failure caused by placement of a glenoid component despite the occurrence of an intraoperative glenoid fracture.

rotator cuff is adequately visualized, inadvertent damage to the rotator cuff by the saw during humeral head resection can be avoided.

Neurovascular Structures

Catastrophic injury to neurovascular structures around the shoulder is exceedingly rare. Transient neuropraxia involving the axillary nerve, however, is one of the most common complications that we observe in unconstrained shoulder arthroplasty (up to 3% of cases).

The neural structures most at risk during unconstrained shoulder arthroplasty are the axillary and musculocutaneous nerves. During primary arthroplasty these nerves should not be at risk for transection when using accepted operative technique. Neuropraxic injury caused by stretch most commonly involves the

axillary nerve, but any nerves within the brachial plexus can be involved. Care should be taken when positioning the patient to maintain the cervical spine in neutral alignment to avoid a stretch injury of the brachial plexus. We have yet to establish risk factors for neuropraxic injury to the axillary nerve. Logic would suggest that patients with the most stiffness creating difficulty in glenoid exposure would be at highest risk for this type of complication. Our clinical experience has not borne this out, however, and currently we are unable to predict which patients are most likely to suffer this complication. Patient education preoperatively is of paramount importance in dealing with neuropraxia because patients are much more accepting if they have heard about the possibility of this complication before surgery. Axillary nerve (and other nerve) neuropraxia is treated by observation, with most patients recovering by 3 to 4 months postoperatively.

Although tearing of the cephalic vein is common and largely without consequence, significant arterial and venous injuries occurring during primary unconstrained shoulder arthroplasty performed for nonfracture indications are exceptionally rare. Injuries to the major upper extremity vessels are generally due to overzealous medial dissection, which is not needed during shoulder arthroplasty. Should one of these injuries occur, after cross-clamping of the injured vessel, emergency intraoperative consultation with a vascular surgeon is required.

POSTOPERATIVE COMPLICATIONS

Postoperative complications are more common than intraoperative complications and occur in up to 20% of cases of unconstrained shoulder arthroplasty.[1] The most common postoperative complications include wound problems (dehiscence, hematoma), glenoid problems, humeral problems, instability, rotator cuff problems, stiffness, and infection.

Wound Problems

Wound problems occur early after unconstrained shoulder arthroplasty. Hematoma is most easily avoided by extensive use of electrocautery during shoulder arthroplasty. Suture ligation, in addition to electrosurgical cauterization, of the anterior humeral circumflex vessels also minimizes the incidence of postoperative wound hematoma. When a hematoma occurs, it is managed by symptomatic nonoperative treatment (warm compresses, pain medication). Operative drainage is reserved for situations in which

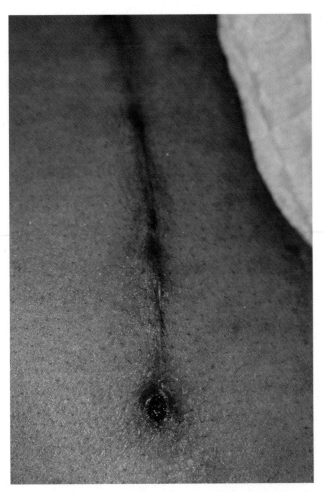

Figure 16-4   Superficial wound dehiscence.

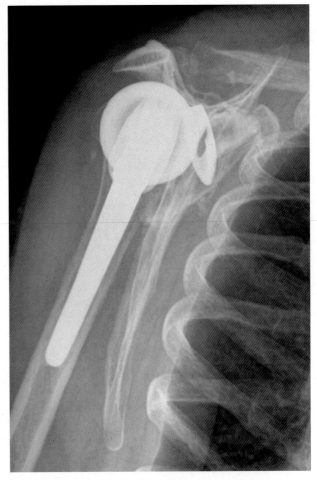

Figure 16-5   Aseptic loosening of a glenoid component.

drainage persists beyond 1 week or infection is suspected (see later) but is rarely necessary.

Wound dehiscence occurs occasionally when susceptible patients have a reaction to dissolving subcutaneous sutures. The presence of minimal serous drainage distinguishes this complication from the more serious deep infection. Superficial wound dehiscence is treated by local wound care, including removal of any residual dissolving suture material and chemical cauterization of any granulating tissue with silver nitrate applicators (Fig. 16-4).

Glenoid Problems

Glenoid problems after unconstrained shoulder arthroplasty are the most common complication necessitating revision surgery. Glenoid complications can develop after both total shoulder arthroplasty and isolated humeral head replacement (hemiarthroplasty). Glenoid component failure after total shoulder arthroplasty can occur as a result of loosening of the glenoid

component from the host bone (Fig. 16-5) or as a result of mechanical breakage of the glenoid implant (Fig. 16-6). Glenoid component problems, when symptomatic, usually require revision surgery (see Section Six).

After hemiarthroplasty, erosion of the remaining glenoid articular cartilage and osseous glenoid can occur. This erosion can take place early or late and is multifactorial in its cause.[11] Successful treatment of glenoid erosion generally requires revision surgery, during which the glenoid is resurfaced (Fig. 16-7).

Humeral Problems

Humeral problems after unconstrained shoulder arthroplasty are rare and can be divided into loosening of the humeral component and periprosthetic humeral fracture. Aseptic loosening of cemented and surface-prepared (grit-blasted, porous-coated, etc.) uncemented unconstrained humeral stems develops in less than 1% of cases. Whenever loosening of a humeral stem occurs, infection must be ruled out (Fig. 16-8; see later). In the

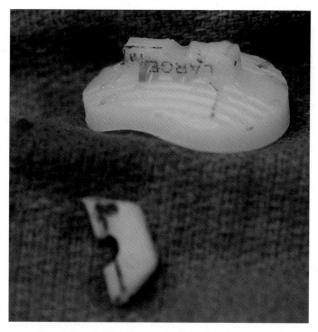

Figure 16-6   Fracture of a glenoid component.

rare instance of symptomatic aseptic loosening of the humeral component, treatment is revision of the humeral stem, usually with a cemented humeral component (see Section Six).

Periprosthetic humeral fractures are more common than loosening of the humeral component and are almost always the result of a fall or similar low-energy trauma (Fig. 16-9). The majority of these fractures occur just distal to the tip of the humeral stem, and most can be treated nonoperatively. Nonoperative treatment consists of fracture bracing, activity modification, pain medication, and frequent radiographic monitoring. If the fracture has not healed within 3 months, we incorporate the use of an external bone stimulator (OL 1000 Bone Growth Stimulator, Donjoy Orthopedics, Vista, CA). Despite these measures, periprosthetic humeral fractures treated nonoperatively may take more than 9 months to heal.[12] Our criteria for recommending operative treatment of periprosthetic fractures (revision surgery; see Section Six) include complete displacement, angulation greater

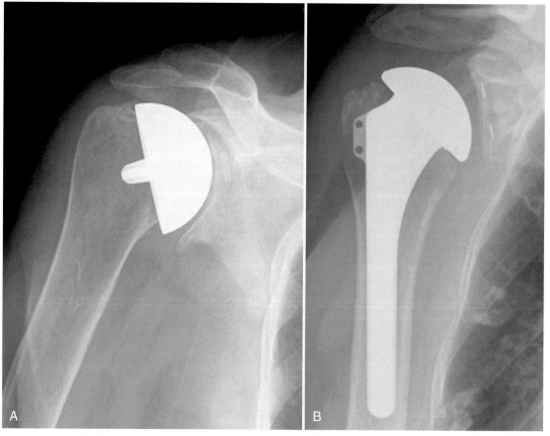

Figure 16-7   Symptomatic glenoid erosion (**A**) necessitating revision surgery for insertion of a glenoid component (**B**).

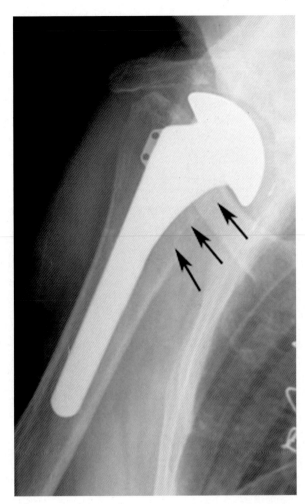

Figure 16-8 Septic loosening of a humeral stem (*arrows*).

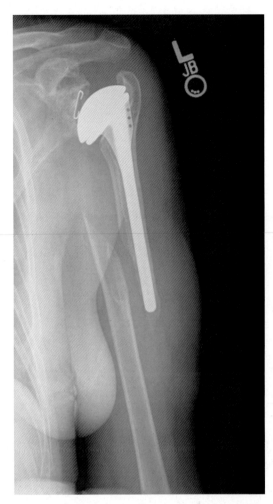

Figure 16-9 Periprosthetic humeral diaphyseal fracture resulting from a fall.

than 30 degrees, loosening of the humeral component, or failure of nonoperative treatment (Fig. 16-10).

Instability

Instability after unconstrained shoulder arthroplasty is usually related to one or more of three factors, including the prosthesis (alignment, size), the capsule, and the rotator cuff. Cases in which prosthetic problems have led to dynamic or static shoulder instability require correction to resolve the instability. Prosthetic problems may be related to the humeral side (excessive retroversion, causing posterior instability; excessive anteversion, causing anterior instability; too small a prosthetic head, causing global instability) or the glenoid side (failure to correct posterior glenoid wear, causing posterior instability). Revision arthroplasty (see Section Six) is the treatment of instability related to a prosthetic problem.

Capsular problems leading to instability are generally related to failure to perform posterior capsulorrhaphy at the time of primary arthroplasty in a patient with posterior glenoid wear and a chronically distended posterior capsule resulting in posterior instability (Fig. 16-11; see Chapter 13). Required treatment consists of revision surgery with performance of posterior capsulorrhaphy (marginally successful) or conversion to a reverse prosthesis (more predictable outcome; Fig. 16-12).

Rotator cuff problems can cause static and dynamic instability. Unconstrained arthroplasty in patients with a compromised rotator cuff often results in static instability (Fig. 16-13). These patients are probably best treated initially with a reverse-design prosthesis to avoid this potential complication. Rarely, in a patient with a previously intact rotator cuff that has undergone unconstrained shoulder arthroplasty, a massive rotator cuff tear will develop and contribute to static instability (Fig. 16-14). These patients, when

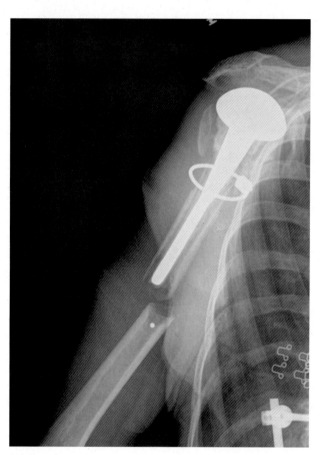

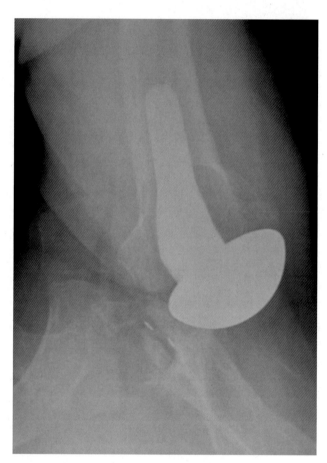

Figure 16-10 Periprosthetic humeral diaphyseal fracture failing 9 months of nonoperative treatment, including use of a bone stimulator.

Figure 16-11 Posterior instability of an unconstrained shoulder arthroplasty.

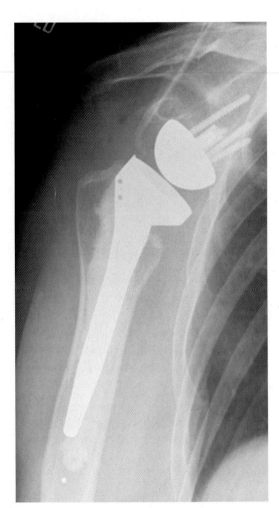

Figure 16-12   Revision of an unconstrained shoulder arthroplasty to a reverse arthroplasty for the treatment of postoperative posterior shoulder instability.

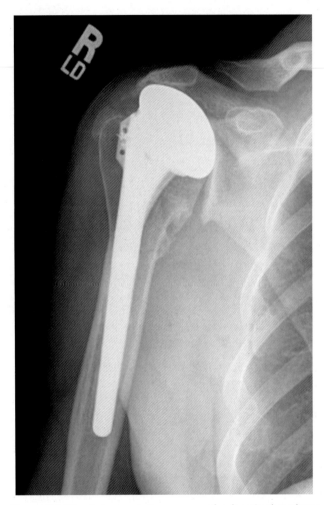

Figure 16-13   Anterosuperior escape of a hemiarthroplasty in a patient with a massive rotator cuff tear.

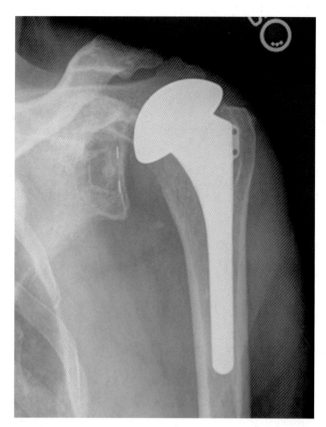

Figure 16-14 Radiograph of a patient who had undergone total shoulder arthroplasty for primary osteoarthritis. The patient did well until a massive degenerative rotator cuff tear developed and led to static proximal migration of the humerus some years after the index arthroplasty.

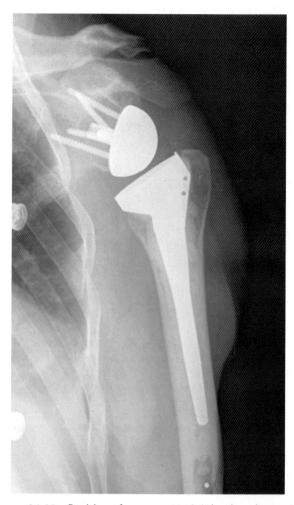

Figure 16-15 Revision of an unconstrained arthroplasty with a reverse prosthesis in a patient with static proximal migration of the humerus.

symptomatic, are best treated by revision to a reverse-design prosthesis (Fig. 16-15).

Dynamic instability after unconstrained shoulder arthroplasty most commonly occurs as anterior instability secondary to failure of the subscapularis repair. If this is diagnosed early, an attempt at subscapularis repair is warranted. Occasionally, failure of the subscapularis repair may be related to implantation of too large a humeral head component (Fig. 16-16). In this situation, subscapularis repair should be accompanied by exchange of the humeral head component for one smaller in size. If diagnosed after 4 to 6 weeks postoperatively, subscapularis repair is not usually possible, and we opt for revision to a reverse-design prosthesis (Fig. 16-17).

Rotator Cuff Problems

Symptomatic problems of the rotator cuff after unconstrained shoulder arthroplasty often result in instability and were described earlier under "Instability." Failure of the subscapularis repair is the most common

postoperative rotator cuff problem that we observe, yet it occurs in less than 3% of cases.[1] When subscapularis failure is minimally symptomatic or asymptomatic, no treatment is indicated. When symptomatic, treatment is indicated as described previously under "Instability."

Isolated internal rotation weakness is not diagnostic of subscapularis failure after unconstrained shoulder arthroplasty. It is common for individuals to lose some internal rotation strength after tenotomy and repair of the subscapularis during shoulder arthroplasty. Subscapularis failure should be documented by computed tomographic arthrography before considering operative treatment of this complication (Fig. 16-18).

Stiffness

Glenohumeral stiffness after unconstrained shoulder arthroplasty is related to capsular contracture or

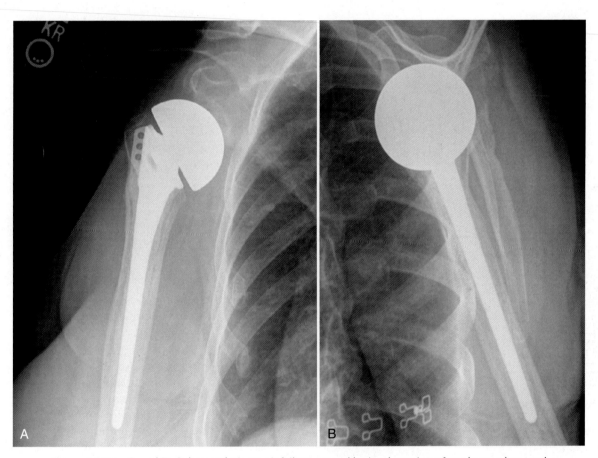

Figure 16-16   **A** and **B,** Subscapularis repair failure caused by implantation of too large a humeral head.

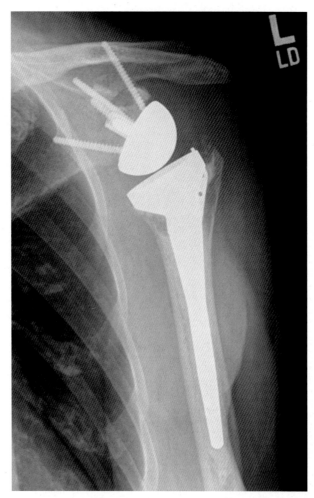

Figure 16-17 Revision arthroplasty with a reverse prosthesis in a patient with dynamic anterior shoulder instability secondary to failure of the subscapularis repair.

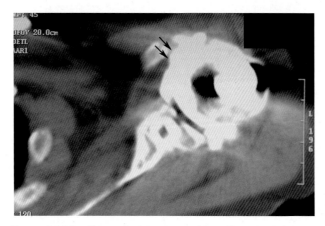

Figure 16-18 Computed tomographic arthrogram demonstrating disruption of the subscapularis (*arrows*).

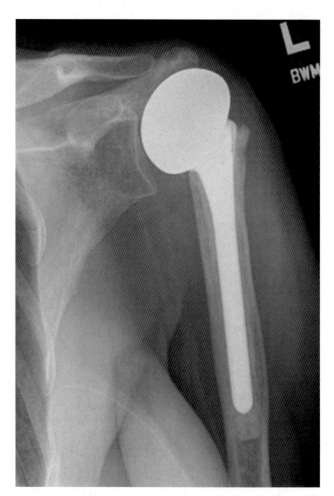

Figure 16-19 Postoperative shoulder stiffness caused by insertion of too large a humeral head component.

the prosthesis (or to both). Prosthetic problems resulting in stiffness are almost always the result of implantation of too large a humeral component (Fig. 16-19). Rehabilitation with capsular stretching can be attempted in an effort to improve mobility. If this fails (no improvement over a 6-month period), revision surgery consisting of downsizing of the humeral head and open release of any capsular contractures that are present is indicated.

Stiffness related to capsular contracture almost always responds to nonoperative management with aquatic-based rehabilitation (see Chapter 43). If a patient shows no improvement in mobility over a 6-month course of rehabilitation and has no obvious prosthetic problem, we will consider the patient a candidate for arthroscopic capsular contracture release.

Infection

Fortunately, infection after shoulder arthroplasty is much less common than infection after hip or knee arthroplasty; it occurs in less than 1% of all cases in our practice. Patients most at risk for infection are those with systemic illness (diabetes mellitus), those with compromised soft tissues (radiation-induced osteonecrosis, post-traumatic arthritis), and those with inflammatory arthropathy (rheumatoid arthritis). These infections are most commonly caused by *Staphylococcus aureus* or *Propionibacterium acnes*. Infections after shoulder arthroplasty can be divided into perioperative (within 6 weeks of surgery) and late (hematogenous) infections.

Early perioperative infections are initially treated by multiple (two or three) irrigation and débridement procedures with retention of the components. At the last planned irrigation and débridement procedure, absorbable antibiotic-impregnated beads (Stimulan, Biocomposites, Inc., Staffordshire, England) are placed in the soft tissues around the shoulder. Consultation with an infectious disease specialist is obtained, and a minimum of 6 weeks of intravenous antibiotics tailored to the specific organism causing the infection (or covering the most likely offending organisms if cultures remain negative despite obvious infection) is usually recommended. If this regimen fails, prosthetic removal ensues as detailed in Section Six.

Late-appearing infections are treated by removal of the prosthesis and intravenous antibiotics as detailed in Section Six. The decision regarding whether to place a revision shoulder arthroplasty or continue with a resection arthroplasty is patient specific.

REFERENCES

1. Walch G, Boileau P: Presentation of the multicentric study. In Walch G, Boileau P, Molé D (eds): 2000 Prostheses d'Epaule . . . Recul de 2 à 10 Ans. Paris, Sauramps Medical, 2001, pp 11-20.
2. Lafosse L, Kempf JF: Omarthrose primitive: Resultants cliniques et radiologiques. In Walch G, Boileau P, Molé D (eds): 2000 Prostheses d'Epaule . . . Recul de 2 à 10 Ans. Paris, Sauramps Medical, 2001, pp 73-85.
3. Gohlke F: Clinical and radiographic results of shoulder arthroplasty in rheumatoid arthritis. In Walch G, Boileau P, Molé D (eds): 2000 Prostheses d'Epaule . . . Recul de 2 à 10 Ans. Paris, Sauramps Medical, 2001, pp 163-169.
4. Versier G, Marchaland JP: Ostéonécorse avasculaire aseptique de la tête humérale (onath): Résultats cliniques et radiologiques des prostheses d'épaule. In Walch G, Boileau P, Molé D (eds): 2000 Prostheses d'Epaule . . . Recul de 2 à 10 Ans. Paris, Sauramps Medical, 2001, pp 127-134.
5. Trojani C, Boileau P, LeHeuc JC, et al: Sequelae of fractures of the proximal humerus: Surgical classification. In Walch G, Boileau P, Molé D (eds): 2000 Prostheses d'Epaule . . . Recul de 2 à 10 Ans. Paris, Sauramps Medical, 2001, pp 271-277.
6. Matsoukis J, Tabib W, Guiffault P, et al: Primary unconstrained shoulder arthroplasty in patients with a fixed anterior glenohumeral dislocation: Results of a multicenter study. J Bone Joint Surg Am 2006;88:547-552.
7. Oudet D, Favard L, Lautmann S, et al: La prosthèse d'épaule aequalis dans les omarthroses avec rupture massive et non réparable de la coiffe. In Walch G, Boileau P, Molé D (eds): 2000 Prostheses d'Epaule . . . Recul de 2 à 10 Ans. Paris, Sauramps Medical, 2001, pp 241-246.
8. Matsoukis J, Tabib W, Guiffault P, et al: Shoulder arthroplasty in patients with a prior anterior shoulder dislocation: Results of a multicenter study. J Bone Joint Surg Am 2003;85:1417-1424.
9. Constant CR, Murley AH: A clinical method of functional assessment of the shoulder. Clin Orthop Relat Res 1987;214:160-164.
10. Constant CR: Assessment of shoulder function. In Gazielly D, Gleyze P, Thomas T (eds): The Cuff. New York, Elsevier, 1997, pp 39-44.
11. Hertel R, Lehmann O: Glenoid erosion after hemiarthroplasty of the shoulder. In Walch G, Boileau P, Molé D (eds): 2000 Prostheses d'Epaule . . . Recul de 2 à 10 Ans. Paris, Sauramps Medical, 2001, pp 417-423.
12. Kumar S, Sperling JW, Haidukewych GH, Cofield RH: Periprosthetic humeral fractures after shoulder arthroplasty. J Bone Joint Surg Am 2004;86:680-689.

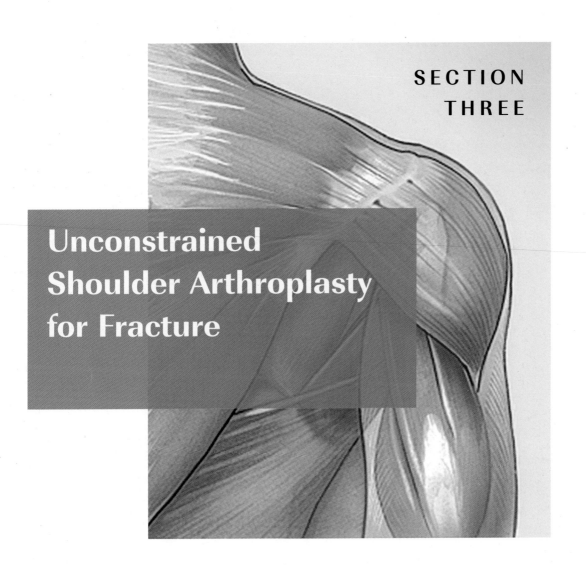

Unconstrained Shoulder Arthroplasty for Fracture

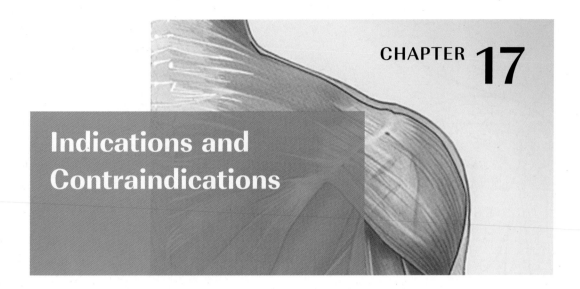

CHAPTER 17

Indications and Contraindications

The use of unconstrained humeral head replacement in acute fracture cases represents perhaps the most difficult indication for shoulder arthroplasty. Patients who are candidates for arthroplasty after proximal humeral fracture tend to be older with age-related osteopenia. Complications, both systemic and shoulder specific, are more common in this patient population than in patients undergoing unconstrained shoulder arthroplasty for chronic conditions. These factors contribute to the difficulty in treating proximal humeral fractures with unconstrained shoulder arthroplasty.

Neer popularized the use of humeral head replacement for the treatment of complex proximal humeral fractures.[1] Neer's classification of these fractures is the most commonly used scheme. Unfortunately, this classification system has been shown to have poor interobserver and intraobserver reliability.[2] Other classification schemes have been introduced, but their complexity has limited their usefulness. For us, the most important, readily observable factor that indicates the need for shoulder arthroplasty after proximal humeral fracture is the condition of the humeral head articular fragment (soft tissue attachments, bone quality, dislocation, head splitting). In all cases in which we are anticipating possible shoulder arthroplasty for the treatment of proximal humeral fracture, we obtain a computed tomogram. Because of the widespread use of Neer's classification scheme, this chapter discusses our indications for unconstrained shoulder arthroplasty based on the condition of the humeral head fragment within the context of the Neer classification as determined by computed tomography.

FOUR-PART PROXIMAL HUMERAL FRACTURES

The most common indication for unconstrained shoulder arthroplasty for proximal humeral fracture is a "four-part" fracture. This refers to a fracture involving four distinct fragments, including a humeral head fragment, a greater tuberosity fragment, a lesser tuberosity fragment, and a humeral shaft fragment (Fig. 17-1). Neer did not consider a fragment to constitute a "part" unless it was displaced greater than 1 cm or angulated more than 45 degrees.[1] We have found strict application of these criteria to be difficult because determination of fragment angulation and even displacement can be complex despite the use of computed tomography. In any fracture that contains fracture lines separating the proximal humerus into four parts for which we plan operative treatment consisting of open reduction and internal fixation, we will be prepared to perform a hemiarthroplasty should the need arise intraoperatively. The two principal circumstances that make us opt for hemiarthroplasty, even in cases in which the tuberosities are displaced less than 1 cm, are when the humeral head fragment is discovered to be completely devoid of soft tissue attachment (Fig. 17-2) and when the bone in the humeral head is too severely osteopenic

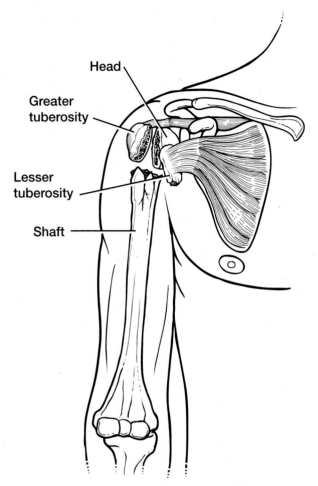

Figure 17-1 Schematic of the typical "four-part" proximal humeral fracture.

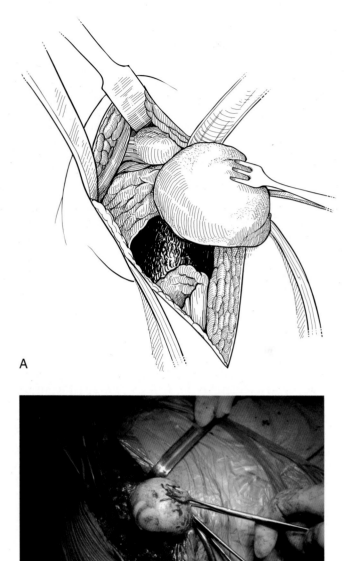

A

B

Figure 17-2 **A** and **B,** Drawing and intraoperative photograph of a humeral head devoid of soft tissue attachment.

to permit any sort of fixation. In cases in which each fragment is clearly displaced more than 1 cm, we plan to perform hemiarthroplasty from the outset (Fig. 17-3).

THREE-PART PROXIMAL HUMERAL FRACTURES

A less common indication for unconstrained shoulder arthroplasty for the treatment of proximal humeral fracture is a "three-part" fracture. This refers to a fracture involving three distinct fragments, including a humeral head fragment, a greater (more common) or lesser (less common) tuberosity fragment, and a humeral shaft fragment (Fig. 17-4). The majority of these fractures can be treated successfully with open reduction and internal fixation. In any fracture that contains fracture lines separating the proximal

humerus into three parts for which we plan operative treatment consisting of open reduction and internal fixation, we will be prepared to perform a hemiarthroplasty should the need arise intraoperatively. The principal circumstance that makes us opt for hemiarthroplasty in three-part fractures, even in cases in which the tuberosities are displaced less than 1 cm, is when the bone in the humeral head is too severely osteopenic to permit any sort of fixation (Fig. 17-5). These cases require osteotomy of the lesser tuberosity at the time of hemiarthroplasty.

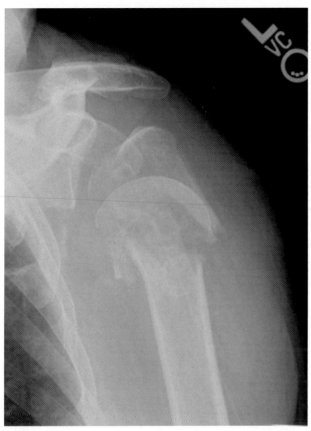

Figure 17-3 Displaced "four-part" proximal humeral fracture.

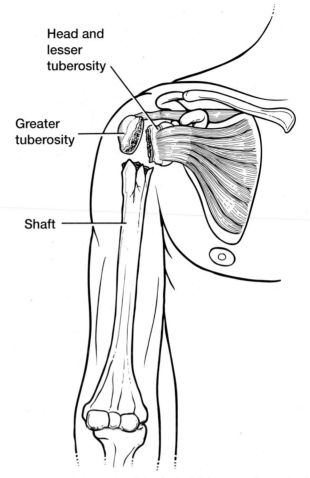

Figure 17-4 Schematic of the typical "three-part" proximal humeral fracture.

FRACTURE-DISLOCATION

Occasionally, a four-part or three-part fracture will be accompanied by dislocation of the humeral head (Fig. 17-6). In these cases we nearly always opt for arthroplasty over open reduction and internal fixation because the humeral head fragment is nearly always devoid of significant soft tissue attachment.

HEAD-SPLITTING FRACTURE

In fractures in which the proximal humeral articular surface has been split, we opt for humeral hemiarthroplasty (Fig. 17-7). These cases nearly always occur with a greater or lesser tuberosity fracture (or both). Occasionally, dislocation of all or part of the proximal humeral articular surface will be present.

SPECIAL SITUATIONS

Severe Osteopenia

An elderly patient with severe osteopenia is occasionally a contraindication to open reduction and internal fixation of a comminuted proximal humeral fracture (Fig. 17-8). Additionally, severe proximal humeral osteopenia may prevent healing of the tuberosities. In our practice, an elderly patient (>75 years) with severe proximal humeral osteopenia and a proximal humeral fracture with indications for replacement is a relative indication for use of a reverse prosthesis combined with fixation of the tuberosities. In this circumstance, in the event that the tuberosities do not heal, elevation may still be possible and prevent the need for further surgery. More discussion of this indication for a reverse prosthesis is provided in Chapter 24.

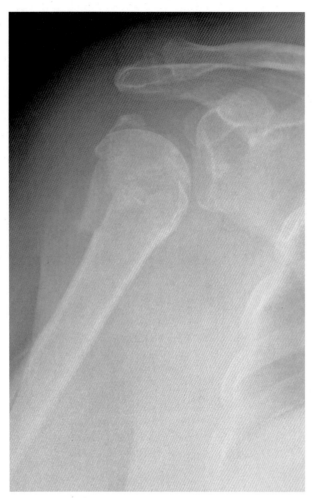

Figure 17-5 Severe osteopenia of the humeral head fragment precluding open reduction and internal fixation in a "three-part" proximal humeral fracture.

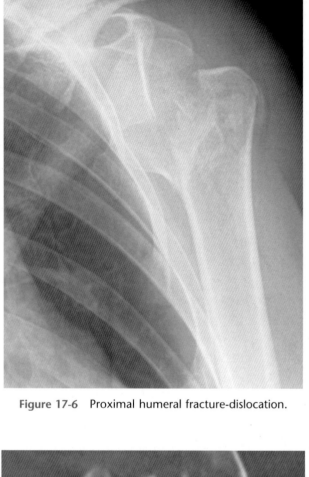

Figure 17-6   Proximal humeral fracture-dislocation.

Neural Injury

Many patients with proximal humeral fractures have signs of neural injury, most commonly deficits of the motor branch of the axillary nerve. These injuries are nearly always neuropraxias that spontaneously recover and do not represent a contraindication to arthroplasty for fracture. The patients need to be educated about this finding, however.

Glenoid Issues

In contrast to unconstrained shoulder arthroplasty performed for chronic conditions, in which we usually resurface the glenoid, we nearly always perform hemiarthroplasty in cases of acute fracture. The only circumstance that we will consider concomitant insertion of a glenoid component is a fracture occurring in the

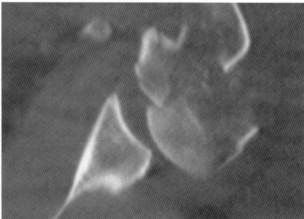

Figure 17-7 Head-splitting fracture of the proximal humerus.

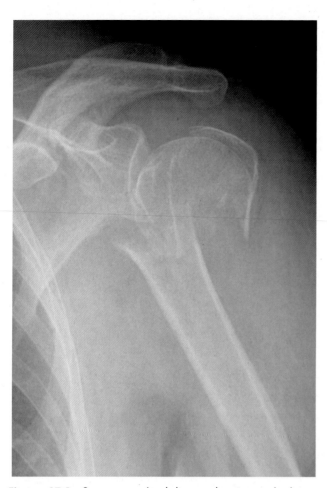

Figure 17-8 Severe proximal humeral osteopenia in an elderly patient with a proximal humeral fracture. In this patient we would consider use of a reverse prosthesis for treatment of the fracture acutely.

presence of end-stage glenohumeral arthritis. In our experience this situation is exceedingly rare.

Although it is true that glenoid erosion will develop in some patients after unconstrained hemiarthroplasty for fracture, the number of patients facing this problem is small relative to those who will experience nonunion or malunion of the tuberosity fragments. If tuberosity fixation failure occurs, the humerus will inevitably subluxate statically. Such subluxation causes nonconcentric loading of a glenoid component if it has been implanted and ultimately leads to failure of the glenoid component via the "rocking horse" phenomenon.[3] Additionally, revision to a reverse prosthesis in a patient with tuberosity fixation failure (our usual treatment in this scenario) is more easily performed if the native glenoid has not been previously violated. For these reasons we prefer isolated humeral hemiarthroplasty in cases in which we use unconstrained shoulder arthroplasty for the treatment of proximal humeral fractures.

Rotator Cuff Pathology

Rarely, a patient with a massive rotator cuff tear that has been relatively asymptomatic will sustain a proximal humeral fracture requiring operative treatment. In this scenario, we opt for use of a reverse prosthesis with excision of the tuberosities if they are devoid of rotator cuff attachment or fixation of the tuberosities if some rotator cuff is still attached.

Table 17-1 CONTRAINDICATIONS TO UNCONSTRAINED SHOULDER ARTHROPLASTY FOR ACUTE PROXIMAL HUMERAL FRACTURES

Contraindication	Absolute or Relative	Comments
Nondisplaced fracture	Absolute	Nonoperative treatment
Fracture amenable to ORIF	Absolute	Should be treated by ORIF
Poor generalized health	Relative	Appropriate perioperative medical treatment required
Active infection	Absolute	
Massive rotator cuff tear	Relative	Glenoid component contraindicated; better suited for reverse prosthesis
Upper motor neuron lesion	Relative	Absolute contraindication if the patient has uncontrolled shoulder spasticity
Poor patient motivation	Relative	May best be treated nonoperatively; consider resection arthroplasty if the shoulder remains symptomatic

ORIF, open reduction with internal fixation.

CONTRAINDICATIONS TO UNCONSTRAINED SHOULDER ARTHROPLASTY FOR FRACTURE

Contraindications to unconstrained shoulder arthroplasty for acute proximal humeral fracture are listed in Table 17-1. Some of these contraindications are absolute, whereas others are relative.

REFERENCES

1. Neer CS II: Displaced proximal humeral fractures: Part 1: classification and evaluation. J Bone Joint Surg Am 1970;52:1077-1089.
2. Siebenrock KA, Gerber C: The reproducibility of classification of fractures of the proximal end of the humerus. J Bone Joint Surg Am 1993;75:1751-1755.
3. Franklin JL, Barrett WP, Jackins SE, Matsen FA III: Glenoid loosening in total shoulder arthroplasty: Association with rotator cuff deficiency. J Arthroplasty 1988;3:39-46.

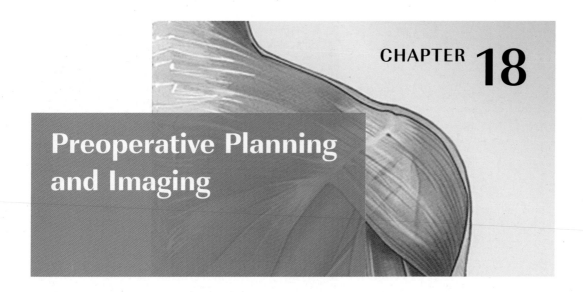

CHAPTER 18

Preoperative Planning and Imaging

Preoperative planning is important for all shoulder arthroplasty indications, but it is most crucial for fracture cases. Although proximal humeral anatomy may be somewhat distorted by prolonged wear and osteophyte formation in cases of chronic disease for which shoulder arthroplasty is performed, most reliable anatomic landmarks remain consistent despite the disease process. In fracture cases, however, these normally reliable landmarks are often displaced, thus making them useless as points of reference. Because of the lack of recognizable landmarks, preoperative planning becomes of paramount importance when attempting to establish the proper position for humeral stem implantation. Thorough preoperative planning minimizes the risk of placing the humeral stem at the incorrect height or version. We have successfully used two techniques to place the humeral stem at the appropriate height. Preoperative planning is of paramount importance for both these techniques and is detailed in this chapter. Additionally, important aspects of the clinical history and physical examination, the radiographic examination, and secondary imaging studies are highlighted.

CLINICAL HISTORY AND EXAMINATION

A thorough history is taken of the antecedent trauma responsible for the fracture. Most often, these proximal humeral fractures are caused by a fall from a standing position. Elucidation of the reason for the fall

should be sought to assist in evaluation of any underlying contributing medical conditions (i.e., syncope as a symptom of cardiac arrhythmia). The presence of any shoulder problems before the fracture should be noted in the history. A previous history of shoulder pathology, such as a massive rotator cuff tear or glenohumeral arthritis, influences surgical decision making (i.e., the type of prosthesis to be implanted, such as an unconstrained fracture prosthesis, reverse shoulder prosthesis, or unconstrained shoulder arthroplasty with a glenoid component).

Physical examination in a patient with an acute proximal humeral fracture is limited so that the patient is not unnecessarily subjected to pain. A detailed neurovascular examination is performed with specific attention to the sensory and motor function of the axillary nerve. The sensory function of the axillary nerve can always be evaluated by testing sensibility to touch of the posterior aspect of the upper part of the arm (superior lateral brachial cutaneous branch of the axillary nerve). Motor function of the axillary nerve may be more difficult to evaluate because pain induced by the fracture may inhibit deltoid contraction. The condition of the soft tissues, particularly anterior at the planned surgical site, is meticulously evaluated.

RADIOGRAPHY

Three radiographic views are obtained in all patients with a proximal humeral fracture. We prefer the same

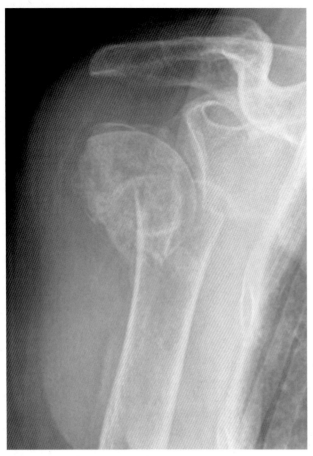

Figure 18-1 Anteroposterior radiograph in a patient with a comminuted proximal humeral fracture.

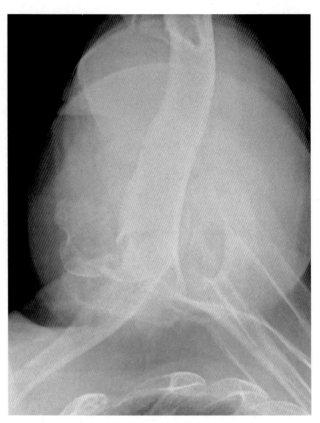

Figure 18-2 Axillary radiograph in a patient with a comminuted proximal humeral fracture.

radiographic views that we obtain for patients being considered for unconstrained shoulder arthroplasty for chronic conditions: an anteroposterior view of the glenohumeral joint with the arm in neutral rotation (Fig. 18-1), an axillary view (Fig. 18-2), and a scapular outlet view (Fig. 18-3). These radiographs are used to evaluate the fracture pattern (two part, three part, four part), the amount of displacement of the fracture fragments, the presence of humeral head dislocation, and the presence of a split in the humeral head fragment. Frequently, the patient has radiographs obtained in an emergency department that are of poor quality. We always repeat these radiographs to obtain better-quality films and to assess for progressive displacement. Once it is determined that the patient is a potential candidate for shoulder hemiarthroplasty, anteroposterior full-length radiographs of both humeri taken with the arm in neutral rotation are obtained for use in preoperative determination of appropriate humeral head height. These radiographs must include the entire length of the humerus and must be controlled for magnification (Fig. 18-4).

SECONDARY IMAGING

Computed tomography is performed in all patients with substantially displaced proximal humeral fractures (Fig. 18-5). This study allows further elucidation of the fracture pattern and assessment of the amount of displacement of the fracture fragments. Additionally, the position of the tuberosities and humeral head is visualized, thereby allowing easier identification at the time of surgery. Any comminution of the tuberosities can be identified with computed tomography as well.

PROSTHETIC POSITIONING WITH ANCILLARY INSTRUMENTATION— THE FRACTURE JIG TECHNIQUE

Placement of the prosthesis at the correct height and version remains one of the most difficult challenges when performing shoulder arthroplasty for fracture. Use of specialized instrumentation enhances the surgeon's ability to place the prosthesis at the correct height and in the correct amount of retroversion.[1] The

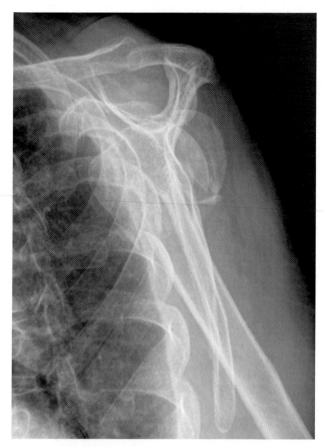

Figure 18-3 Scapular outlet radiograph in a patient with a comminuted proximal humeral fracture.

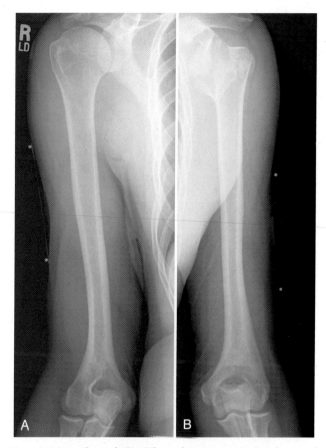

Figure 18-4 A and **B,** Bilateral anteroposterior humeral radiographs that have been controlled for magnification.

fracture jig references the humeral epicondyles to allow intraoperative estimation of proper prosthetic height and retroversion. More importantly, the fracture jig permits trial reduction of the glenohumeral joint and reduction of the tuberosities before final cementation of the humeral implant, thus allowing adjustment of prosthetic position.

When preoperative planning is performed for the fracture jig technique, only the anteroposterior full-length humeral radiograph of the unaffected arm is required. From this radiograph the length of the humerus from the superior aspect of the greater tuberosity to the transepicondylar axis is measured and normalized for magnification. This measurement is obtained by first establishing the prosthetic axis proximally within the humeral canal. We do this by measuring the center point of the proximal diaphysis at two locations and connecting these points with a line running the length of the humerus (Fig. 18-6). Next, a line perpendicular to the prosthetic axis is drawn at the level of the greater tuberosity (Fig. 18-7). A third line intersecting the prosthetic axis is drawn at the transepicondylar axis of the distal humerus (Fig. 18-8).

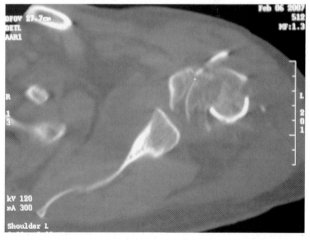

Figure 18-5 Computed tomogram of a comminuted proximal humeral fracture being evaluated for hemiarthroplasty.

The distance between the greater tuberosity and the transepicondylar axis is measured in centimeters along the prosthetic axis (Fig. 18-9). This value is corrected for magnification if necessary (a digital radiography system does this step automatically at our institution)

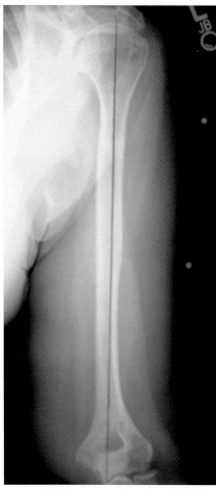

Figure 18-6 Establishing the prosthetic axis for the fracture jig technique.

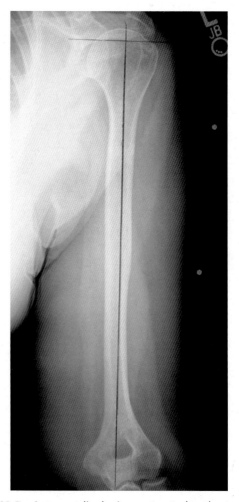

Figure 18-7 A perpendicular is constructed to the prosthetic axis at the level of the greater tuberosity.

by using the mathematical formula shown in the example in Figure 18-10. This measurement, once corrected for radiographic magnification, provides an estimated height at which to set the fracture jig during the procedure.

PROSTHETIC POSITIONING WITHOUT ANCILLARY INSTRUMENTATION— THE GOTHIC ARCH TECHNIQUE

Although the fracture jig technique has proved valuable in improving prosthetic positioning during shoulder hemiarthroplasty performed for fracture, it does have certain disadvantages. First, many surgeons consider the instrumentation bulky and awkward. Second, lack of familiarity with the instrumentation combined with the infrequency with which hemiarthroplasty is performed for fracture by many surgeons has pre-

vented them from using the fracture jig technique. Finally, the body habitus (obesity or soft tissue swelling from trauma) of many patients limits the usefulness of the fracture jig because their humeral epicondyles are not readily palpable and the large amount of soft tissue between the fracture jig and the humerus allows the fracture jig to be positioned improperly initially or to translate during the procedure. As a result of these concerns, Sumant "Butch" Krishnan has developed a technique for prosthetic positioning that we have found useful and reproducible; he terms the technique "restoration of the Gothic arch."[2]

When using this technique it is necessary to perform preoperative planning with anteroposterior radiographs of the affected and unaffected humeri. Use of the radiograph of the unaffected humerus is similar to the technique involving the fracture jig. From this radiograph, the length of the humerus from the supe-

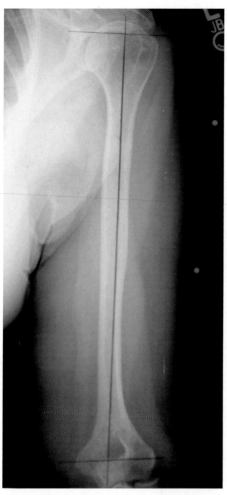

Figure 18-8 A line is drawn at the transepicondylar axis of the distal humerus intersecting the prosthetic axis.

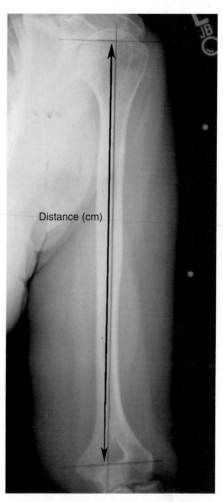

Figure 18-9 The distance between the greater tuberosity and the transepicondylar axis is measured in centimeters along the prosthetic axis.

rior aspect of the humeral head to the transepicondylar axis is measured and normalized for magnification. This measurement is obtained by first establishing the prosthetic axis proximally within the humeral canal. This is done by measuring the center point of the proximal diaphysis at two locations and connecting these points with a line running the length of the humerus. Next, a line perpendicular to the prosthetic axis is drawn at the superior aspect of the humeral head (Fig. 18-11). A third line intersecting the prosthetic axis is drawn at the transepicondylar axis of the distal humerus. The distance between the superior aspect of the humeral head and the transepicondylar axis is measured in centimeters along the prosthetic axis (Fig. 18-12). Just as with the fracture jig technique, this value is corrected for magnification if necessary (a digital radiography system does this step automatically at our institution) by using the mathematical formula shown in the example in Figure 18-10.

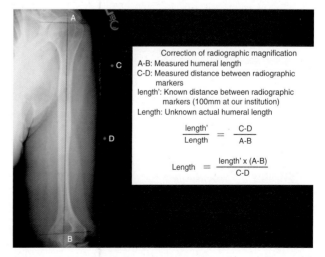

Correction of radiographic magnification
A-B: Measured humeral length
C-D: Measured distance between radiographic markers
length': Known distance between radiographic markers (100mm at our institution)
Length: Unknown actual humeral length

$$\frac{\text{length}'}{\text{Length}} = \frac{\text{C-D}}{\text{A-B}}$$

$$\text{Length} = \frac{\text{length}' \times (\text{A-B})}{\text{C-D}}$$

Figure 18-10 Example of correction for radiographic magnification.

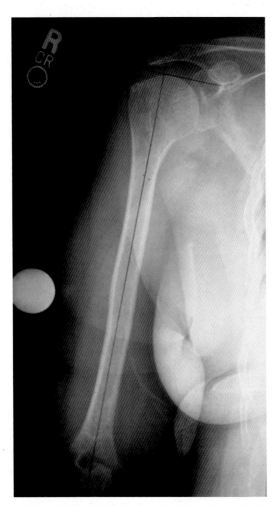

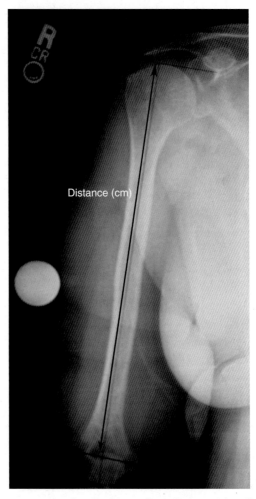

Figure 18-11 When using the Gothic arch technique, a perpendicular to the prosthetic axis is drawn at the superior aspect of the humeral head.

Figure 18-12 In the Gothic arch technique, the distance between the superior aspect of the humeral head and the transepicondylar axis is measured in centimeters along the prosthetic axis.

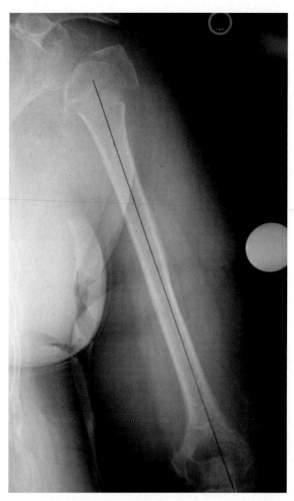

Figure 18-13 By using an anteroposterior humeral radiograph of the affected extremity, the prosthetic axis and transepicondylar axis are established for the Gothic arch technique.

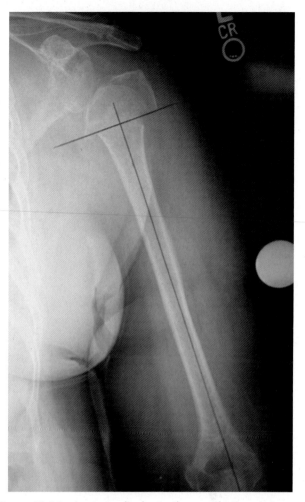

Figure 18-14 A perpendicular to the prosthetic axis is constructed at the level of the fracture medially for the Gothic arch technique.

By using the anteroposterior humeral radiograph of the affected extremity, the prosthetic axis and transepicondylar axis are established (Fig. 18-13). A line perpendicular to the prosthetic axis is drawn at the level of the fracture medially (Fig. 18-14). The distance between the medial fracture line and the transepicondylar axis (residual humeral length) is measured and corrected for magnification if necessary (Fig. 18-15). In cases in which the greater tuberosity is visible as a single fragment, the length of the greater tuberosity is measured and corrected for magnification (Fig. 18-16). The difference between humeral length measured on the unaffected radiograph and residual humeral length measured on the affected radiograph is calculated (Fig. 18-17). This difference is marked on the humeral implant to establish the height at which the humeral stem should be positioned with respect to the medial fracture line (Fig. 18-18). The length of the greater tuberosity, when available, is used as a checkrein. When the length of the greater tuberosity is added to length of the residual humerus, the sum should be approximately 3 to 5 mm less than the humeral length measured on the radiograph of the unaffected humerus (Fig. 18-19).

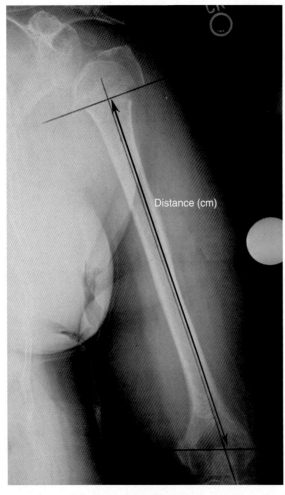

Figure 18-15 The distance between the medial fracture line and the transepicondylar axis (residual humeral length) is measured and corrected for magnification, if necessary.

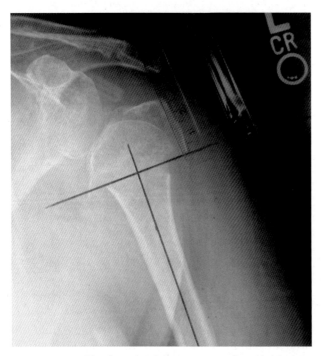

Figure 18-16 The length of the greater tuberosity is measured and corrected for magnification.

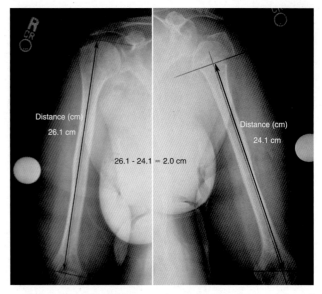

Figure 18-17 The difference between the humeral length measured from the unaffected radiograph and the residual humeral length measured from the affected radiograph is calculated.

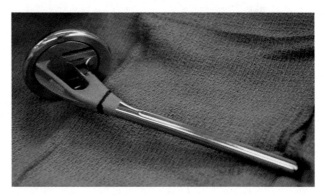

Figure 18-18 The difference between the humeral length measured on the unaffected humeral radiograph and the residual humeral length measured on the affected humeral radiograph is marked on the humeral implant to establish the height at which the humeral stem should be positioned with respect to the medial fracture line.

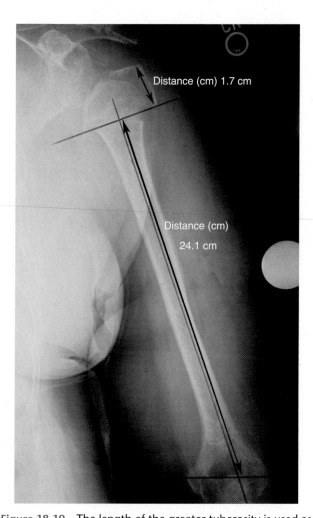

Distance (cm) 1.7 cm

Distance (cm)
24.1 cm

Figure 18-19   The length of the greater tuberosity is used as a checkrein. When the greater tuberosity length is added to the residual humeral length measured on the affected humeral radiograph, this calculation should be approximately 3 to 5 mm less than the humeral length measured on the unaffected humeral radiograph.

REFERENCES

1. Boileau P, Coste JS, Ahrens PM, Staccini P: Prosthetic shoulder replacement for fracture: Results of the multicentre study. In Walch G, Boileau P, Molé D (eds): 2000 Prosthèses d'Epaule . . . Recul de 2 à 10 Ans. Paris, Sauramps Medical, 2001, pp 561-578.
2. Krishnan SG, Pennington SD, Burkhead WZ, Boileau P: Shoulder arthroplasty for fracture: Restoration of the "gothic arch." Tech Shoulder Elbow Surg 2005;6:57-66.

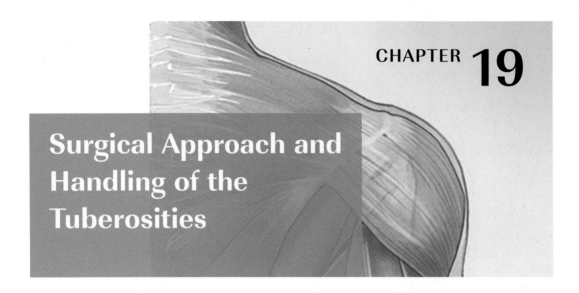

CHAPTER 19

Surgical Approach and Handling of the Tuberosities

SURGICAL APPROACH

When performing shoulder arthroplasty for fracture, operating room setup, anesthesia, patient positioning, surgical site preparation, and sterile draping (Chapters 3 and 4) are essentially the same as for nonfracture cases, with a few exceptions. Draping of the patient differs slightly in fracture cases in which use of the fracture jig for prosthetic positioning is planned, in that the stockinet covers only the forearm so that the elbow and humeral epicondyles are easily accessible to use as reference points in judging prosthetic retroversion. When use of the fracture jig is planned, the epicondyles are palpated and marked with a surgical marking pen (Fig. 19-1).

A standard deltopectoral approach is used for exposure just as in arthroplasty cases performed for chronic conditions. The skin incision starts at the tip of the coracoid process and extends distally and laterally approximately 10 to 15 cm, depending on the size of the patient. A needle tip electrocautery is used for deep dissection throughout the procedure to minimize hemorrhage. The interval between the deltoid and pectoralis major is identified by locating the cephalic vein. Once the cephalic vein is identified, it is retracted laterally with the deltoid muscle. The superior centimeter of the pectoralis major tendon is divided with the electrocautery to further enhance exposure. A self-retaining deltopectoral retractor is placed to maintain exposure during the procedure. The conjoined tendon is identified and traced to its insertion on the coracoid

process. The tip of a Hohmann-type retractor is placed behind the base of the coracoid process to provide proximal retraction. With the arm abducted and externally rotated, the apex formed by the insertion of the coracoacromial ligament and the conjoined tendon onto the coracoid process is identified. The conjoined tendon is retracted medially to expose the proximal humeral fracture (Fig. 19-2).

IDENTIFICATION AND HANDLING OF THE TUBEROSITY

A Cobb elevator is used to perform blunt dissection and begin the process of identification of the tuberosities (Fig. 19-3). In the prototypical four-part fracture pattern, the lesser tuberosity with the attached subscapularis represents one fragment, the greater tuberosity with the attached posterior superior rotator cuff represents a second fragment, the humeral head represents a third fragment, and the humeral shaft represents the final fragment. A variety of combinations exist; however, the most common fracture pattern for which arthroplasty is indicated involves these major fracture fragments. Control of the lesser tuberosity is achieved by identifying the tuberosity and subscapularis tendon anteriorly in the shoulder just posterior to the conjoined tendon. Stay sutures of no. 1 polyester are placed through the subscapularis tendon just medial to its osseous insertion on the lesser tuberosity.

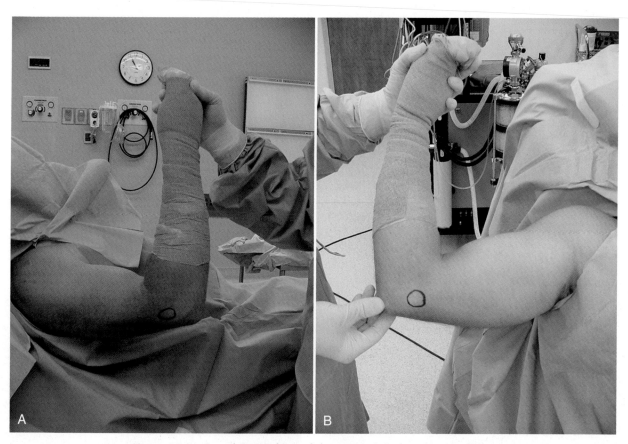

Figure 19-1 **A** and **B,** Marking of the patient's humeral epicondyles.

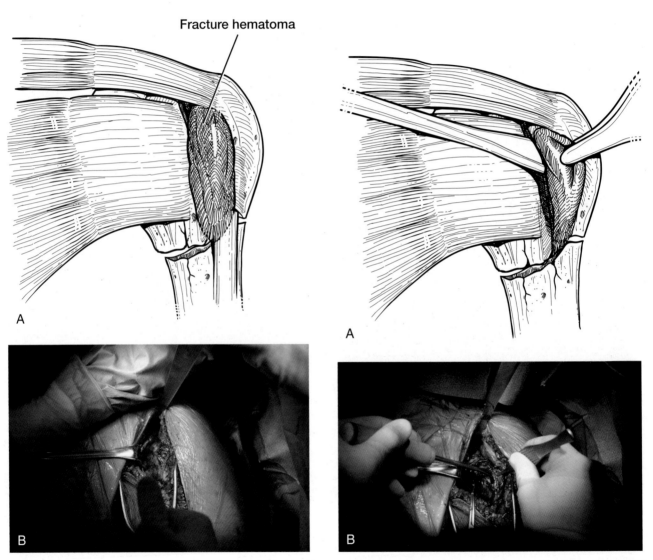

Fracture hematoma

A

A

B

B

Figure 19-2 **A** and **B,** Identification of the proximal humeral fracture.

Figure 19-3 **A** and **B,** Development of fracture planes with a Cobb elevator.

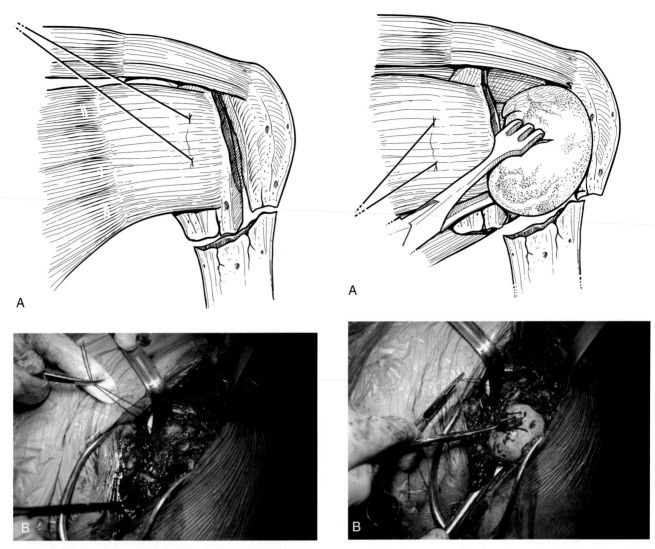

Figure 19-4 **A** and **B**, Control of the lesser tuberosity with stay sutures placed through the subscapularis tendon.

Figure 19-5 **A** and **B**, Removal of the humeral head fragment.

One suture is placed superiorly and a second suture is placed inferiorly if necessary (Fig. 19-4). Sutures are not placed through the lesser tuberosity because it is usually osteopenic and does not support transosseous sutures sufficiently. These sutures will also aid in retracting the lesser tuberosity to gain access to the humeral head fragment. The humeral head fragment is identified and may be dislocated or split into two or more fragments. The humeral head is removed with locking forceps (Lahey type) and kept on the sterile field for later use as bone graft material (Fig. 19-5).

Removal of the humeral head facilitates identification of the greater tuberosity, which is located posteriorly in the shoulder. Frequently, especially in elderly patients in whom these fractures are most common, the greater tuberosity is a mere shell of thin cortical bone and must be handled with care to avoid further fracture (Fig. 19-6). Control of the greater tuberosity

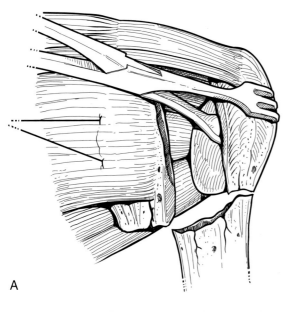

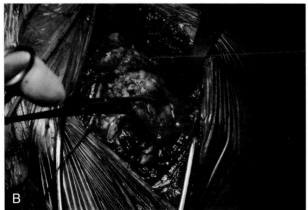

Figure 19-6 **A** and **B,** Thin shell of cortical bone representing what remains of the greater tuberosity after a proximal humeral fracture.

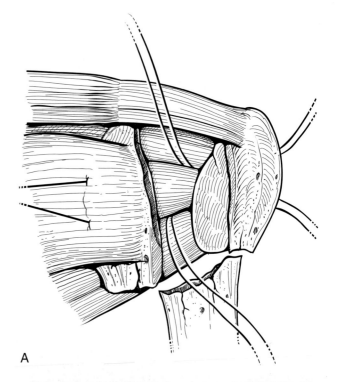

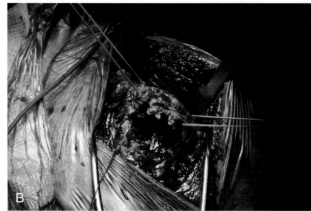

Figure 19-7 **A** and **B,** Control of the greater tuberosity by passing no. 2 braided permanent suture through the rotator cuff tendons just medial to their insertion on the greater tuberosity.

and attached posterior superior rotator cuff is obtained by passing no. 2 braided permanent suture through the rotator cuff tendons just medial to their insertion on the greater tuberosity. A large curved free needle is loaded with two strands of suture and passed through the rotator cuff at the junction of the supraspinatus and infraspinatus. A second free needle loaded with two strands of suture is passed through the rotator cuff at the junction of the infraspinatus and teres minor

(Fig. 19-7). These sutures provide immediate control of the greater tuberosity and are used later for fixation of both the greater and lesser tuberosities. As with the lesser tuberosity, sutures are not placed through the greater tuberosity because it is usually osteopenic and does not support transosseous sutures sufficiently. Occasionally, it is necessary to temporarily grasp the greater tuberosity with Lahey forceps to provide traction and enable suture placement. This should always

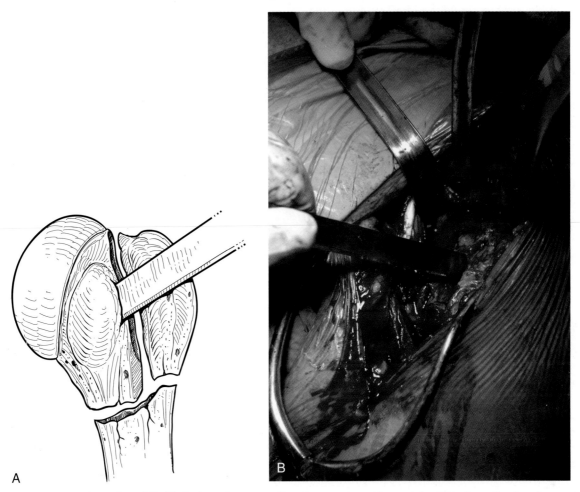

Figure 19-8 A and **B,** Technique for separating the greater or lesser tuberosity from the head fragment with an osteotome.

be done gently and with great care to avoid further fracture of the tuberosity.

Rarely, hemiarthroplasty is indicated in patients in whom the greater or lesser tuberosity remains attached to the humeral head (fracture-dislocation, head-splitting fracture). In these cases the tuberosity must be detached from the humeral head fragment. A 1-inch osteotome is used while leaving as much bone with the tuberosity fragment as possible (Fig. 19-8). The tuberosity is then handled as with a four-part fracture, as described earlier.

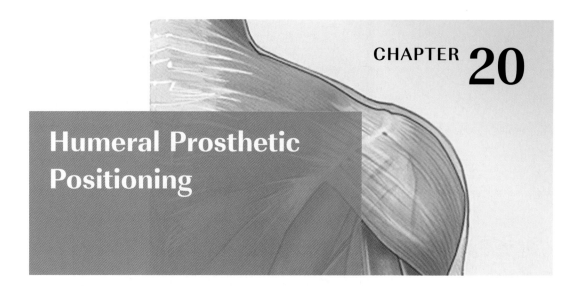

CHAPTER **20**

Humeral Prosthetic Positioning

Humeral prosthetic positioning remains the most difficult step in performing unconstrained shoulder arthroplasty for fracture. Placing the humeral component excessively proud or in excessive retroversion may result in loss of fixation and subsequent migration of the greater tuberosity (Figs. 20-1 and 20-2). The complication of tuberosity migration has been found to be a key factor in poor results after unconstrained shoulder arthroplasty performed for the treatment of proximal humeral fractures.[1] This chapter details humeral prosthetic positioning with each of the techniques described in Chapter 18.

IDENTIFICATION AND PREPARATION OF THE HUMERAL DIAPHYSIS

After control of both tuberosities has been achieved, the humeral shaft is identified. The humeral shaft is progressively reamed until the reamer that is used corresponds to the diameter of the prosthesis to be implanted (Fig. 20-3). Using the largest diaphyseal reamer that is possible to advance down the humeral canal without difficulty avoids selecting too small a diameter of the humeral implant, which can inadvertently be positioned in valgus or varus (Fig. 20-4). Because most of these patients are severely osteopenic, however, no effort is made to force too large a reamer down the humeral canal for fear of iatrogenic fracture. The bicipital groove is located and two 2-mm holes are drilled in the humeral shaft approximately 1 cm distal to the fracture site, one on each side of the bicipital groove, for use later in tuberosity fixation (Fig. 20-5). The intra-articular portion of the long head of the biceps, which is frequently at least partially torn, is excised, and suture tenodesis of the remaining stump to the pectoralis major tendon is carried out with no. 1 nonabsorbable braided suture in a figure-of-eight stitch as described in Chapter 5.[2]

SELECTION OF THE HUMERAL IMPLANT

The trial humeral implant is then assembled by selecting a stem with a diameter corresponding to the largest diaphyseal reamer used and a head size corresponding to the size of the removed head fracture fragment. The humeral head fragment is usually slightly ovoid and has a lesser and greater diameter. A head size corresponding to the lesser diameter is selected to avoid insertion of too large a component, which can lead to nonunion of the tuberosities (Fig. 20-6). The prosthetic system that we use allows variation of the posterior and medial offset of the humeral head seen in normal anatomy. The "R" and "L" positions correspond to the average anatomic posterior and medial offset of a given head size for a right and left shoulder, respectively (Fig. 20-7). The variable offset is set to the "R" or "L" position, depending on whether surgery is being performed on the right or left shoulder. Once selected, the trial implant is attached to the prosthetic holder (Fig. 20-8).

PROSTHETIC POSITIONING WITH ANCILLARY INSTRUMENTATION— THE FRACTURE JIG TECHNIQUE

Placement of the prosthesis at the correct height and version remains one of the most difficult challenges

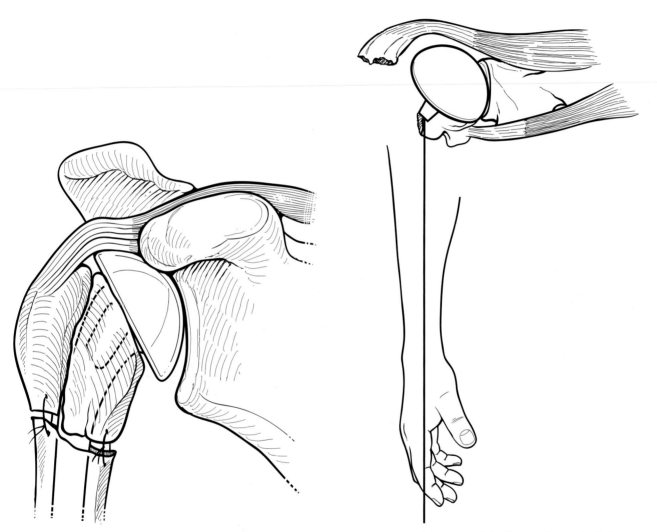

Figure 20-1 Placement of the humeral prosthesis excessively proud can result in loss of greater tuberosity fixation.

Figure 20-2 Placement of the humeral prosthesis in excessive retroversion can result in loss of greater tuberosity fixation.

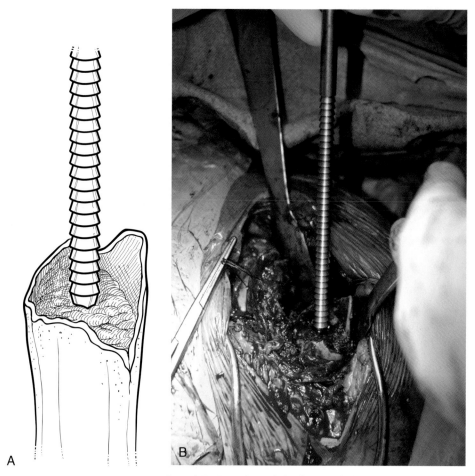

Figure 20-3   **A** and **B,** Reaming of the humeral shaft.

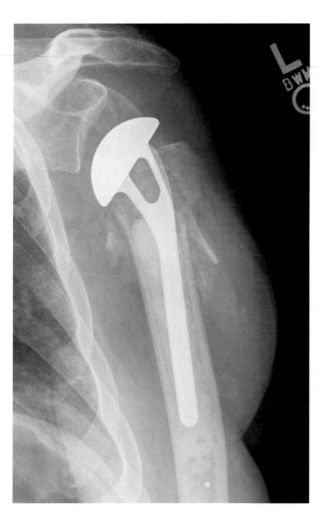

Figure 20-4 Radiograph of a humeral implant placed in valgus. Use of a larger-diameter implant would potentially have avoided this problem.

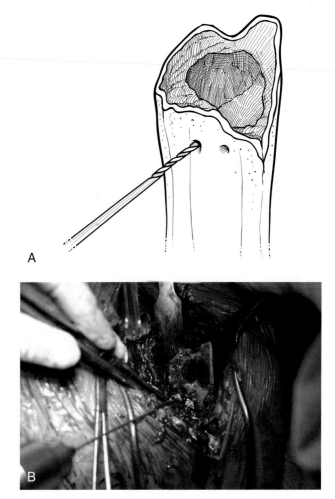

Figure 20-5 **A** and **B,** Holes are drilled on each side of the bicipital groove in the humeral shaft for later fixation of the tuberosities.

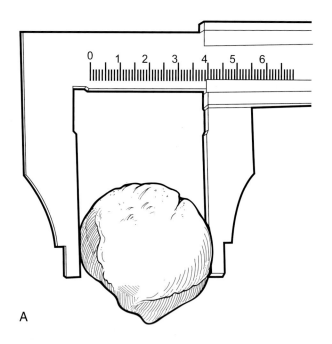

A

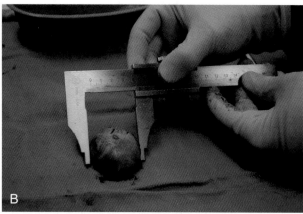

B

Figure 20-6 **A** and **B,** Selection of the appropriate humeral head prosthetic diameter. The lesser diameter from the native humeral head is selected.

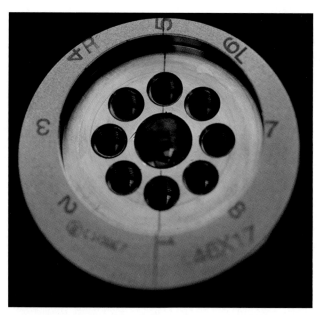

Figure 20-7 "R" and "L" positions on the prosthetic humeral head correspond to the average anatomic posterior and medial offset of a given head size for a right and left shoulder, respectively.

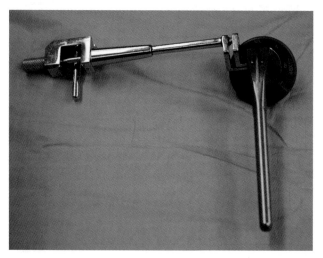

Figure 20-8 Trial implant attached to the prosthetic holder.

when performing shoulder arthroplasty for fracture. Use of ancillary instrumentation enhances the surgeon's ability to place the prosthesis at the correct height and in the correct amount of retroversion. The fracture jig references the humeral epicondyles to allow intraoperative estimation of proper prosthetic height and retroversion. More importantly, the fracture jig permits trial reduction of the glenohumeral joint and reduction of the tuberosities before final cementation of the humeral implant, thereby allowing adjustment of prosthetic position.

Selection of appropriate humeral height is initiated preoperatively by evaluating the length of the uninjured humerus from the superior aspect of the greater tuberosity to the transepicondylar axis radiographi-

cally, as described in Chapter 18. This measurement provides an estimated height at which to set the fracture jig during the procedure (Fig. 20-9). Appropriate humeral retroversion is provided by the protractor component of the fracture jig and is usually between 20 and 30 degrees relative to the transepicondylar humeral axis (Fig. 20-10).

After diaphyseal preparation is complete, the fracture jig is applied. The arm and forearm component is

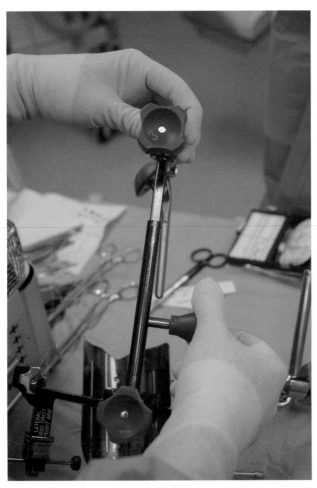

Figure 20-9 Adjustment of humeral prosthetic height with the fracture jig.

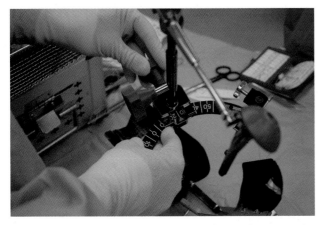

Figure 20-10 Adjustment of humeral prosthetic version with the fracture jig.

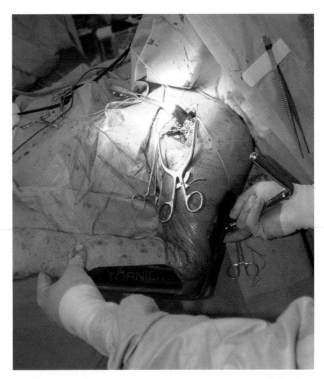

Figure 20-11 The arm and forearm component of the fracture jig is applied to the patient's upper extremity.

secured to the patient with a disposable elastic bandage while taking care to ensure that the patient's extremity is well seated in the device (Fig. 20-11). The selected trial stem is connected to the remainder of the fracture jig. The fracture jig's height is initially based on preoperative radiographs of the contralateral humerus, and the retroversion is set at 25 degrees. The trial stem is placed in the humeral shaft, and the two portions of the fracture jig (the portion attached to the stem and the portion attached to the patient) are linked but not tightened (Fig. 20-12). The glenohumeral joint is reduced, and the surgeon positions the epicondylar pads of the fracture jig over the medial and lateral humeral epicondyles (Fig. 20-13). When the surgeon is satisfied with the position of the fracture jig, an assistant tightens the linking bar to secure the position of the prosthesis (Fig. 20-14).

After the linking bar of the fracture jig has been tightened, minor adjustments can be made in prosthetic position based on intraoperative observations. Measurements made from preoperative radiographs provide guidelines but should not be followed blindly. Although theoretically the preoperative measurements should be very accurate, anatomic factors such as soft tissue interposed between the fracture jig and osseous reference points introduce some inaccuracies. The preoperatively measured height provides a starting point

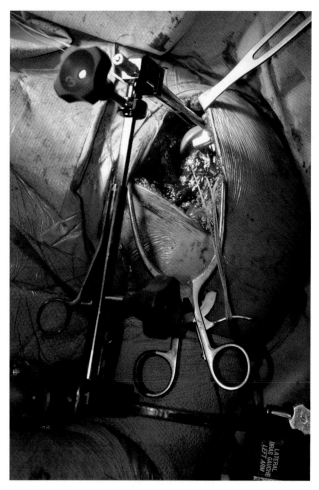

Figure 20-12 The trial stem is placed in the humeral shaft and the two portions of the fracture jig are linked but not tightened.

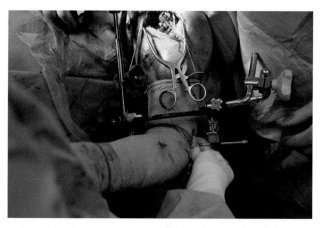

Figure 20-13 The surgeon positions the epicondylar pads of the fracture jig over the medial and lateral humeral epicondyles.

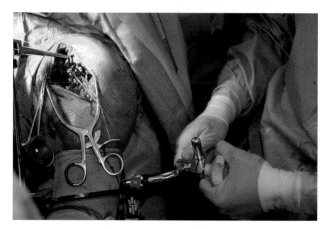

Figure 20-14 An assistant tightens the linking bar to secure the position of the prosthesis.

for establishing prosthetic positioning but must usually be adjusted in accordance with intraoperative observations. Helpful anatomic landmarks for establishing correct prosthetic height are the superior medial aspect of the humeral shaft and the inferior medial aspect of the humeral head fracture fragment. The amount of nonarticular surface attached to the inferior medial aspect of the humeral head fragment can be noted and a similar gap left between the inferior aspect of the humeral head component and the superior medial aspect of the native humeral shaft (Fig. 20-15). Also helpful is reduction of the greater and lesser tuberosities around the trial prosthesis to judge prosthetic height. The tuberosities should be readily reducible to the humeral diaphysis (Fig. 20-16). Adjustment of the height setting on the fracture jig is based on these observations. We have attempted to use intraoperative fluoroscopy with this technique; however, the abun-

dance of metallic artifact introduced by the fracture jig prohibits reproducible use of image-assisted prosthetic positioning (Fig. 20-17).

Prosthetic version is judged and adjusted so that it matches the trial reduction of the glenohumeral joint. With the arm in neutral rotation, the prosthetic humeral head should be directed into the center of the glenoid. Adjustment of the protractor component of the fracture jig allows the introduction of more or less humeral retroversion based on these observations. Once the surgeon is satisfied with the position of the trial implant, the trial implant and prosthetic holding arm are removed while the rest of the fracture jig is left in place. The actual humeral implant is attached to the prosthetic holding arm in preparation for implantation.

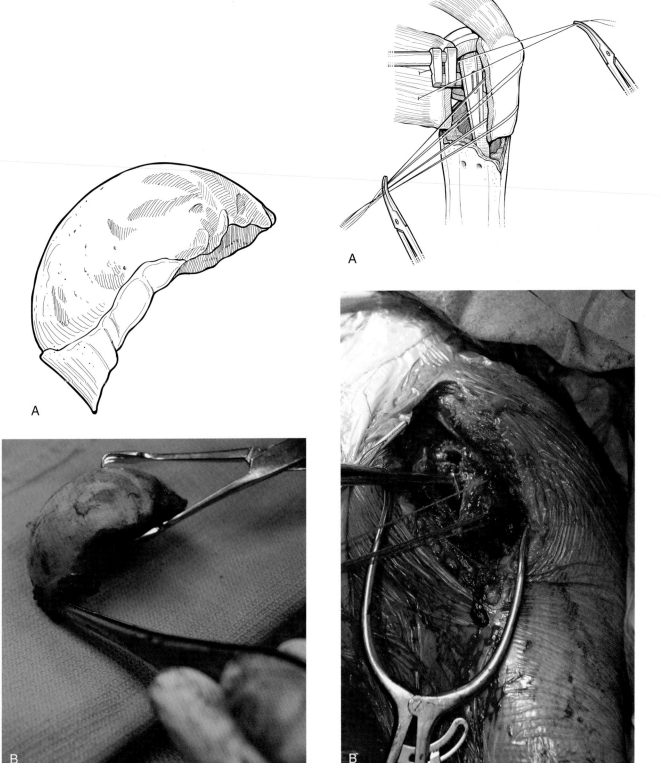

Figure 20-15   **A** and **B,** The amount of nonarticular surface attached to the inferior medial aspect of the humeral head fragment can be noted and a similar gap left between the inferior aspect of the humeral head component and the superior medial aspect of the native humeral shaft.

Figure 20-16   **A** and **B,** Trial reduction of the greater and lesser tuberosities.

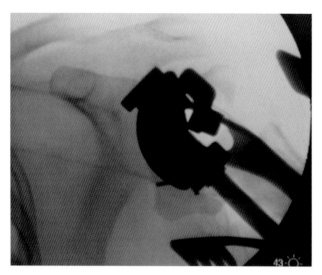

Figure 20-17   Fluoroscopic evaluation of the position of the humeral implant with the fracture jig in place. The abundance of metallic artifact created by the fracture jig limits the usefulness of fluoroscopy when using the fracture jig.

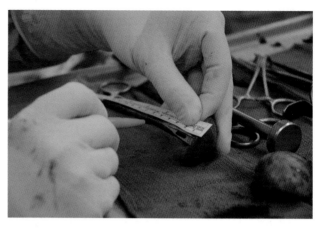

Figure 20-18   When using the Gothic arch technique, the position on the humeral trial implant that should correspond to the position of the medial aspect of the fracture is marked.

PROSTHETIC POSITIONING WITHOUT ANCILLARY INSTRUMENTATION— THE GOTHIC ARCH TECHNIQUE

An alternative to the fracture jig technique is the Gothic arch technique.[3] In this technique, prosthetic height is based on preoperative planning, as described in Chapter 18. With these calculations the position on the humeral trial implant that should correspond to the position of the medial aspect of the fracture is marked (Fig. 20-18). The trial humeral implant is placed in the humeral canal at the desired height with the prosthetic holder. Humeral retroversion is set between 20 and 30 degrees by judging the angle formed by the prosthetic holder and the forearm (Fig. 20-19). The glenohumeral joint is reduced while the trial implant is held at the desired height and version with the prosthetic holder. The humeral head should be directed into the center of the glenoid fossa with the arm held in neutral rotation. Once proper version is determined, an electrocautery is used to mark the position of the prosthetic fin on the humeral diaphysis (Fig. 20-20). An assistant can reduce the tuberosities around the trial implant, thereby further confirming appropriate prosthetic position (Fig. 20-21). Finally, intraoperative fluoroscopy can be used to help confirm appropriate prosthetic position. Because the plastic trial humeral head is radiolucent, we use the actual humeral implant when judging prosthetic position with fluoroscopy (Fig. 20-22). Once prosthetic position is found acceptable, the implant is removed, the appro-

priate height is marked on the implant, and the humeral implant is attached to the prosthetic holder (Fig. 20-23).

IMPLANTATION OF THE HUMERAL COMPONENT

A cement restrictor is placed in the humeral canal to create a 1-cm distal cement mantle (Fig. 20-24). Two strands of no. 2 nonabsorbable braided suture are passed in an outside-to-inside direction through one of the holes previously drilled in the humeral shaft adjacent to the bicipital groove. These sutures are then passed from inside to outside though the other hole previously drilled in the humeral shaft adjacent to the bicipital groove (Fig. 20-25). The humeral canal is irrigated and dried thoroughly. Bone cement (we prefer to use DePuy 2 bone cement [DePuy, Inc., Warsaw, IN] because of its accelerated curing time of less than 8 minutes) is mixed and introduced into the humeral shaft with a catheter tip syringe.

With the fracture jig technique, the humeral implant attached to the prosthetic holding arm is inserted into the humeral shaft, and the prosthetic holding arm is attached to the fracture jig. The glenohumeral joint is reduced and a trial reduction of the tuberosities is performed to ensure that prosthetic position is acceptable (Fig. 20-26). Minor adjustments can be made in prosthetic position with the fracture jig if necessary.

In the Gothic arch technique, the humeral implant attached to the prosthetic holder is introduced into the humeral shaft to the appropriate level marked on

Text continued on p. 197

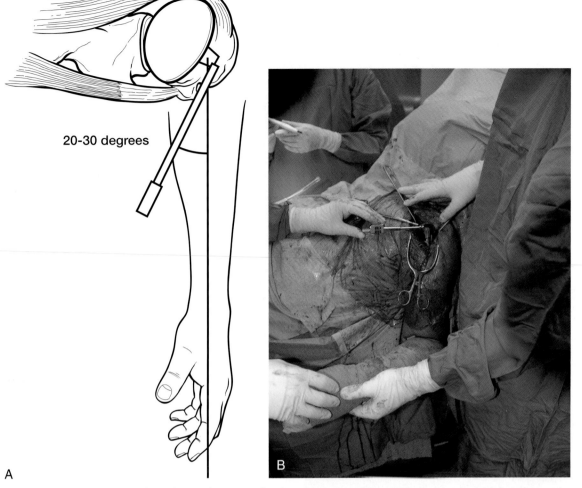

Figure 20-19 **A** and **B,** Humeral retroversion is set between 20 and 30 degrees by judging the angle formed by the prosthetic holder and the forearm.

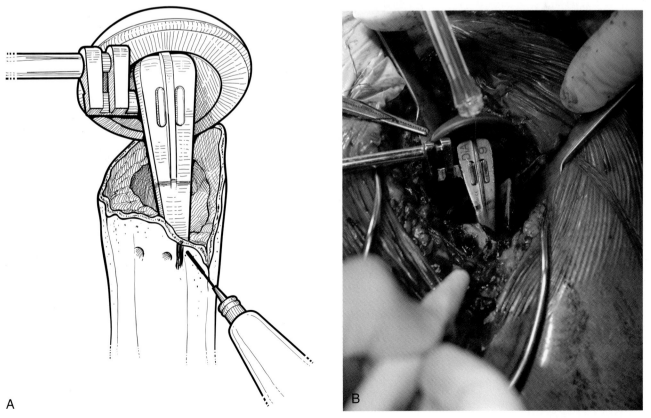

Figure 20-20 **A** and **B,** Once proper version is determined, the diaphysis is marked with an electrocautery.

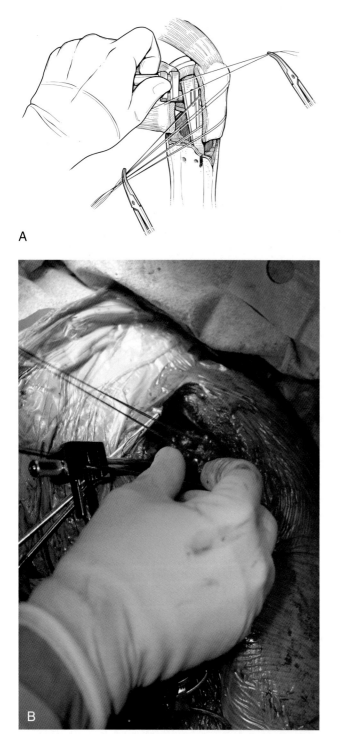

Figure 20-21   **A** and **B,** Trial reduction of the tuberosities by an assistant while the trial prosthesis is held with the prosthesis holder by the surgeon.

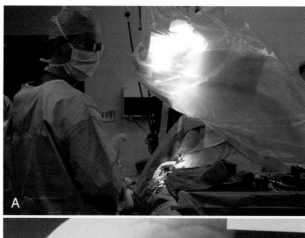

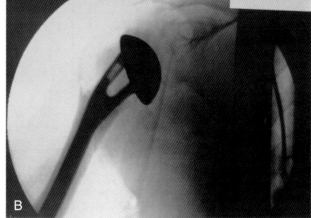

Figure 20-22   **A** and **B,** Evaluation of humeral trial position via intraoperative fluoroscopy.

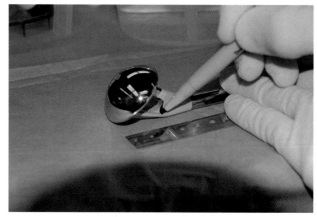

Figure 20-23   The final humeral implant is marked at the level that should correspond to the medial fracture line.

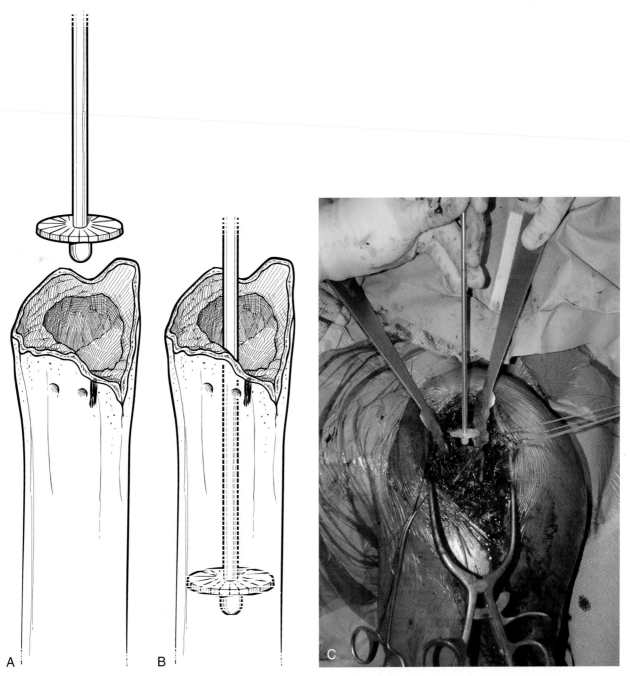

Figure 20-24   A to **C,** Placement of a diaphyseal cement restrictor to create a 1-cm distal cement mantle.

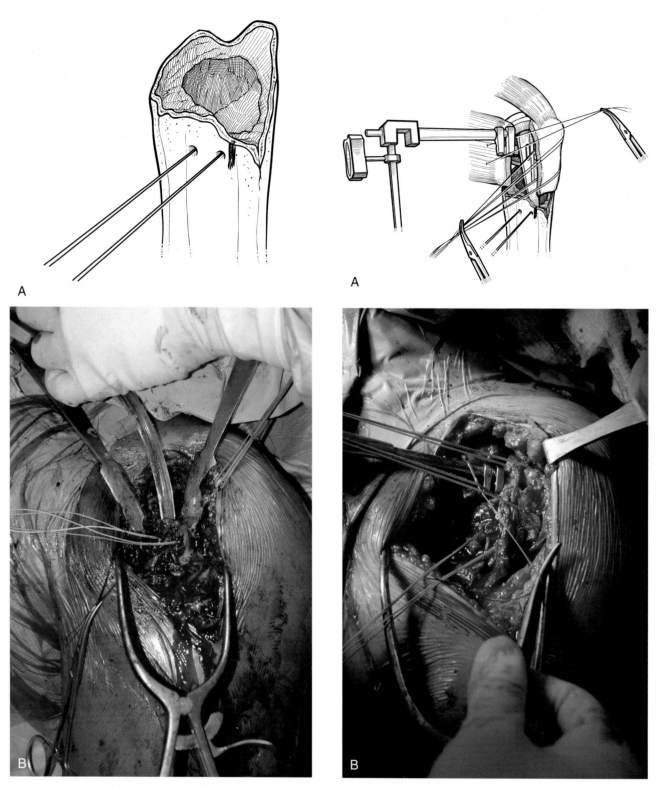

Figure 20-25   A and **B,** Two strands of no. 2 nonabsorbable braided suture are passed in an outside-to-inside direction through one of the holes previously drilled in the humeral shaft adjacent to the bicipital groove. These sutures are then passed from inside to outside through the other hole previously drilled in the humeral shaft adjacent to the bicipital groove.

Figure 20-26   A and **B,** Reduction of the glenohumeral joint with a trial reduction of the greater and lesser tuberosities via the fracture jig technique.

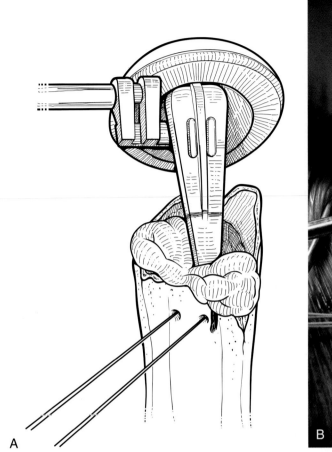
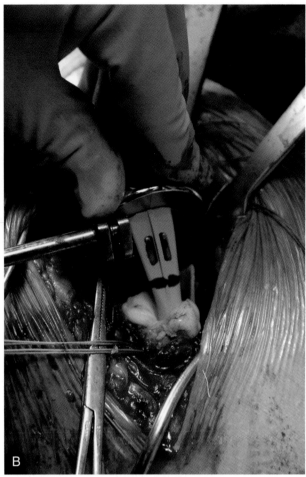

Figure 20-27   **A** and **B,** Implantation of the humeral prosthesis at the appropriate height via the Gothic arch technique.

the implant and at the version marked on the humeral diaphysis (Fig. 20-27). The position of the prosthesis is continually checked to ensure that no movement occurs as the cement cures.

All excess cement is removed with special attention to removing cement in the fenestration of the prosthesis and at the diaphyseal fracture site. Once the appropriate prosthetic position is confirmed and excess cement has been removed, the cement is allowed to fully cure, thus completing insertion of the humeral component.

REFERENCES

1. Boileau P, Coste JS, Ahrens PM, Staccini P: Prosthetic shoulder replacement for fracture: Results of the multi-centre study. In Walch G, Boileau P, Molé D (eds): 2000 Prothèses d'Epaule . . . Recul de 2 à 10 Ans. Paris, Sauramps Medical, 2001, pp 561-578.
2. Dines D, Hersch J: Long head of the biceps lesions after shoulder arthroplasty. Paper presented at the 8th International Congress on Surgery of the Shoulder, April 2001, Cape Town, South Africa.
3. Krishnan SG, Pennington SD, Burkhead WZ, Boileau P: Shoulder arthroplasty for fracture: Restoration of the "gothic arch." Tech Shoulder Elbow Surg 2005;6:57-66.

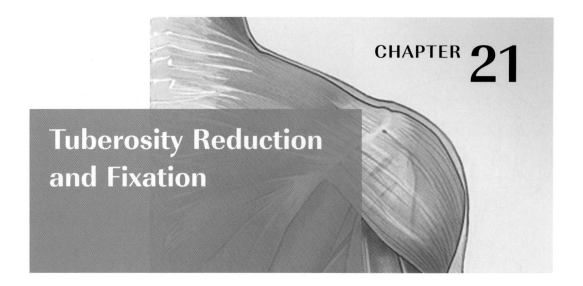

CHAPTER 21

Tuberosity Reduction and Fixation

Greater and lesser tuberosity complications are primary obstacles to achieving a satisfactory result after unconstrained arthroplasty for the treatment of proximal humeral fractures.[1] Tuberosity malunion and nonunion are situations to be avoided. The first step in avoiding these complications is placement of the tuberosities at their correct anatomic location through proper preoperative planning and accurate humeral prosthetic positioning (Chapters 18 and 20). The second step in avoiding these complications is through tuberosity fixation. Tuberosity fixation consists of two major components: use of a reliable and reproducible suture fixation technique to provide initial fracture stability, and use of bone graft to assist in tuberosity healing and provide long-term fracture stability. This chapter details our preferred tuberosity fixation technique and the use of bone graft to enhance tuberosity position and healing.

PREPARATION OF BONE GRAFT

Autogenous bone graft is taken from the humeral head fragment and serves two purposes. First, the bone graft enhances healing between the greater and lesser tuberosities and between the tuberosities and the humeral diaphysis. Second, because the greater tuberosity fragment is often no more than a thin shell of bone, the bone graft acts to position the greater tuberosity laterally in a more anatomic position.

A specially designed bone graft cutter is used to harvest bone graft plugs from the humeral head fragment. The thumbscrew of the bone graft cutter is completely recessed, and the cutting edge is advanced through the humeral head from cancellous surface to articular surface with a mallet (Figs. 21-1 and 21-2). After the cutting edge of the bone graft cutter has been advanced completely through the humeral head, the remaining humeral head is removed from the cutter and preserved. The thumbscrew of the bone graft cutter is advanced slightly to extrude just the portion of the bone graft plug covered with articular cartilage (Fig. 21-3). The articular cartilage is removed from the bone graft plug with a large biting rongeur (Fig. 21-4). The bone graft plug is then fully extruded from the bone graft cutter (Fig. 21-5). This process is repeated for a second bone graft plug.

The remaining cancellous bone in the humeral head fragment is removed with a large biting rongeur and morselized (Fig. 21-6). Care is taken to not include articular cartilage in the morselized bone graft. One of the bone graft plugs is gently impacted into the fenestration of the humeral prosthesis that had previously been cemented into place, as described in Chapter 20 (Fig. 21-7).

TECHNIQUE FOR REDUCTION AND FIXATION OF THE TUBEROSITIES

Fixation of the tuberosities is achieved with a reproducible suture fixation technique consisting of four horizontal cerclage sutures (two around the greater tuberosity and two around the greater and lesser tuberosities) and two vertical cerclage sutures (Fig. 21-8). The sutures to be used for horizontal cerclage were previously placed when control of the greater tuberosity was initially achieved (Chapter 19) and consist of two strands of no. 2 braided permanent suture placed through the rotator cuff at the junction of the supra-

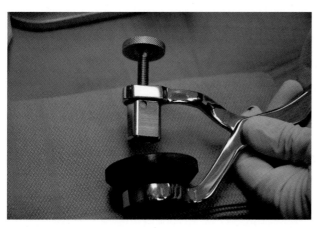

Figure 21-1 Bone graft cutter with the thumbscrew completely recessed.

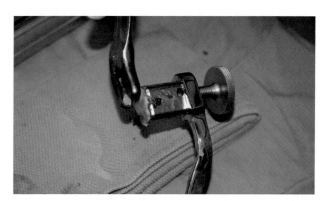

Figure 21-4 The articular cartilage is removed from the bone graft plug with a large biting rongeur.

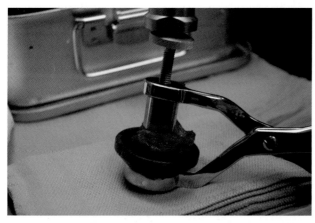

Figure 21-2 Advancing the bone graft cutter through the humeral head.

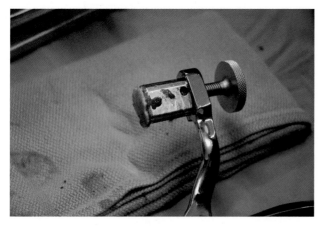

Figure 21-5 Bone graft plug harvested with the bone graft cutter.

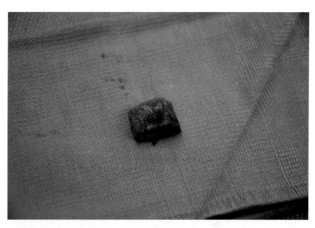

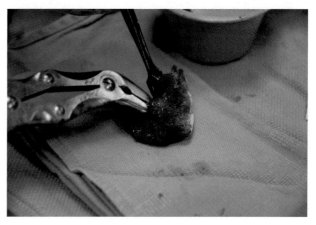

Figure 21-3 The thumbscrew of the bone graft cutter is advanced slightly to extrude just the portion of the bone graft plug covered with articular cartilage.

Figure 21-6 Removal of any remaining cancellous bone from the humeral head fragment.

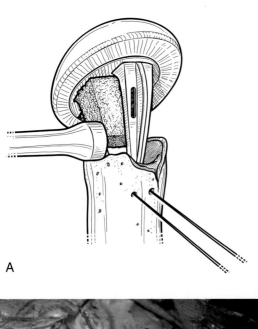

A

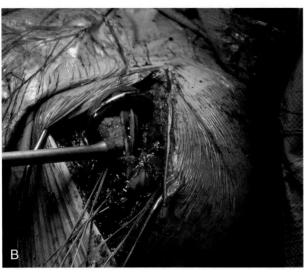

B

Figure 21-7   A and **B,** Placement of the first bone graft plug into the fenestration of the humeral prosthesis.

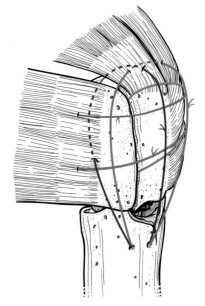

Figure 21-8   Overview of the suture fixation technique used for the greater and lesser tuberosities.

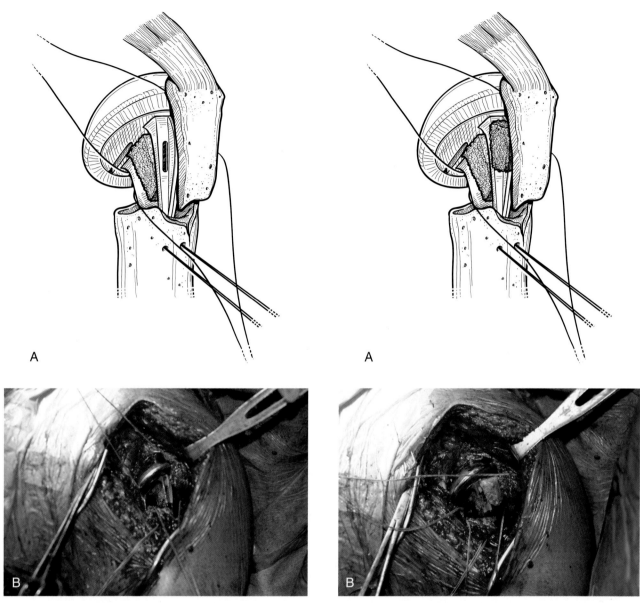

Figure 21-9 **A** and **B,** The sutures controlling the greater tuberosity are passed around the smooth polished medial aspect of the prosthetic neck.

Figure 21-10 **A** and **B,** A bone graft plug is placed lateral to the neck of the prosthesis to accommodate for bone loss in the greater tuberosity and place the greater tuberosity in a more anatomic lateral position.

spinatus and infraspinatus and two strands of no. 2 braided permanent suture placed through the rotator cuff at the junction of the infraspinatus and teres minor. The vertical cerclage sutures consist of the two strands of no. 2 nonabsorbable braided suture placed in the humeral diaphysis before humeral implant cementation, as described in Chapter 20.

The sutures controlling the greater tuberosity are passed around the smooth polished medial aspect of the prosthetic neck (Fig. 21-9). The second of the two bone graft plugs is placed lateral to the neck of the prosthesis to accommodate for bone loss in the greater tuberosity and to place the greater tuberosity in a more anatomic lateral position (Fig. 21-10). The morselized

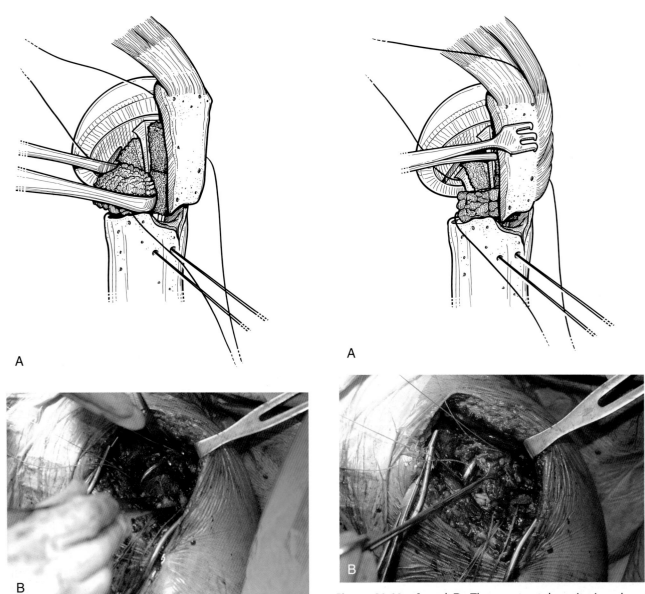

A

B

Figure 21-11 **A** and **B,** Morselized bone graft is placed along the diaphyseal fracture line to promote healing of the greater and lesser tuberosities to the humeral shaft.

A

B

Figure 21-12 **A** and **B,** The greater tuberosity is reduced into position lateral to the second bone graft plug with Lahey forceps.

bone graft is placed along the diaphyseal fracture line to promote healing of the greater and lesser tuberosities to the humeral shaft (Fig. 21-11). The greater tuberosity is gently grasped with Lahey forceps and reduced into position lateral to the second bone graft plug (Fig. 21-12). Two of the sutures controlling the greater tuberosity, one superior and one inferior, are tied to fixate the greater tuberosity (Fig. 21-13). The remaining two sutures, one superior and one inferior, are passed through the subscapularis tendon just

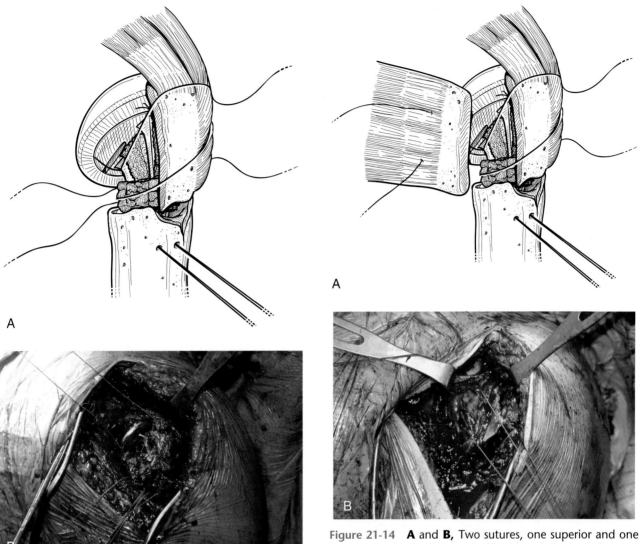

Figure 21-13 **A** and **B,** Two of the sutures controlling the greater tuberosity, one superior and one inferior, are tied to fixate the greater tuberosity.

Figure 21-14 **A** and **B,** Two sutures, one superior and one inferior, are passed through the subscapularis tendon just medial to its osseous insertion on the lesser tuberosity.

medial to its osseous insertion on the lesser tuberosity (Fig. 21-14). The lesser tuberosity is reduced with the previously placed stay sutures, and the circumferential sutures are tied to secure the tuberosity (Fig. 21-15). Tuberosity fixation is completed with the two sutures previously placed through drill holes in the humeral diaphysis. One suture is passed through the subscapularis and supraspinatus tendons just medial to their

osseous insertion and then tied (Fig. 21-16). The second suture is passed through the infraspinatus and supraspinatus tendons just medial to their osseous insertion and then tied (Fig. 21-17). Security of the tuberosities must be evaluated by checking the mobility of the shoulder after tuberosity repair. The tuberosities and prosthetic humeral head implant should move as one unit.

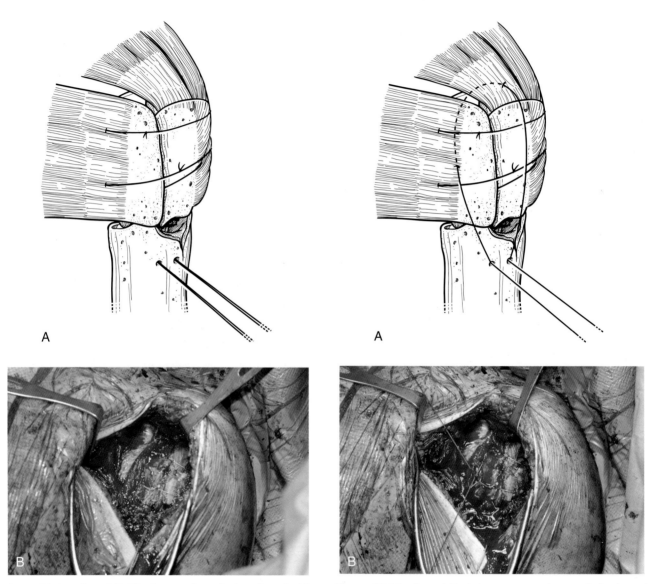

A

A

B

B

Figure 21-15   **A** and **B,** The lesser tuberosity is reduced with the previously placed stay sutures, and the circumferential sutures are tied to secure the tuberosity.

Figure 21-16   **A** and **B,** A transosseous humeral diaphyseal suture is passed through the subscapularis and supraspinatus tendons just medial to their osseous insertion and then tied.

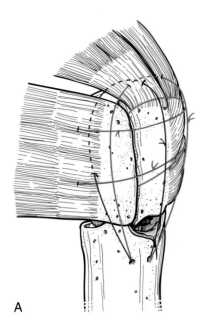

A

REFERENCE

1. Boileau P, Coste JS, Ahrens PM, Staccini P: Prosthetic shoulder replacement for fracture: Results of the multicentre study. In Walch G, Boileau P, Molé D (eds): 2000 Prosthèses d'Epaule . . . Recul de 2 à 10 Ans. Paris, Sauramps Medical, 2001, pp 561-578.

B

Figure 21-17 A and **B,** A second transosseous humeral diaphyseal suture is passed through the infraspinatus and supraspinatus tendons just medial to their osseous insertion and then tied.

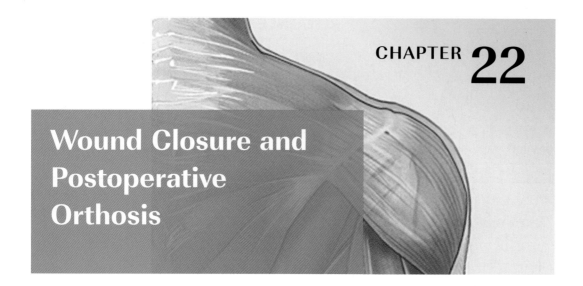

Wound Closure and Postoperative Orthosis

The final steps of the operative procedure are wound closure and placement of the postoperative orthosis. The major difference from patients undergoing unconstrained shoulder arthroplasty performed for chronic disease is the type of postoperative orthosis used.

TECHNIQUE FOR WOUND CLOSURE

After fixation of the tuberosities, the wound is irrigated with 800 mL of antibiotic-impregnated sterile saline (50,000 units bacitracin per liter sterile normal saline) via a bulb syringe. The wound is checked to ensure that adequate hemostasis has been achieved. An electrocautery is used as necessary to minimize any residual hemorrhage. A drain is not routinely used. However, some patients, particularly those with a history of anticoagulant therapy, may have substantial bleeding from fractured bone surfaces. In this circumstance we consider the use of a medium closed wound suction drain (Bard, Inc., Covington, GA) for 24 hours after surgery (Fig. 22-1). The drain is placed deep to the deltopectoral interval with the trocar provided and exits the skin approximately 3 cm distal to the terminal extent of the skin incision (Fig. 22-2). The proximal extent of the drain tubing is trimmed with heavy scissors to allow the proximal tip of the drain to reach the superior aspect of the humerus (Fig. 22-3). Care is taken to not cut the drain tubing through a side portal because this risks fracture of the drain during removal (Fig. 22-4). Uncut half-inch Steri-Strips are applied immediately to secure the drain distally to skin (Fig. 22-5).

Wound closure is performed in the same manner as described for unconstrained arthroplasty (Chapter 15). We do not close the deltopectoral interval but initiate our closure with the overlying fascial layer. This layer is reapproximated with no. 0 braided absorbable suture in an interrupted figure-of-eight technique. If a drain has been placed, care is taken to avoid passing a suture through or around the drain. Always check that the drain slides freely after sutures are placed in the fascia. The subcutaneous fascia is reapproximated with 2-0 braided absorbable suture via an interrupted figure-of-eight technique. The skin is reapproximated with 3-0 undyed absorbable monofilament suture in a subcuticular running closure.

The occlusive draping is removed adjacent to the incision, and the skin is cleansed of blood with a saline-soaked sponge and then dried. Half-inch Steri-Strips are placed over the incision. Sterile gauze is placed over the incision and a sterile absorbent pad is placed over the gauze. The dressing is secured with 3-inch foam tape. The remaining surgical drapes are then removed.

The dressing is maintained in place until postoperative day 3, at which time it is removed. If a drain has been used, the distal extent of the dressing is loosened to allow drain removal with removal of the drain Steri-Strips the morning after surgery. After removal of the dressing on postoperative day 3, the patient is allowed to shower, but submerging the incision in a bathtub is prohibited until 2 weeks postoperatively. The Steri-Strips are progressively removed by the patient as they lose their adhesion to the skin.

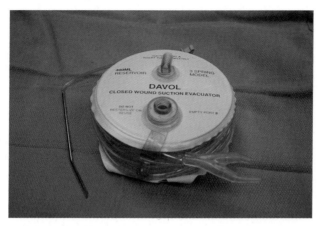

Figure 22-1 The type of medium suction drain used in select fracture cases.

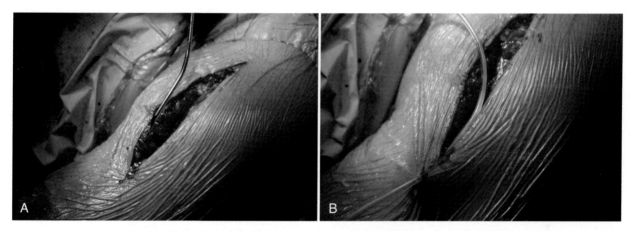

Figure 22-2 **A** and **B,** Placement of the drain with the trocar provided.

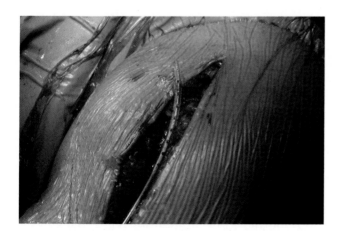

Figure 22-3 Proximal extent of the drain.

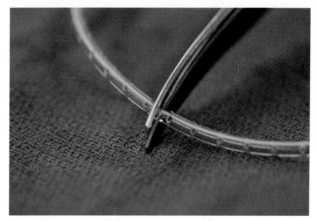

Figure 22-4 Care is taken to not cut the drain tubing through a side portal because this risks fracture of the drain during removal.

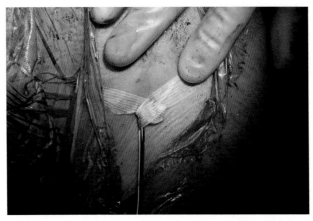

Figure 22-5   Uncut half-inch Steri-Strips are used immediately to secure the drain distally to the skin.

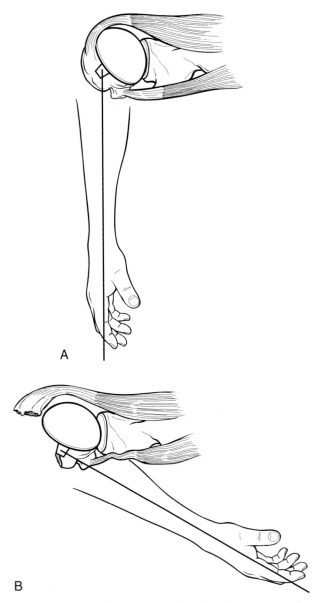

Figure 22-7   A and **B,** Tension placed on the greater tuberosity repair when positioning the arm in internal rotation.

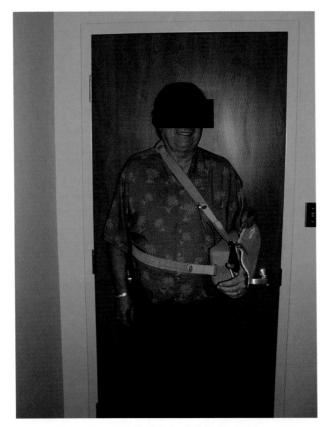

Figure 22-6   Neutral rotation sling used after shoulder arthroplasty for fracture.

POSTOPERATIVE ORTHOSIS

The postoperative orthosis is placed immediately after the dressing in the operating room and consists of a neutral-rotation sling (Fig. 22-6). This sling avoids internal rotation, a situation that places increased tension on the greater tuberosity fixation (Fig. 22-7). The sling is maintained for 4 to 6 weeks to protect the tuberosity repair. In patients with good bone quality and secure tuberosity fixation, the sling is discontinued at 4 weeks. In patients with poor bone quality or less secure tuberosity fixation (or both), the sling is maintained until 6 weeks postoperatively. Patients are allowed to remove the sling only for hygiene and rehabilitation exercises. Patients are discouraged from internally rotating or adducting the arm before the postoperative orthosis has been discontinued because of the potential for tuberosity migration.

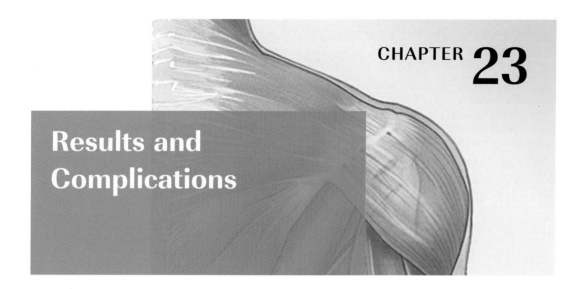

CHAPTER 23

Results and Complications

The results of unconstrained shoulder arthroplasty for fracture have been reported by multiple investigators. The overall results have been very disappointing and are not comparable to those obtained for chronic conditions such as primary osteoarthritis. The advances in unconstrained arthroplasty implants and techniques for fracture described in this section have greatly improved the results. To our knowledge, the largest reported database of results of unconstrained shoulder arthroplasty for fracture was presented in Nice, France, in 2001.[1] Because of the large number of patients enrolled, this multicenter study has allowed meaningful conclusions to be made about the outcomes and complications of unconstrained shoulder arthroplasty for the treatment of fracture. Our results have largely mirrored those reported in the Nice study. This chapter reports the results of unconstrained shoulder arthroplasty for the treatment of proximal humerus fractures by drawing from information in the Nice database and our arthroplasty database that was prospectively established in 2003. Additionally, the most frequent complications and their treatment are outlined.

RESULTS

The results of unconstrained shoulder arthroplasty for fracture are largely related to two prognostic factors: age and the presence of tuberosity complications (nonunion, malunion). These two factors are related in that older patients are more likely to have osteopenia of the tuberosities and hence complications with tuberosity healing. Although age-related osteopenia is beyond the surgeon's control, advances in prosthetic design and tuberosity fixation techniques continue to

decrease the rate of tuberosity-related complications. Table 23-1 details the results of unconstrained shoulder arthroplasty in the treatment of proximal humeral fracture.[2] This table expresses the results in terms of active mobility; patient satisfaction; the Constant score, a shoulder-specific outcomes device incorporating pain, mobility, activity, and strength; and the age- and gender-adjusted Constant score.[3,4]

INTRAOPERATIVE COMPLICATIONS

Intraoperative complications are uncommon during unconstrained shoulder arthroplasty for proximal humeral fractures and are usually related to neurovascular injury or iatrogenic humeral shaft fracture.

Neurovascular Structures

Catastrophic injury to neurovascular structures around the shoulder, though rare, are more common during performance of shoulder arthroplasty for fracture than for performance of shoulder arthroplasty for nonfracture indications. Many patients with proximal humeral fractures suffer neuropraxic injury to the axillary nerve, and this should be documented on clinical examination before surgery. Additionally, the implications of axillary nerve injury secondary to fracture should be discussed with the patient extensively before surgery. Treatment of axillary nerve injury is observation, with less than 2% of patients sustaining a permanent axillary nerve deficit.[5]

Vascular injuries during unconstrained shoulder arthroplasty performed for fracture most often involve injury to the axillary artery. Such injury is usually a

Table 23-1   RESULTS OF UNCONSTRAINED SHOULDER ARTHROPLASTY IN THE TREATMENT OF PROXIMAL HUMERAL FRACTURES

Series	Absolute Constant Score (Points) (Postoperative)	Adjusted Constant Score (%) (Postoperative)	Active Forward Flexion (Degrees) (Postoperative)	Active External Rotation (Degrees) (Postoperative)	Excellent/ Good Subjective Results (%)
Nice multicenter study (*n* = 300)[2]	54	74	103	21	39
Authors' prospective database (*n* = 21)	48	61	97	27	75

consequence of overzealous medial dissection or retraction (or both), combined with vasculature that has been compromised by aging (plaques, calcification). Should one of these injuries occur after cross-clamping of the injured structure, emergency intraoperative consultation with a vascular surgeon is required.

Humeral Shaft Fracture

Intraoperative humeral shaft fractures are very rare when performing unconstrained shoulder arthroplasty for the treatment of proximal humeral fractures. Stiffness is rarely a problem in these cases, thus minimizing the torsional stress placed on the humeral shaft during manipulation of the arm. More commonly, humeral injury occurs during reaming of the humeral shaft. The diaphyseal cortex in many elderly patients is very thin and hence has an increased risk of diaphyseal penetration. When this complication occurs, it is often unrecognized (Fig. 23-1).

POSTOPERATIVE COMPLICATIONS

Postoperative complications are much more common than intraoperative complications and occur in more than 50% of cases of unconstrained shoulder arthroplasty performed for fracture.[5] Most complications involve the greater or lesser tuberosities (or both) but also may include wound problems (dehiscence, hematoma), glenoid problems, humeral problems, instability, stiffness, and infection.

Tuberosity Complications

Nonunion and malunion of the greater and lesser tuberosities are the most common complications after

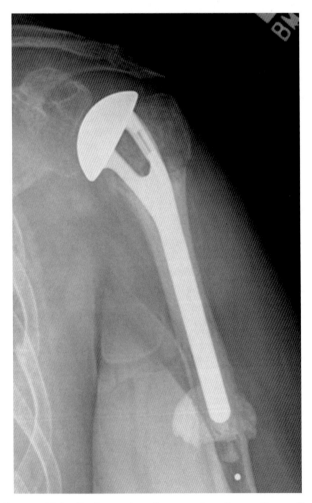

Figure 23-1 Radiograph of cement extravasation after unrecognized diaphyseal perforation during insertion of a humeral stem for a proximal humeral fracture.

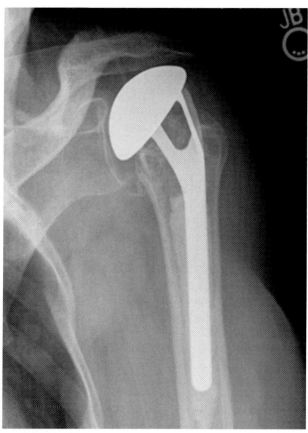

Figure 23-2 Migration of the greater tuberosity after unconstrained shoulder arthroplasty performed for a proximal humeral fracture.

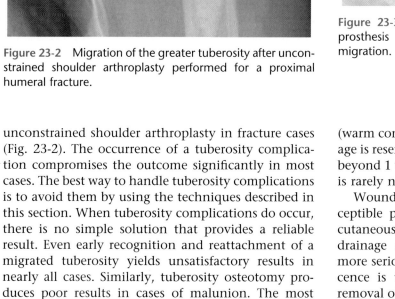

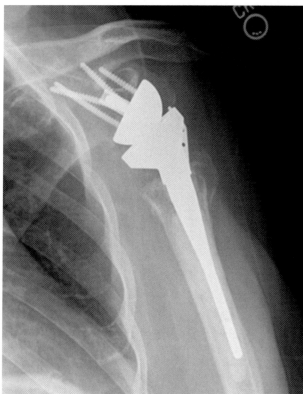

Figure 23-3 Revision of a hemiarthroplasty to a reverse prosthesis for the treatment of greater tuberosity migration.

unconstrained shoulder arthroplasty in fracture cases (Fig. 23-2). The occurrence of a tuberosity complication compromises the outcome significantly in most cases. The best way to handle tuberosity complications is to avoid them by using the techniques described in this section. When tuberosity complications do occur, there is no simple solution that provides a reliable result. Even early recognition and reattachment of a migrated tuberosity yields unsatisfactory results in nearly all cases. Similarly, tuberosity osteotomy produces poor results in cases of malunion. The most predictable results are obtained with revision arthroplasty to a reverse prosthesis in these cases (Fig. 23-3; see Section Six).

Wound Problems

Wound problems occur early after unconstrained shoulder arthroplasty for fracture. Hematoma is most easily avoided by extensive use of electrocautery during the procedure. When a hematoma occurs, it is managed by symptomatic nonoperative treatment

(warm compresses, pain medication). Operative drainage is reserved for situations in which drainage persists beyond 1 week or infection is suspected (see later) and is rarely necessary.

Wound dehiscence occurs occasionally when susceptible patients have a reaction to dissolving subcutaneous sutures. The presence of minimal serous drainage distinguishes this complication from the more serious deep infection. Superficial wound dehiscence is treated with local wound care, including removal of any residual dissolving suture material and chemical cauterization of any granulating tissue with silver nitrate applicators.

Glenoid Problems

Glenoid problems after unconstrained shoulder arthroplasty for fracture are exceedingly rare. After hemiarthroplasty for fracture, erosion of the glenoid articular cartilage and osseous glenoid can occur. Successful treatment of glenoid erosion usually requires revision surgery with resurfacing of the glenoid.

Humeral Diaphysis Problems

Humeral diaphysis problems after unconstrained shoulder arthroplasty for fracture, as in unconstrained shoulder arthroplasty for chronic conditions, are rare and consist of loosening of the humeral component or periprosthetic humeral fracture.

Aseptic loosening of the humeral stem occurs more frequently in fracture cases than in nonfracture cases, mainly because of the lack of metaphyseal support of the implant. Use of cement is always indicated in fracture cases to help prevent this potential complication. Whenever a humeral stem loosens, infection must be ruled out (see later). In the rare instance of symptomatic aseptic loosening of the humeral component, treatment is revision of the humeral stem, often with a reverse prosthesis, because this complication is generally accompanied by tuberosity nonunion (see Section Six).

Periprosthetic humeral fractures are almost always the result of a fall or similar low-energy trauma. The majority of these fractures occur just distal to the tip of the humeral stem, and most can be treated nonoperatively. Nonoperative treatment consists of fracture bracing, activity modification, pain medication, and frequent radiographic monitoring. If the fracture has not healed within 3 months, we incorporate the use of an external bone stimulator (OL 1000 Bone Growth Stimulator, Donjoy Orthopedics, Vista, CA). Despite these measures, periprosthetic humeral fractures treated nonoperatively may take longer than 9 months to heal.[6] Our criteria for recommending operative treatment of periprosthetic fractures (revision surgery; see Section Six) include complete displacement, angulation of greater than 30 degrees, loosening of the humeral component, or failure of nonoperative treatment.

Instability

Instability after unconstrained shoulder arthroplasty for fracture is usually related to tuberosity nonunion or, less commonly, prosthetic malalignment. Tuberosity nonunion may result in static migration of the humerus superiorly or anterosuperiorly, similar to the situation in a patient with rotator cuff tear arthropathy who has undergone hemiarthroplasty. In most cases, reattachment of the tuberosities does not resolve the instability, so we treat these patients by revision to a reverse-design prosthesis (Fig. 23-4; see Section Six).

Less commonly, prosthetic malposition will lead to instability despite healing of the tuberosities. The instability is caused by version malalignment (excessive retroversion causing posterior instability or excessive anteversion causing anterior instability) or by the humeral stem's being implanted at an improper level with the humeral shaft (Fig. 23-5). In this scenario, revision of the humeral stem to change prosthetic position is necessary (see Section Six). If the prosthetic malalignment has resulted in wear of the glenoid cartilage, resurfacing of the glenoid should be considered as well.

Stiffness

Glenohumeral stiffness is a common complication after unconstrained shoulder arthroplasty for fracture and is related to capsular contracture or the prosthesis (or both). Prosthetic problems resulting in stiffness are almost always the result of implantation of too large a humeral component or placement of the humeral component in the wrong position, as described earlier. Rehabilitation with capsular stretching can be attempted in an effort to improve mobility. If rehabilitation fails (no improvement over a 6-month period), revision surgery is indicated, consisting of realignment of the humeral component or downsizing of the humeral head with open release of any capsular contractures that are present.

Stiffness related to capsular contracture almost always responds to nonoperative management with aquatic-based rehabilitation (see Chapter 43). If the patient shows no improvement in mobility over a 6-month course of rehabilitation and has no obvious prosthetic problem, we consider the patient a candidate for arthroscopic capsular contracture release.

Infection

Infection after shoulder arthroplasty for fracture is rare, though more common than with other indications for primary arthroplasty. Patients most at risk for infection are those with systemic illness (diabetes mellitus) and those with compromised soft tissues (open fractures). These infections are most commonly caused by *Staphylococcus aureus* or *Propionibacterium acnes*. Infections after shoulder arthroplasty can be divided into perioperative (within 6 weeks of surgery) and late (hematogenous) infections.

Early perioperative infections are initially treated with multiple (two or three) irrigation and débridement procedures and retention of the humeral component if the tuberosity repair remains intact. At the last planned irrigation and débridement procedure, absorbable antibiotic-impregnated beads (Stimulan, Biocomposites, Inc., Staffordshire, England) are placed in the soft tissues around the shoulder. Consultation with an infectious disease specialist is obtained, and a

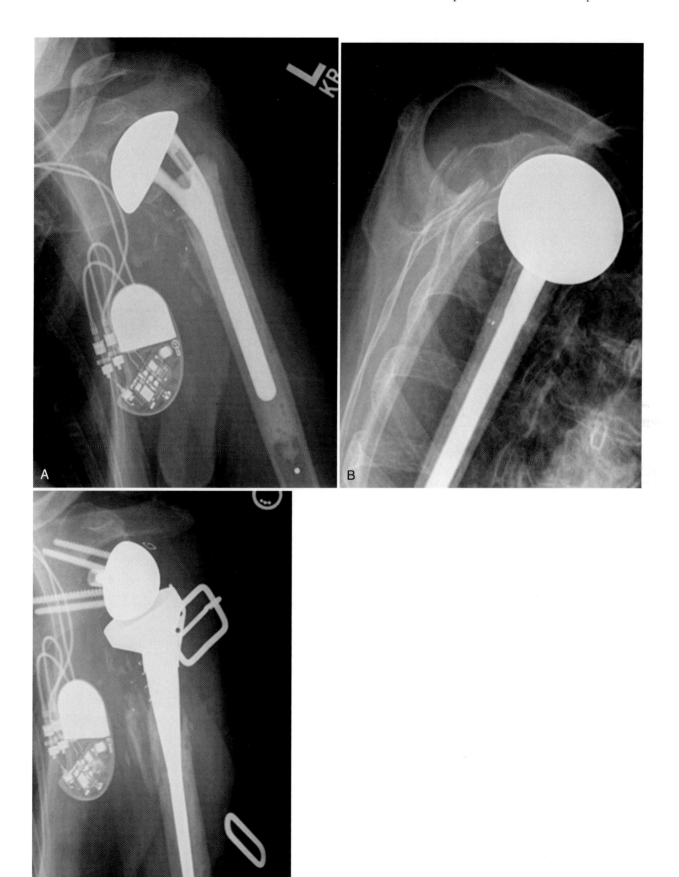

Figure 23-4 A to **C,** Anterosuperior instability of a hemiarthroplasty used in the treatment of a proximal humeral fracture necessitated revision with a reverse prosthesis.

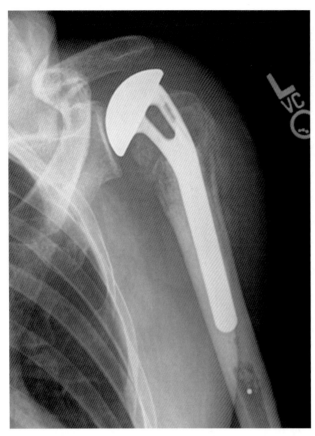

Figure 23-5 A humeral stem implanted too proximally within the humeral shaft resulted in instability.

minimum of 6 weeks of intravenous antibiotics tailored to the specific organism causing the infection (or covering the most likely offending organisms, if cultures remain negative despite obvious infection) is usually recommended. If this regimen fails or if the tuberosity repair fails because of the infection, the humeral component is removed and the patient is treated in the same manner as for a late-appearing infection.

Late-appearing infections are treated by removal of the prosthesis and intravenous antibiotics, as detailed in Section Six. The decision whether to perform a revision shoulder arthroplasty or continue with a resection arthroplasty is patient specific.

REFERENCES

1. Walch G, Boileau P: Presentation of the multicentric study. In Walch G, Boileau P, Molé D (eds): 2000 Prosthèses d'Epaule . . . Recul de 2 à 10 Ans. Paris, Sauramps Medical, 2001, pp 11-20.
2. Hubert L, Dayez J: Results of the standard Aequalis prosthesis for proximal humeral fractures: The entire series. In Walch G, Boileau P, Molé D (eds): 2000 Prosthèses d'Epaule . . . Recul de 2 à 10 Ans. Paris, Sauramps Medical, 2001, pp 527-529.
3. Constant CR, Murley AH: A clinical method of functional assessment of the shoulder. Clin Orthop Relat Res 1987;214:160-164.
4. Constant CR: Assessment of shoulder function. In Gazielly D, Gleyze P, Thomas T (eds): The Cuff. New York, Elsevier, 1997, pp 39-44.
5. Schild F, Burger B, Willems J: Complications of prostheses for fractures. In Walch G, Boileau P, Molé D (eds): 2000 Prosthèses d'Epaule . . . Recul de 2 à 10 Ans. Paris, Sauramps Medical, 2001, pp 539-544.
6. Kumar S, Sperling JW, Haidukewych GH, Cofield RH: Periprosthetic humeral fractures after shoulder arthroplasty. J Bone Joint Surg Am 2004;86:680-689.

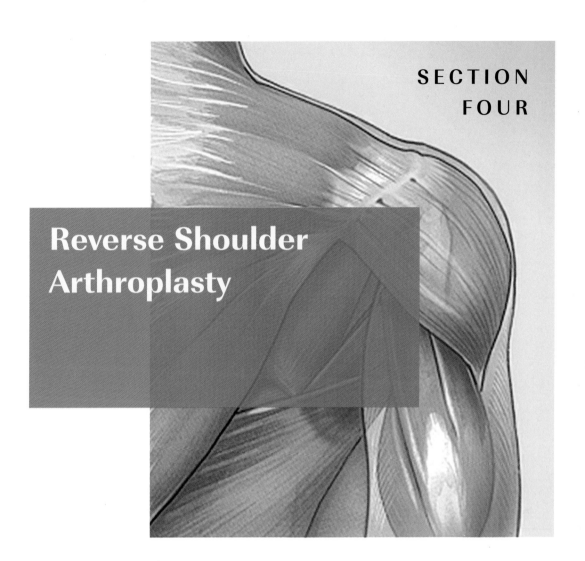

SECTION FOUR

Reverse Shoulder Arthroplasty

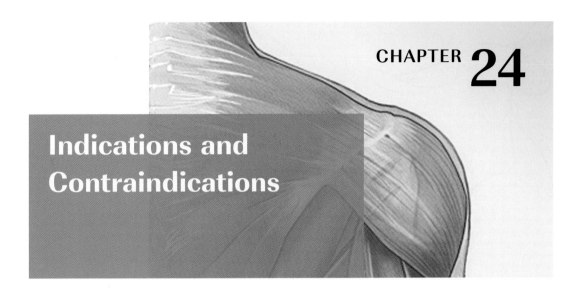

CHAPTER 24

Indications and Contraindications

Reintroduction of reverse-design shoulder arthroplasty has added a powerful device to the shoulder surgeon's armamentarium. Reverse ball-and-socket shoulder prostheses were initially introduced in the 1960s to treat patients with glenohumeral arthritis and massive rotator cuff tears. The concept of these and subsequent devices is to resolve upward migration of the humeral head and thereby restore the normal deltoid moment arm. This allows the deltoid to power active elevation of the arm (Fig. 24-1). The problem with the initial designs was early loosening of the glenoid caused by the action of deltoid forces on the laterally offset center of glenohumeral rotation (Fig. 24-2). These failures eventually resulted in abandonment of these early prosthetic designs.

In 1987, Paul Grammont introduced a reverse-design prosthesis that used a "glenosphere" component fixated over the scapular neck. In an effort to overcome the failures that had plagued earlier attempts, Grammont's design placed the center of glenohumeral rotation within the bone of the glenoid instead of lateral to it (Fig. 24-3).[1] Most available reverse prostheses take advantage of Grammont's ingenuity.

The reverse prosthesis was originally introduced to treat rotator cuff tear arthropathy. The reverse prosthesis resurfaces the glenohumeral joint with a total shoulder arthroplasty to treat the arthritis component and restores normal deltoid tension to allow active elevation, goals that are infrequently accomplished with conventional unconstrained hemiarthroplasty. Because the results from this implant were observed to be good and the complication rate low for this select indication, indications were expanded as experience broadened. Currently, a reverse prosthesis is considered in a patient who has severe rotator cuff dysfunction but would otherwise be a candidate for unconstrained shoulder arthroplasty. This chapter details the specific indications for which we use a reverse prosthesis as a primary shoulder arthroplasty. Another application for a reverse prosthesis is revision arthroplasty. We cover that scenario in Section Six.

ROTATOR CUFF TEAR ARTHROPATHY (GLENOHUMERAL OSTEOARTHRITIS WITH MASSIVE ROTATOR CUFF TEAR)

Rotator cuff tear arthropathy was initially described by Neer and consists of a massive irreparable rotator cuff tear combined with glenohumeral arthritis and, in the late stages, humeral head osteonecrosis.[2] This entity has gradually expanded to include all patients with massive rotator cuff tears and glenohumeral arthritis, even in the absence of humeral head osteonecrosis. Although we believe that rotator cuff tear arthropathy as described by Neer and glenohumeral osteoarthritis with a massive rotator cuff tear are two distinct entities, the clinical scenarios are sufficiently similar that we consider them together both in our practice and in this textbook.

Rotator cuff tear arthropathy (glenohumeral osteoarthritis with a massive rotator cuff tear) is the single most common indication for which we perform reverse shoulder arthroplasty. This indication

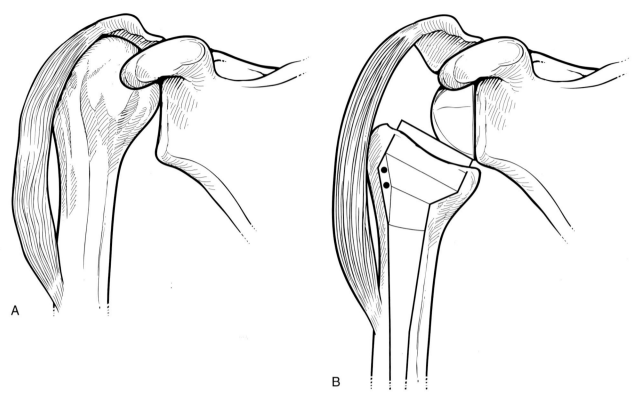

Figure 24-1 **A** and **B,** Restoration of deltoid tension with a reverse-design prosthesis.

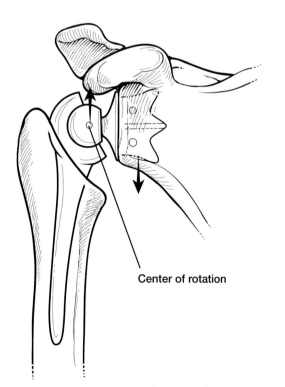

Center of rotation

Figure 24-2 Forces acting on the glenoid fixation causing loosening of early reverse prosthetic designs.

accounts for nearly half of our cases of reverse shoulder arthroplasty.

Clinical Findings

Clinical findings in patients with glenohumeral osteoarthritis and a massive rotator cuff tear are variable and depend on both the degree of arthritis and the specific tendons of the rotator cuff that are torn. Most patients demonstrate some glenohumeral crepitus with stiffness. Additionally, acromiohumeral crepitus may be present.

Testing of the individual rotator cuff tendons will typically demonstrate obvious insufficiency. Rotator cuff insufficiency may involve the posterior superior rotator cuff (supraspinatus, infraspinatus, teres minor), the anterior superior rotator cuff (supraspinatus, subscapularis), or the entire rotator cuff. Additionally, the long head of the biceps tendon is often ruptured, as demonstrated by the characteristic deformity of the upper part of the arm. Chapter 7 details clinical testing of the rotator cuff.

Imaging Findings

Plain radiography demonstrates loss of the normal glenohumeral joint space. Humeral head osteophytes

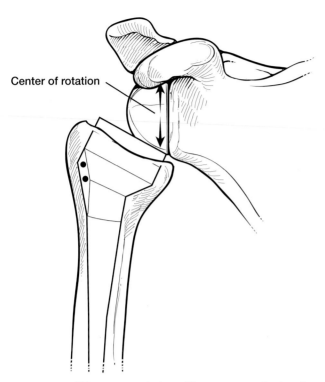

Figure 24-3 "Grammont-designed" reverse prosthesis using a medialized center of rotation to decrease the risk of loosening of the glenoid component.

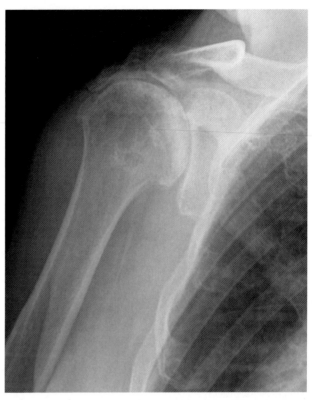

Figure 24-4 Radiograph demonstrating superior migration of the humeral head in a patient with osteoarthritis and a massive rotator cuff tear involving the posterior superior rotator cuff.

may or may not be present. Static migration of the humeral head is almost always present. In patients with insufficiency of the posterior superior rotator cuff, the humeral head migration occurs in a superior direction (Fig. 24-4). In patients with insufficiency of the anterior superior rotator cuff, static anterior migration may be apparent on just the axillary radiograph (Fig. 24-5). Less frequently, the patient may demonstrate only dynamic migration of the humeral head as a result of rotator cuff insufficiency. Acromial changes on radiographs of patients with no apparent static superior humeral head migration may show evidence of this dynamic instability (Fig. 24-6). Patients with osteoarthritis and a massive rotator cuff tear will frequently have osseous wear on the undersurface of the acromion, on the superior glenoid, or on both (Fig. 24-7). Less frequently, insufficiency fractures of the acromion may be caused by wear (Fig. 24-8). These stress fractures, however, do not contraindicate use of a reverse prosthesis.

Secondary imaging studies (computed tomographic arthrography, magnetic resonance imaging) will always show rotator cuff tears involving more than one

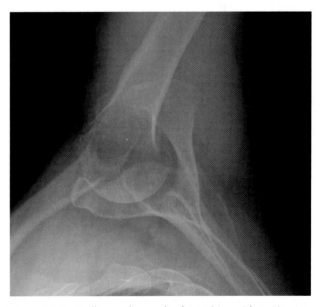

Figure 24-5 Axillary radiograph of a patient with static anterior migration of the humeral head caused by chronic anterior superior rotator cuff insufficiency.

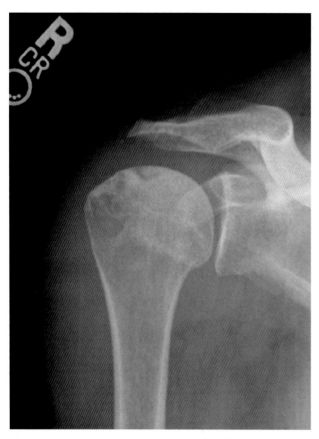

Figure 24-6 Acromial changes mirroring the radius of curvature of the humeral head in a patient with chronic rotator cuff insufficiency and only mild chronic humeral head superior migration.

tendon (Fig. 24-9). The rotator cuff muscle belly of the torn tendons shows fatty infiltration (Fig. 24-10). In cases with long-standing rotator cuff tears involving the infraspinatus in which the teres minor is intact, the teres minor muscle belly may demonstrate compensatory hypertrophy (Fig. 24-11).

Secondary imaging studies can confirm osseous wear (glenoid, acromion) in patients with glenohumeral osteoarthritis and a massive rotator cuff tear. Coronal sections of computed tomography or magnetic resonance imaging have been used to classify superior glenoid wear (Fig. 24-12).[3]

Special Considerations

We emphasize that this patient group (osteoarthritis with a massive rotator cuff tear/rotator cuff tear arthropathy) consists only of individuals with *glenohumeral* osteoarthritis and massive *irreparable* rotator cuff tears involving *more than one* rotator cuff tendon. Patients with glenohumeral osteoarthritis and rotator cuff tears limited to the supraspinatus tendon do not fit this criterion and are best treated with other options

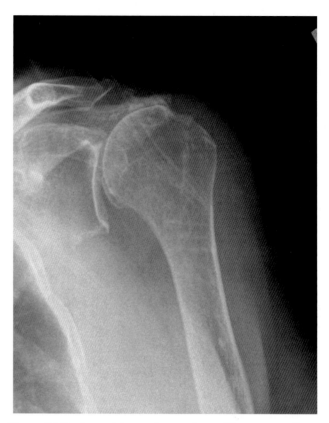

Figure 24-7 Acromial wear in a patient with rotator cuff tear arthropathy.

(nonoperative, unconstrained total shoulder arthroplasty). Furthermore, patients with massive irreparable rotator cuff tears *without* glenohumeral arthritis do not fit in this group and are rarely treated with a reverse prosthesis.

RHEUMATOID ARTHRITIS (INFLAMMATORY ARTHROPATHY) WITH MASSIVE ROTATOR CUFF TEAR

More than 10% of patients considered for shoulder arthroplasty with an underlying diagnosis of rheumatoid arthritis have a large tear of the rotator cuff that contraindicates unconstrained total shoulder arthroplasty.[4] These patients are candidates for either reverse shoulder arthroplasty (our preferred treatment) or unconstrained hemiarthroplasty (our preferred treatment only in cases of severe osseous insufficiency).

Clinical Findings

Clinical findings in patients with rheumatoid arthritis and a massive rotator cuff tear include glenohumeral

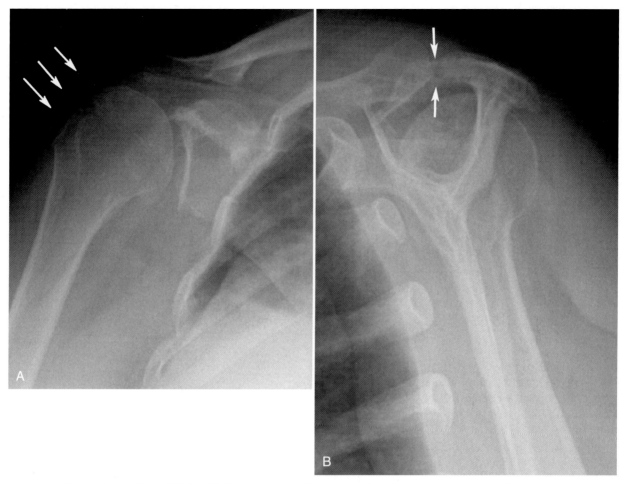

Figure 24-8 **A** and **B,** Insufficiency fracture of the acromion (*arrows*) in a patient with rotator cuff tear arthropathy.

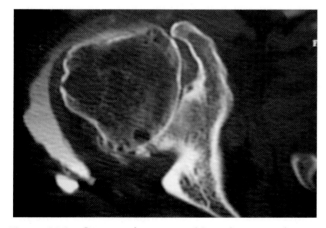

Figure 24-9 Computed tomographic arthrogram demonstrating a massive rotator cuff tear with glenohumeral arthritis.

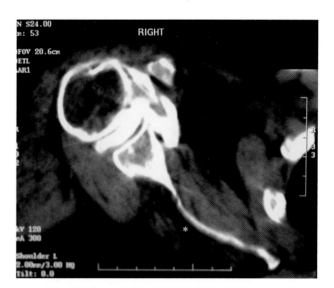

Figure 24-10 Computed tomographic arthrogram demonstrating severe fatty infiltration of the infraspinatus (*asterisk*). Compare with the normal subscapularis.

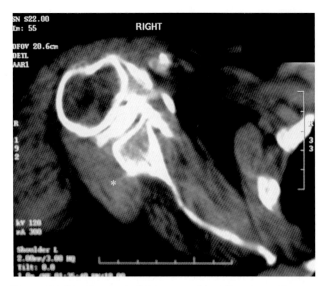

Figure 24-11 Computed tomographic arthrogram demonstrating hypertrophy of the teres minor in a patient with infraspinatus insufficiency (*asterisk*).

crepitus and stiffness. Acromiohumeral crepitus may be present. Testing of the individual rotator cuff tendons will typically demonstrate obvious insufficiency. The rotator cuff insufficiency may involve the posterior superior rotator cuff (supraspinatus, infraspinatus, teres minor), the anterior superior rotator cuff (supraspinatus, subscapularis), or all of the rotator cuff tendons. Additionally, the long head of the biceps tendon is often ruptured, as demonstrated by the characteristic deformity of the upper part of the arm. Chapter 7 details clinical testing of the rotator cuff.

Imaging Findings

Plain radiography demonstrates loss of the normal glenohumeral joint space. Humeral head osteophytes are rarely seen (Fig. 24-13). Static migration of the humeral head is almost always present. In patients with insufficiency of the posterior superior rotator cuff, the humeral head migration occurs in a superior direction (Fig. 24-14). In patients with insufficiency of the anterior superior rotator cuff, static anterior migration may be apparent on the axillary radiograph only. Patients with rheumatoid arthritis and a massive rotator cuff tear may have severe osseous wear on the undersurface of the acromion, on the superior glenoid, or on both (Fig. 24-15). Additionally, severe destruction of the humeral head may be present (Fig. 24-16).

As in cases of rotator cuff tear arthropathy, secondary imaging studies (computed tomographic arthrography, magnetic resonance imaging) will show rotator cuff tears involving more than one tendon in all cases. The rotator cuff muscle belly of the torn tendons shows fatty infiltration.

Osseous wear/destruction (glenoid, acromion, humeral head) is seen on secondary imaging studies. Severe loss of glenoid bone with glenoid protrusion morphology may be present (Fig. 24-17).

Special Considerations

As in cases of osteoarthritis with a massive rotator cuff tear/rotator cuff tear arthropathy, we emphasize that use of a reverse prosthesis in rheumatoid arthritis should be reserved for patients with *glenohumeral* osteoarthritis and massive *irreparable* rotator cuff tears involving *more than one* rotator cuff tendon. Patients with inflammatory arthritis and rotator cuff tears limited to the supraspinatus tendon do not fit this criterion and are best treated with other options (nonoperative treatment or unconstrained total shoulder arthroplasty).

PROXIMAL HUMERAL NONUNION

Post-traumatic proximal humerus fracture problems include proximal humeral nonunion and malunion. In certain cases, severe loss of proximal humeral bone prohibits the preferred treatment of proximal humeral nonunion—operative fixation and bone grafting. Proximal humeral bone loss often results from osteopenia, failed attempts at previous operative treatment, or a combination of the two. Previously, no good solution was available for use in these difficult cases. Because unconstrained shoulder arthroplasty with attempted fixation of the residual tuberosities has largely been unsatisfactory in the treatment of this problem, we now consider this a reasonable indication for use of a reverse prosthesis, provided that no other reasonable option can reliably provide pain relief and return of function (Fig. 24-18).

PROXIMAL HUMERAL MALUNION

Many cases of glenohumeral arthritis with proximal humeral malunion are treatable by unconstrained shoulder arthroplasty (see Chapter 6). Certain cases, however, yield unpredictable results with unconstrained arthroplasty, and the use of reverse shoulder arthroplasty may be indicated. Specifically, in cases of severe malunion in which distorted proximal humeral anatomy prohibits insertion of an unconstrained

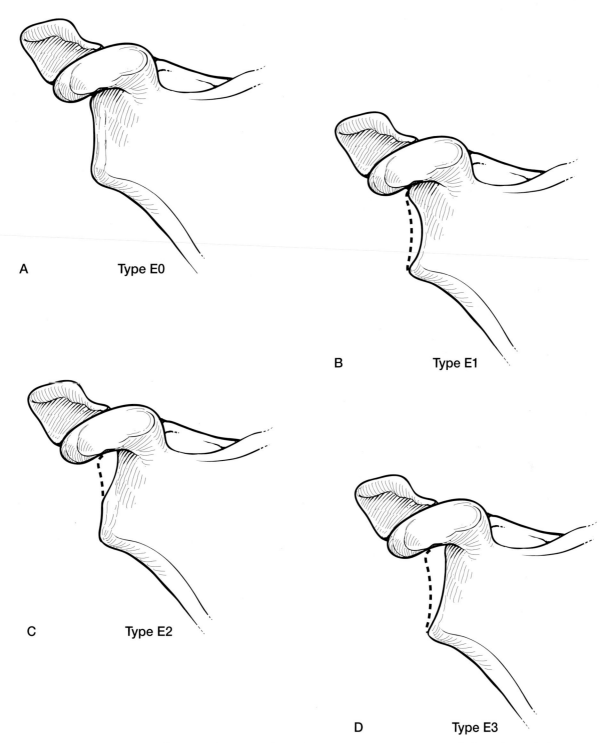

Figure 24-12   Classification of superior glenoid wear. **A,** E0 represents normal glenoid morphology. **B,** E1 represents central glenoid wear. **C,** E2 represents superior glenoid wear with superior biconcavity. **D,** E3 represents severe superior glenoid wear with a superiorly oriented glenoid morphology. (From Oudet D, Favard L, Lautmann S, et al: La prosthèse d'épaule Aequalis dans les omarthroses avec rupture massive et non réparable de la coiffe. In Walch G, Boileau P, Molé D [eds]: 2000 Prosthèses d'Epaule . . . Recul de 2 à 10 Ans. Paris, Sauramps Medical, 2001, pp 241-246.)

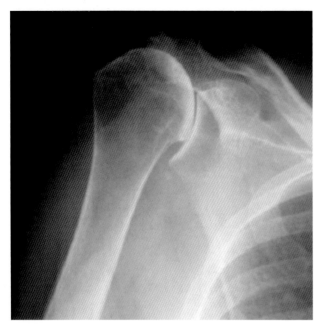

Figure 24-13 Radiograph of a patient with rheumatoid arthritis demonstrating a paucity of osteophytes.

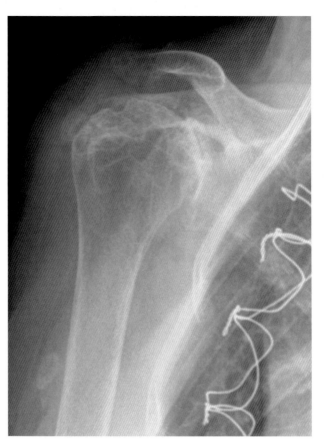

Figure 24-15 Severe osseous wear of both the glenoid and acromion occurring in a patient with rheumatoid arthritis and a massive rotator cuff tear.

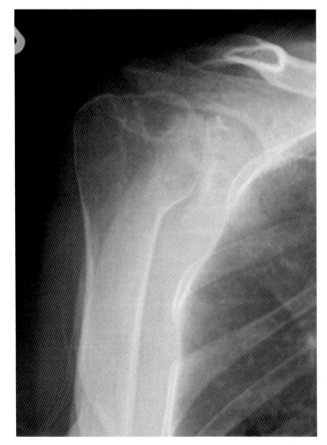

Figure 24-14 Radiograph of a patient with rheumatoid arthritis and a massive posterior superior rotator cuff tear demonstrating superior migration of the humeral head.

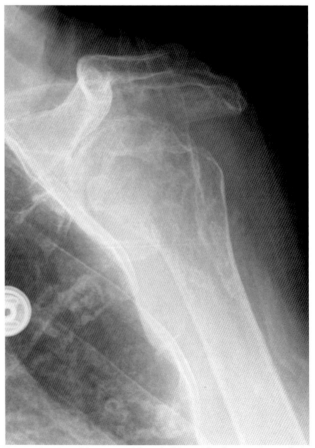

Figure 24-16 Rheumatoid arthritis with destruction of the humeral head.

humeral implant without disruption of the rotator cuff (Fig. 24-19) or in cases in which the proximal humeral malunion is accompanied by a massive irreparable rotator cuff tear, shoulder arthroplasty with a reverse prosthesis may be the best operative option.

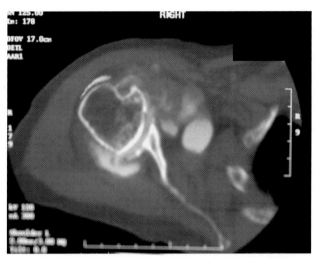

Figure 24-17 Computed tomogram demonstrating severe glenoid bone loss in a patient with rheumatoid arthritis and a massive rotator cuff tear.

Clinical Findings

Clinical findings in patients with proximal humeral malunion are variable. In patients with distortion of proximal humeral anatomy caused by malunion, shoulder stiffness may be exceptionally severe and attributable to mechanical impingement, subdeltoid contracture, and subacromial contracture, in addition to the glenohumeral incongruity and glenohumeral capsular contractures seen in primary osteoarthritis. Rotator cuff testing may be normal or compromised by pain or rotator cuff tearing, or both.

Imaging Findings

Plain radiography demonstrates loss of the normal glenohumeral joint space. Other radiographic findings are variable and depend on the severity of the proximal humeral malunion.

Secondary imaging studies (computed tomographic arthrography, magnetic resonance imaging), like plain radiography, show variable findings, depending on the deformity present. The rotator cuff may be compromised on secondary imaging studies.

Special Considerations

We perform unconstrained total shoulder arthroplasty in cases of post-traumatic arthritis in which the rotator

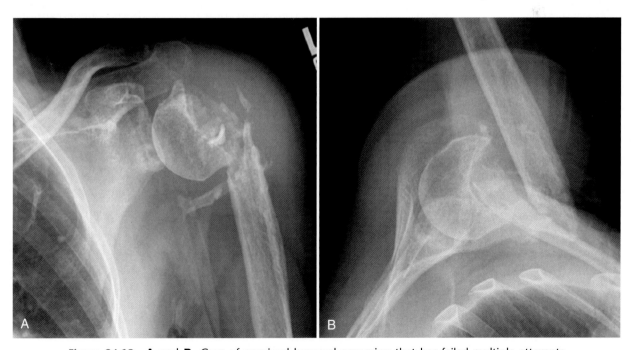

Figure 24-18 A and **B,** Case of proximal humeral nonunion that has failed multiple attempts at open reduction and internal fixation. The remaining proximal humerus is insufficient to allow successful fixation.

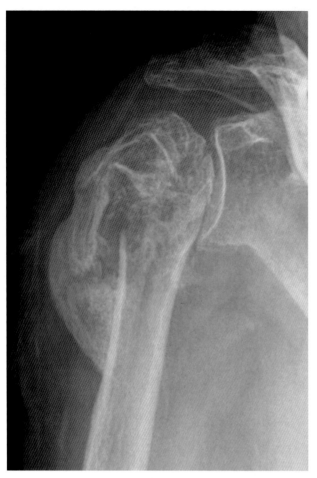

Figure 24-19 Post-traumatic arthritis in a patient with a severe malunion of the proximal humerus. Use of an unconstrained arthroplasty in this patient would require either violation of the rotator cuff or greater tuberosity osteotomy. We prefer the use of a reverse-design prosthesis in this scenario.

cuff is competent and the proximal humeral anatomy allows insertion of an unconstrained humeral component. In patients with rotator cuff insufficiency or in those who would require a greater tuberosity osteotomy to perform humeral arthroplasty, we opt for a reverse-design prosthesis (see Fig. 24-19).

MASSIVE ROTATOR CUFF TEAR WITH CHRONIC PSEUDOPARALYSIS BUT WITHOUT GLENOHUMERAL OSTEOARTHRITIS

A rare and somewhat controversial indication for reverse shoulder arthroplasty is a massive irreparable rotator cuff tear with chronic pseudoparalysis but no glenohumeral arthritis. In such cases, the massive

rotator cuff tear leads to an inability to counteract the glenohumeral shear forces of the deltoid and prevents active elevation of the arm. Pain may or may not be a complaint in this subset of patients. Neurologic examination and neurodiagnostic testing, if performed, are normal. Patients have usually failed prolonged (>6 months) attempts at rehabilitation with physical therapy. In these cases we will offer the patient a reverse prosthesis, provided that no other reasonable option is available.

Clinical Findings

Patients with chronic pseudoparalysis have a normal neurologic examination. Anterosuperior escape of the humeral head may be palpable on attempts at active arm elevation. Rotator cuff testing will usually indicate which rotator cuff musculotendinous units are compromised. The subscapularis is generally torn in patients with chronic pseudoparalysis and seems to play a major role in the ongoing inability to elevate the arm.

Imaging Findings

Plain radiography demonstrates maintenance of the normal glenohumeral joint space. Static migration of the humeral head is almost always present. In patients with insufficiency of the posterior superior rotator cuff, the humeral head migration occurs in a superior direction (Fig. 24-20). In patients with insufficiency of the anterior superior rotator cuff, static anterior migration may be apparent on the axillary radiograph only. Osseous wear is uncommon in this indication.

As in cases of rotator cuff tear arthropathy, secondary imaging studies (computed tomographic arthrography, magnetic resonance imaging) will show rotator cuff tears involving more than one tendon in all cases. The subscapularis is usually involved in the rotator cuff tear. The rotator cuff muscle belly of the torn tendons shows marked fatty infiltration.

Special Considerations

Most patients with massive irreparable rotator cuff tears and pseudoparalysis can be treated effectively without reverse shoulder replacement. We institute a physical therapy program in all of these patients, as well as symptomatic nonoperative treatment (analgesics, modalities, corticosteroid injections). After 6 months, if still unable to actively elevate the arm, the patient is considered a candidate for reverse shoulder arthroplasty, provided that no contraindications exist.

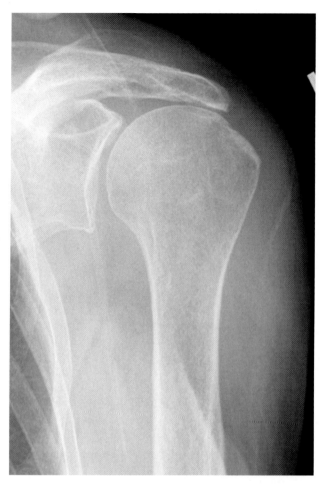

Figure 24-20 Proximal migration of the humeral head in a patient with a massive irreparable rotator cuff tear but without glenohumeral arthritis.

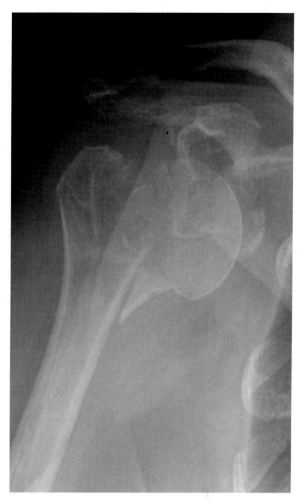

Figure 24-21 Radiograph of a 93-year-old active patient with age-related osteopenia and a four-part fracture-dislocation of the proximal humerus. We believe that this patient is best treated with a reverse prosthesis.

If the patient is able to elevate the arm but it remains painful, the patient is considered for other nonarthroplasty interventions, such as arthroscopic débridement with biceps tenotomy or tendon transfer.

ACUTE FRACTURE

Elderly patients (>75 years) with severe osteopenia who have complex proximal humeral fractures that would normally be an indication for replacement with a hemiarthroplasty (see Chapter 17) may be candidates for treatment with a reverse prosthesis (Fig. 24-21). In these difficult cases, even a perfectly performed hemiarthroplasty with fixation of the tuberosities may result in tuberosity nonunion and migration because of impaired healing imparted by osteopenia and local biology. In these cases we may opt for a reverse prosthesis combined with fixation of the tuberosities as

described in Chapter 21. In this scenario, in the event that the tuberosities do not heal, the patient still obtains reasonable pain relief and some active elevation, and the need for further surgery is therefore minimized.

FIXED GLENOHUMERAL DISLOCATION

Our outcomes using unconstrained shoulder arthroplasty for the treatment of fixed glenohumeral dislocations in elderly patients have been disappointing because we have observed a high rate of recurrent instability.[5] For this reason, we now use a reverse prosthesis as our implant of choice for fixed glenohumeral dislocations in elderly patients.[6]

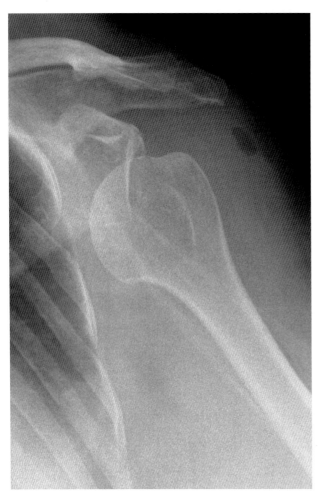

Figure 24-22 Fixed anterior dislocation in an elderly patient.

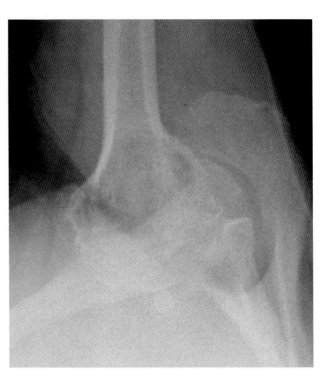

Figure 24-23 Axillary radiograph demonstrating a fixed anterior dislocation of the glenohumeral joint with severe loss of the anterior glenoid.

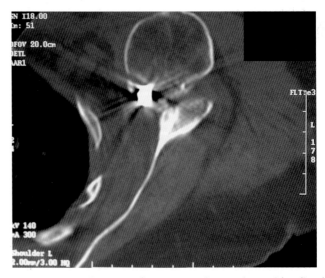

Figure 24-24 Computed tomogram in a patient with a fixed anterior dislocation and severe anterior glenoid bone erosion.

Clinical Findings

Patients with fixed glenohumeral dislocation have very limited active mobility of the involved shoulder. Findings are invariably consistent with massive rotator cuff tearing. Special attention should be paid to the neurologic examination, specifically axillary nerve function. Glenohumeral crepitus is usually present with shoulder motion.

Imaging Findings

Plain radiography demonstrates dislocation of the glenohumeral joint (Fig. 24-22). Axillary radiography may be difficult to perform because of the dislocation. If obtained, the axillary radiograph may demonstrate substantial wear of the osseous glenoid (Fig. 24-23).

Secondary imaging studies almost always demonstrate a massive rotator cuff tear. Frequently, erosion of the anterior or posterior glenoid occurs as a result of the chronic articulation of the dislocated humeral head (Fig. 24-24). Additionally, the humeral head may be eroded from this pathologic articulation (Fig. 24-25).

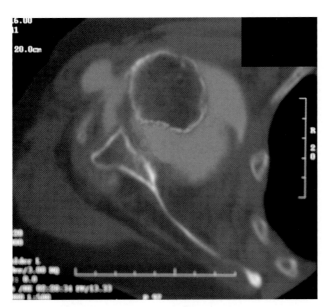

Figure 24-25 Computed tomogram in a patient with a fixed anterior dislocation and osseous erosion of the humeral head.

Special Considerations

Implantation of a reverse prosthesis in this subset of patients is technically difficult. Glenoid bone grafting may be required to address anterior or posterior glenoid bone loss.

POSTINFECTIOUS ARTHROPATHY

Postinfectious arthropathy can occur after a rotator cuff repair that subsequently became infected (Fig. 24-26). In this scenario, the rotator cuff repair usually fails and may result in rotator cuff insufficiency, similar to that observed in rotator cuff tear arthropathy. In cases of postinfectious arthropathy coupled with severe rotator cuff dysfunction, a reverse prosthesis is our implant of choice. Just as with postinfectious arthropathy and a competent rotator cuff, successful shoulder arthroplasty in these patients depends on complete eradication of the previous infection before shoulder arthroplasty is undertaken. Our approach for workup of these patients is detailed in the postinfectious arthropathy section of Chapter 6.

TUMOR

Tumors about the shoulder girdle are an exceptionally rare indication for reverse shoulder arthroplasty. In

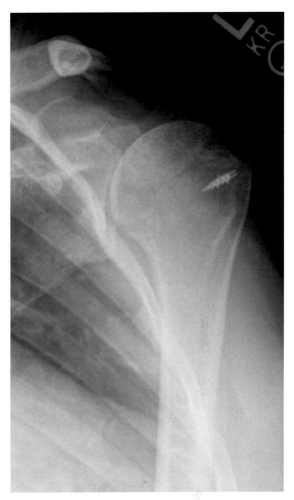

Figure 24-26 Radiograph of a patient with postinfectious arthropathy after failed rotator cuff repair.

our practice we infrequently assist in reconstruction of the shoulder after tumor resection by an orthopedic oncologic surgeon. If resection requires removal of the rotator cuff or tuberosities (or both) and leaves the humeral diaphysis and glenoid, a reverse prosthesis can be considered in the reconstruction (Fig. 24-27).[7]

CONTRAINDICATIONS TO REVERSE SHOULDER ARTHROPLASTY

Contraindications to reverse shoulder arthroplasty are listed in Table 24-1. Some of these contraindications are absolute, whereas others are relative.

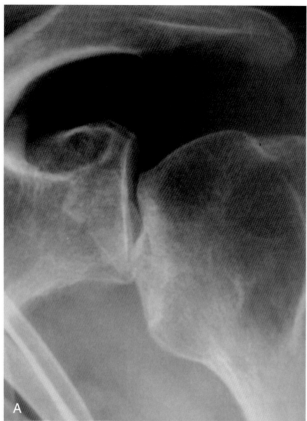
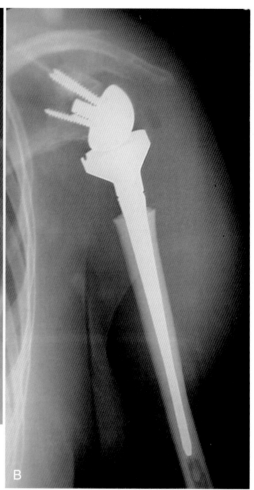

Figure 24-27 **A** and **B,** Radiographs of a patient with a desmoid tumor of the shoulder girdle. The patient underwent reconstruction with a reverse prosthesis after tumor resection.

Table 24-1	**CONTRAINDICATIONS TO REVERSE SHOULDER ARTHROPLASTY**	
Contraindication	**Absolute or Relative**	**Comments**
Poor generalized health	Relative	Appropriate perioperative medical treatment required
Active infection	Absolute	
Axillary nerve palsy	Absolute	Better suited for resection arthroplasty or arthrodesis
Deltoid insufficiency	Absolute	
Insufficient humeral bone stock	Absolute	
Insufficient glenoid bone stock	Absolute	Glenoid component contraindicated. Better suited for hemiarthroplasty
Ankylosed shoulder	Absolute	
Previous shoulder arthrodesis	Absolute	
Upper motor neuron lesion	Relative	Absolute contraindication if the patient has uncontrolled shoulder spasticity
Poor patient motivation	Absolute	

REFERENCES

1. Grammont PM, Baulot E: Delta shoulder prosthesis for rotator cuff rupture. Orthopedics 1993;16:65-68.
2. Neer CS 2nd, Craig EV, Fukuda H: Cuff tear arthropathy. J Bone Joint Surgery Am 1983;65:1232-1244.
3. Oudet D, Favard L, Lautmann S, et al: La prosthèse d'épaule Aequalis dans les omarthroses avec rupture massive et non réparable de la coiffe. In Walch G, Boileau P, Molé D (eds): 2000 Prosthèses d'Epaule . . . Recul de 2 à 10 Ans. Paris, Sauramps Medical, 2001, pp 241-246.
4. Vandermaren C, Docquier P: Shoulder arthroplasty in rheumatoid arthritis: Influence of the rotator cuff on the results. In Walch G, Boileau P, Molé D (eds): 2000 Prosthèses d'Epaule . . . Recul de 2 à 10 Ans. Paris, Sauramps Medical, 2001, pp 177-182.
5. Matsoukis J, Tabib W, Guiffault P, et al: Primary unconstrained shoulder arthroplasty in patients with a fixed anterior glenohumeral dislocation: Results of a multicenter study. J Bone Joint Surg Am 2006;88:547-552.
6. Cortés ZE, Edwards TB, Elkousy HA, Gartsman GM: Reverse total shoulder arthroplasty as treatment for fixed anterior shoulder dislocation. Paper presented at a conference titled Treatment of Complex Shoulder Problems, January 2005, Tampa, FL.
7. Sikka RS, Voran M, Edwards TB, et al: Desmoid tumor of the subscapularis presenting as isolated loss of shoulder external rotation: A report of two cases. J Bone Joint Surg Am 2004;86:159-164.

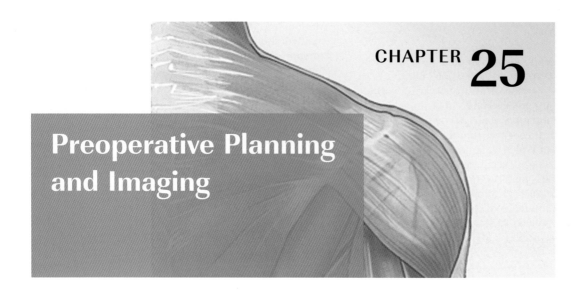

CHAPTER 25

Preoperative Planning and Imaging

Reintroduction of the reverse-design prosthesis has allowed surgeons to treat complicated shoulder pathology for which no good solution existed before availability of this implant. The severity and diversity of shoulder pathology treatable with a reverse prosthesis make preoperative planning even more important in these cases than with primary unconstrained shoulder arthroplasty. Candidates for a reverse prosthesis may include patients with substantial proximal humeral or glenoid bone loss, or both. Because of the complex nature of many of these cases, preoperative planning should be done well in advance of the surgical procedure and not be an afterthought the morning of surgery. As with unconstrained shoulder arthroplasty, preoperative planning for reverse shoulder arthroplasty requires that the surgeon review the patient's clinical history and physical examination, radiographs, and secondary imaging studies. This chapter outlines our approach to preoperative planning for reverse shoulder arthroplasty.

CLINICAL HISTORY AND EXAMINATION

The same type of clinical history and physical examination is used for candidates for reverse shoulder arthroplasty as for candidates for unconstrained shoulder arthroplasty (see Chapter 7). Because most candidates for reverse shoulder arthroplasty have a compromised rotator cuff, it is important to obtain a detailed history of the patient's complaints (pain only; weakness only; pain and weakness; pain, weakness, and stiffness).

Any previous surgery, especially attempts at rotator cuff repair and fracture surgery, merits special consid-

eration. The type of surgical approach (arthroscopic or open) should be noted. Previous open surgery may compromise deltoid function to a degree that contraindicates use of a reverse prosthesis.

As with unconstrained shoulder arthroplasty, any symptoms of previous infection, especially in patients who have undergone surgery or injections, should be investigated further. If patients have a history of infection after shoulder surgery or have had symptoms suggestive of infection (systemic fevers; shoulder warmth, redness), a preoperative infection workup is indicated. The workup includes hematologic evaluation with a complete blood cell count and differential, a sedimentation rate, and C-reactive protein. Additionally, fluoroscopically guided shoulder aspiration is performed and the specimen submitted for aerobic, anaerobic, fungal, and mycobacterial culture. If the findings are suggestive or diagnostic of infection, shoulder arthroplasty is postponed or canceled until infectious disease consultation is obtained and the infection is appropriately treated.

Any medical history of systemic illness (diabetes mellitus, cardiac problems) should be considered in the preoperative planning. Although these factors may not affect the actual surgical procedure, they may necessitate special considerations in the patient's postoperative care. The availability of appropriate care of these systemic illnesses, including the availability of consultants, should be confirmed before surgery.

All of our patients undergo a thorough shoulder examination, much of which is detailed in Chapter 7. The visual appearance of the shoulder yields useful information in candidates for reverse shoulder arthroplasty. The presence and location of surgical scars are noted (Fig. 25-1). In thin patients, anterosuperior

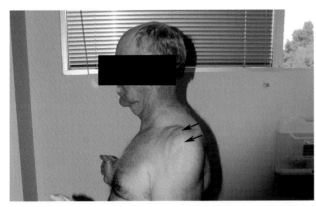

Figure 25-1 Scar from a previous open rotator cuff repair (*arrows*) in a candidate for implantation of a reverse prosthesis.

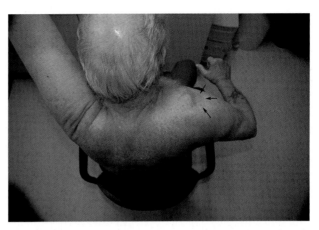

Figure 25-3 Patient with previous surgery involving detachment of the deltoid (*arrows*).

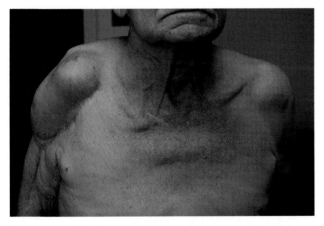

Figure 25-2 Obvious anterior superior escape of the humeral head.

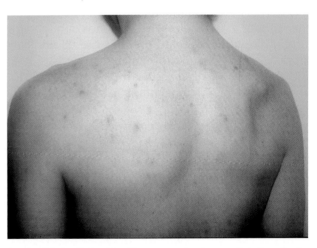

Figure 25-4 Patient with supraspinatus and infraspinatus atrophy.

escape of the humeral head caused by anterior superior rotator cuff deficiency may be obvious (Fig. 25-2) or may be noted only when the patient attempts arm elevation or abduction. Special attention should be paid to the condition of the deltoid, especially if it has previously been surgically violated (Fig. 25-3). The condition of the deltoid is best evaluated by asking the patient to push against your hand to observe an isometric contraction. Any areas of deltoid origin that may not have healed to the acromion after a previous operation should be noted. Atrophy of the supraspinatus and infraspinatus should be noted as well (Fig. 25-4).

Both active and passive mobility is recorded, as detailed in Chapter 7. The presence of glenohumeral crepitus with motion is recorded, as is any discrepancy in active and passive mobility. Special attention should be paid to evaluation of the deltoid muscle. If deltoid contractility appears to be compromised, additional

evaluation with electromyography and nerve conduction studies should be performed before further consideration for implantation of a reverse prosthesis.

Rotator cuff examination consists of testing each tendon of the rotator cuff by isolating it as much as possible. Jobe's test is used to test supraspinatus integrity.[1] The infraspinatus is tested by the external rotation lag sign and external rotation strength with the arm at the side.[2] The horn blower's sign is used to test the teres minor.[3] The subscapularis is tested with the belly press test and, when mobility allows, the lift-off test.[4] Performance of the various rotator cuff tests is depicted in Chapter 7.

The results of the clinical history and examination are documented in the patient's chart and reviewed well in advance of surgery as part of preoperative planning. Findings are discussed with the patient in terms of postoperative outcome and patient expectations.

For example, it is important for patients without posterior rotator cuff function (no infraspinatus or teres minor) to understand that the operation will not restore their ability to actively externally rotate the arm.

RADIOGRAPHY

Radiographs are obtained in all patients who are being considered as candidates for reverse shoulder arthroplasty. An anteroposterior view of the glenohumeral joint with the arm in neutral rotation, an axillary view, and a scapular outlet view are the views that we use for all shoulder arthroplasty patients. The anteroposterior radiograph is used to evaluate the glenohumeral joint space, the presence of humeral and glenoid osteophytes, the size of the humeral canal, the presence of any loose bodies, the existence of any deformity of the humeral shaft, the presence of any static superior migration of the humeral head (Fig. 25-5), and the presence of any superior glenoid wear (Fig. 25-6). The axillary radiograph is used to evaluate the

glenohumeral joint space, the presence of anterior or posterior humeral head subluxation, and the presence of osseous glenoid wear and dysplasia. The scapular outlet radiograph is used to evaluate the condition of the acromion (thin, fractured, deficient); the presence of anterior, posterior, or superior humeral head subluxation (Fig. 25-7); the presence of loose bodies in the subscapularis recess; and the existence of any deformity of the humeral shaft.

Ideally, these radiographs are taken with magnification and fluoroscopic control. Some patients come to our clinic with radiographs taken by a referring physician. If these radiographs are judged to be of sufficient quality, are less than 6 months old, and do not show any unusual circumstances (excessively small humeral intramedullary canal), they are not repeated. In all other cases, radiographs are repeated with magnification and fluoroscopically controlled techniques.

In patients demonstrating proximal humeral bone loss from causes such as fracture nonunion, bilateral,

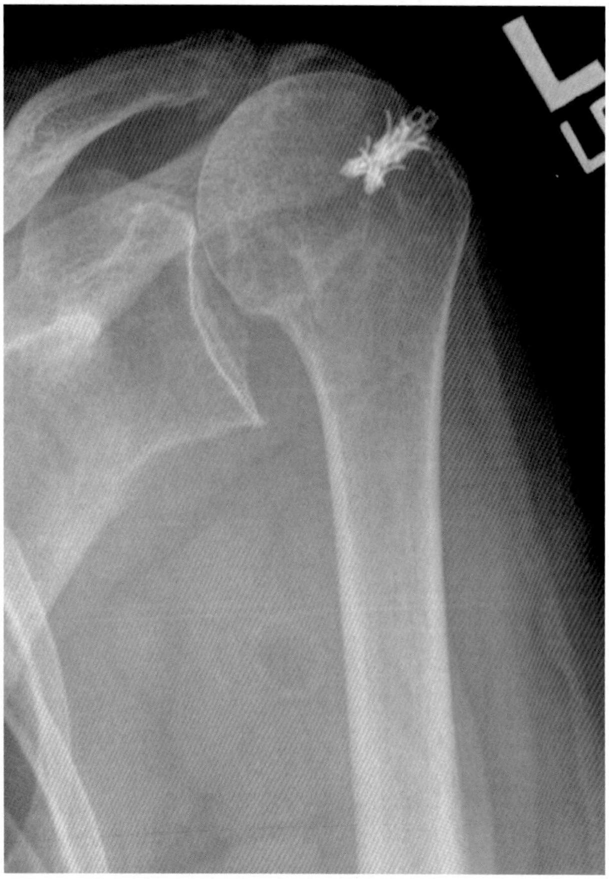

Figure 25-5 Static superior migration of the humeral head.

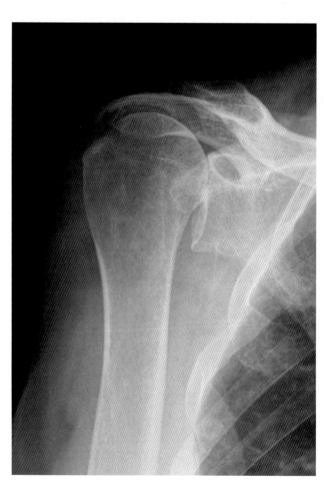

Figure 25-6 Superior glenoid wear from static superior humeral head migration.

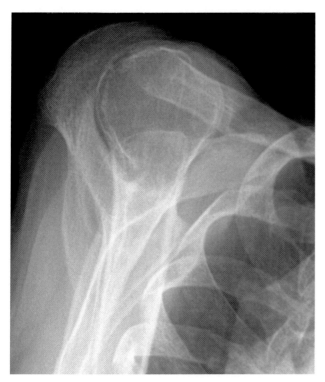

Figure 25-7 Superior humeral head migration demonstrated on an outlet radiograph.

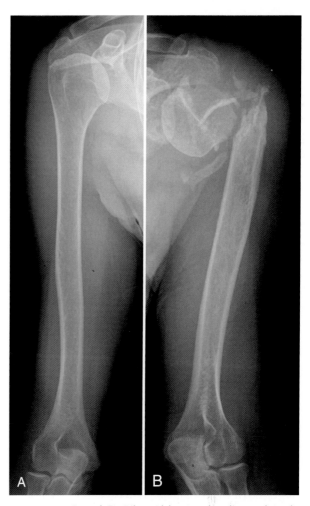

Figure 25-8 **A** and **B,** Bilateral humeral radiographs taken to help estimate the level at which the humeral component should be implanted in a patient with severe proximal humeral bone loss.

full-length, magnification-controlled anteroposterior humeral radiographs are obtained (Fig. 25-8). These radiographs are used to help select the height at which to implant the humeral stem.

Most reverse shoulder arthroplasty prosthetic systems have radiographic templates available for preoperative planning (Fig. 25-9). For routine causes such as rotator cuff tear arthropathy, we do not routinely use preoperative radiographic templating because we have not found it to be useful. In cases of proximal humeral bone loss, preoperative radiographic templating is done on full-length humeral radiographs. The desired position of the reverse prosthesis is templated on the radiograph of the unaffected humerus, and the level of the metaphyseal-diaphyseal junction of the humeral component is marked (Fig. 25-10). The distance from the transepicondylar axis at the elbow to this point is measured (Fig. 25-11). A mark is made at the same distance from the transepicondylar axis on the affected radiograph. A second mark is made at the most proximal extent of the humeral shaft (Fig. 25-12). The distance between the desired prosthetic level at the metaphyseal-diaphyseal junction and the proximal extent of the humeral shaft is measured (Fig. 25-13). A ruler is used during surgery to measure the distance and mark the level on the humeral stem for

the desired prosthetic position (Fig. 25-14). This technique of preoperative planning provides only a guideline and may be superseded by intraoperative observations. In general, intraoperative deltoid tension is more important in determining the correct prosthetic position than preoperative radiographic templating is. Preoperative planning does, however, provide a starting point for establishing proper prosthetic height.

Rarely, proximal humeral bone loss (previous trauma, tumor) is sufficiently severe to necessitate use of a custom implant or proximal humeral composite bone graft. Templates are useful to determine whether existing prefabricated implants are sufficient or a custom-manufactured implant is required (Fig. 25-15).

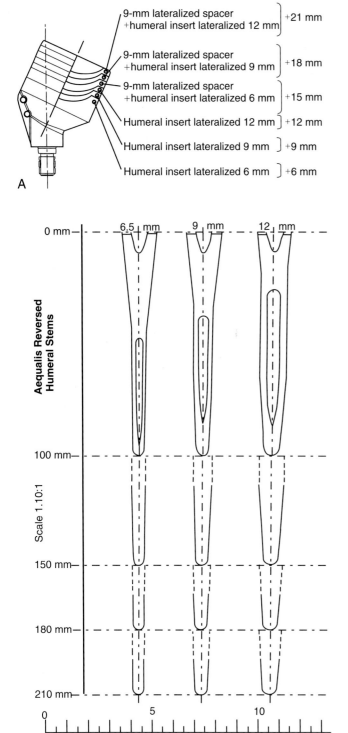

Aequalis Reversed Metaphysis 36 mm

9-mm lateralized spacer
+humeral insert lateralized 12 mm } +21 mm

9-mm lateralized spacer
+humeral insert lateralized 9 mm } +18 mm

9-mm lateralized spacer
+humeral insert lateralized 6 mm } +15 mm

Humeral insert lateralized 12 mm] +12 mm

Humeral insert lateralized 9 mm] +9 mm

Humeral insert lateralized 6 mm] +6 mm

A

Figure 25-9   **A** and **B,** Radiographic templates for preoperative planning of reverse shoulder arthroplasty.

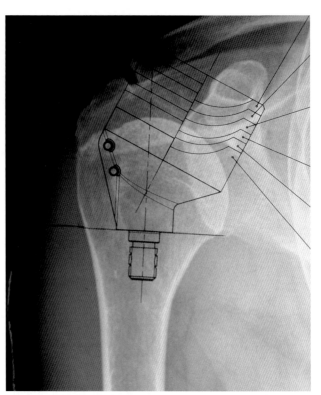

Figure 25-10   The desired position of a reverse prosthesis is templated on the unaffected humeral radiograph, and the level of the metaphyseal-diaphyseal junction of the humeral component is marked.

SECONDARY IMAGING

A secondary imaging study is obtained in all patients before reverse shoulder arthroplasty to evaluate the rotator cuff and osseous morphology. As with unconstrained shoulder arthroplasty, our preferred secondary imaging modality in most cases is computed tomographic arthrography. If a patient has a previous magnetic resonance imaging scan that allows sufficient evaluation of the osseous structures and rotator cuff and is less than 6 months old, we will not order additional secondary imaging. In the scenario of a patient with possible deltoid muscle detachment from previous open rotator cuff surgery, our imaging modality of choice becomes magnetic resonance imaging, which in our experience more easily shows deltoid pathology.

On a computed tomogram (or magnetic resonance image), axial glenoid morphology is classified according to the system of Walch and colleagues, as described in Chapter 7.[5] The axial sections of the secondary imaging scan are used to measure the depth of the glenoid vault to determine whether sufficient bone exists to implant the 15-mm peg of the reverse pros-

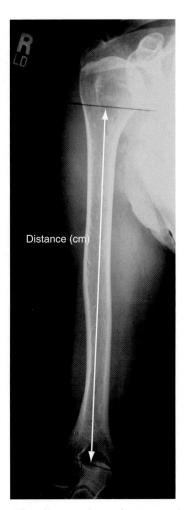

Figure 25-11 The distance from the transepicondylar axis at the elbow to the level of the metaphyseal-diaphyseal junction of the humeral component is measured.

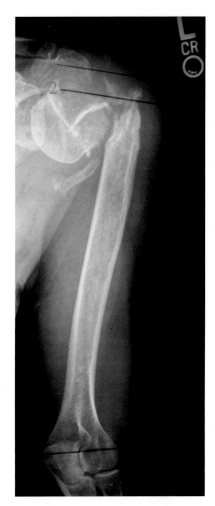

Figure 25-12 A mark (1) is made at the same distance from the transepicondylar axis on the affected radiograph. A second mark (2) is made at the most proximal extent of the humeral shaft.

thesis base plate (Fig. 25-16). Additionally, coronal glenoid morphology is classified as described by Sirveaux and associates (Fig. 25-17).[6] In this system, type E0 represents no glenoid wear, type E1 represents central glenoid wear, type E2 represents superior glenoid wear with superior biconcavity, and type E3 represents severe superior glenoid wear extending inferiorly and reorienting the glenoid surface to a superiorly tilted position. In cases of severe superior glenoid bony wear, a superior bone graft may be necessary to reorient the glenoid to a neutral or inferiorly directed position (Fig. 25-18).

The rotator cuff is next evaluated with secondary imaging modalities, including assessment of tendinous integrity and evaluation of muscle quality (fatty infiltration). In addition, the condition of the long head of the biceps tendon is noted, particularly its

position (centered, subluxated, dislocated, ruptured), to assist in identifying it at the time of surgery. Each tendon of the rotator cuff is individually evaluated with the secondary imaging study. Even though tears or fatty infiltration of the rotator cuff (or both) may not contraindicate use of a reverse prosthesis, knowledge of the status of the rotator cuff assists in determination of the postoperative prognosis. Moreover, a completely nonfunctioning posterior rotator cuff may be an indication for use of a latissimus dorsi transfer with the reverse prosthesis to better restore postoperative external rotation, although the usefulness of this adjunctive procedure is not yet well established in this scenario.

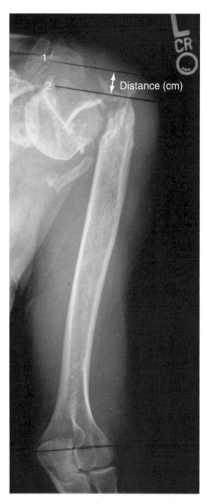

Figure 25-13 The distance between the desired prosthetic level at the metaphyseal-diaphyseal junction (1) and the proximal extent of the humeral shaft (2) is measured.

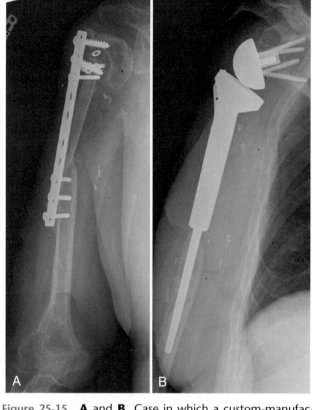

Figure 25-15 **A** and **B,** Case in which a custom-manufactured implant was required to accommodate for severe proximal humeral bone loss.

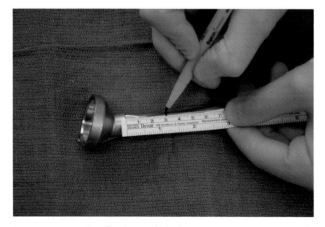

Figure 25-14 A ruler is used during surgery to measure the distance and mark on the humeral stem the level for the desired prosthetic position.

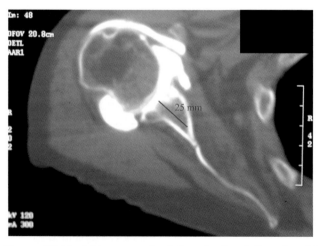

Figure 25-16 Measurement of the depth of the glenoid vault with a computed tomogram preoperatively to determine whether the glenoid is sufficient for implantation of the reverse prosthesis base plate.

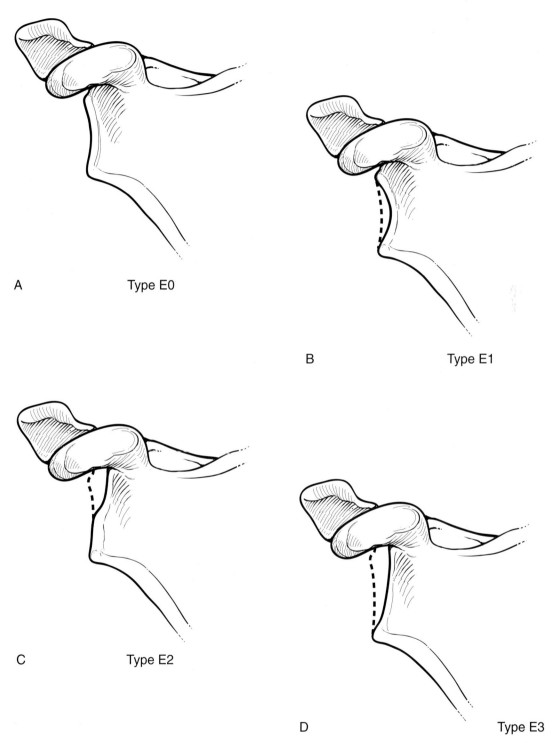

A   Type E0

B   Type E1

C   Type E2

D   Type E3

Figure 25-17 Classification of coronal glenoid morphology. **A,** Type E0 represents no glenoid wear. **B,** Type E1 represents central glenoid wear. **C,** Type E2 represents superior glenoid wear with superior biconcavity. **D,** Type E3 represents severe superior glenoid wear extending inferiorly and reorienting the glenoid surface to a superiorly tilted position.

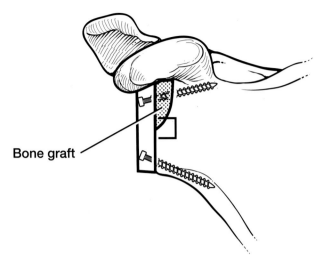

Bone graft

Figure 25-18   In cases of severe superior glenoid bony wear, a superior bone graft may be necessary to reorient the glenoid to a neutral or inferiorly directed position.

REFERENCES

1. Jobe FW, Jobe C: Painful athletic injuries of the shoulder. Clin Orthop Relat Res 1983;173:117-124.
2. Hertel R, Ballmer FT, Lambert SM, et al: Lag signs in the diagnosis of rotator cuff rupture. J Shoulder Elbow Surg 1996;5:307-313.
3. Gerber C, Vinh TS, Hertel R, Hess CW: Latissimus dorsi transfer for the treatment of massive tears of the rotator cuff: A preliminary report. Clin Orthop Relat Res 1988;232:51-61.
4. Gerber C, Krushell RJ: Isolated rupture of the tendon of the subscapularis muscle: Clinical features in 16 cases. J Bone Joint Surg Br 1991;73:389-394.
5. Walch G, Badet R, Boulahia A, Khoury A: Morphologic study of the glenoid in primary glenohumeral osteoarthritis. J Arthroplasty 1999;14:756-760.
6. Sirveaux F, Favard L, Oudet D, et al: Grammont inverted total shoulder arthroplasty in the treatment of glenohumeral osteoarthritis with massive rupture of the cuff: Results of a multicentre study of 80 shoulders. J Bone Joint Surg Br 2004;86:388-395.

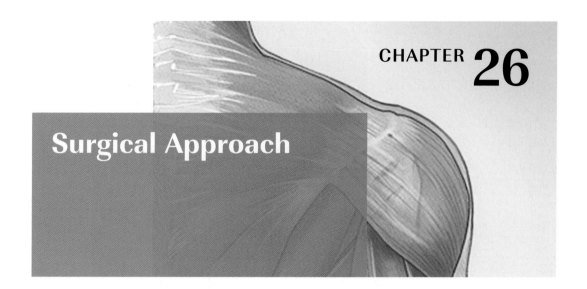

CHAPTER 26

Surgical Approach

Two surgical approaches have been described for implantation of a reverse prosthesis. The anterior superior approach was initially used because it makes use of the rotator cuff defect. More recently, the deltopectoral approach has been used for insertion of a reverse prosthesis. We perform all reverse prostheses through the deltopectoral approach, which is our preferred approach for five reasons:

1. **Deltoid violation.** A reverse prosthesis relies on the deltoid muscle to power elevation of the arm. The anterior superior approach violates the deltoid muscle, which may be a problem.
2. **Level of humeral resection.** Glenoid exposure when using the anterior superior approach may require more resection of the proximal humerus than when using the deltopectoral approach. During the anterior superior approach, the humerus is retracted inferiorly to obtain access to the glenoid. If glenoid exposure is inadequate after appropriate soft tissue release, the only solution to enhance glenoid exposure is resection of more of the proximal humerus. More bone resection may make proper deltoid tensioning difficult and lead to weakness in elevation.
3. **Glenoid component positioning.** It is generally agreed that the reverse glenoid component should be placed inferiorly on the glenoid face to help prevent impingement of the humeral component on the scapula and subsequent scapular notching. The need to retract the humerus inferiorly to access the glenoid with the anterior

superior approach creates more difficulty in getting the glenoid component aligned with the inferior aspect of the glenoid face. Debate exists on whether inferior tilt should be introduced during glenoid reaming so that the glenoid component is positioned to better avoid scapular notching. However, it is agreed that superior tilt should be avoided. Using the anterior superior approach risks inadvertently placing the glenoid component in a superiorly tilted position, which risks glenoid failure (Fig. 26-1).

4. **Extensile exposure.** The deltopectoral approach can easily be extended into an anterolateral approach to the humerus, whereas the axillary nerve limits distal extension of the anterior superior approach. Review of a consecutive series of 100 reverse prostheses performed at Texas Orthopedic Hospital demonstrated that the underlying etiology necessitated a more extensile exposure than what could be obtained with an anterior superior approach in 36 cases (18 nonunion/malunion, 17 revision, 1 fixed dislocation requiring anterior glenoid reconstruction with iliac crest autograft).
5. **Familiarity.** One third of our shoulder replacements involve the use of a reverse prosthesis. The other two thirds use an unconstrained device implanted through a deltopectoral approach. We are very comfortable performing unconstrained shoulder arthroplasty through a deltopectoral approach and do not substantially change this approach when implanting a reverse prosthesis.

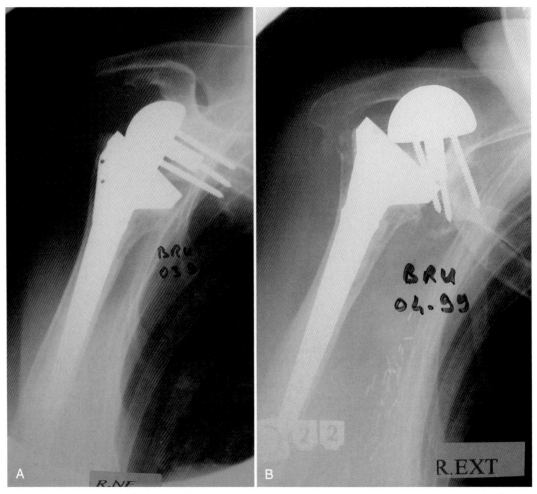

Figure 26-1   A, Radiograph of a reverse prosthesis implanted through an anterior superior approach with the glenoid component inadvertently inserted with a superior tilt. **B,** This malpositioned implant eventually failed.

TECHNIQUE FOR THE DELTOPECTORAL APPROACH

The deltopectoral approach used for implantation of a reverse prosthesis is nearly identical to the deltopectoral approach used for unconstrained shoulder arthroplasty described in Chapter 8. The skin incision, subcutaneous dissection, development of the deltopectoral interval, identification of the conjoined tendon and coracoid process, and retractor placement proceed as detailed in Chapter 8 and shown in Figures 8-1 through 8-6.

With the arm abducted and externally rotated, the apex formed by the insertion of the coracoacromial ligament and the conjoined tendon onto the coracoid process is identified. The coracoacromial ligament is sectioned just lateral to its insertion on the coracoid with a needle tip electrocautery to enhance exposure

of the superiorly migrated humeral head (Fig. 26-2). This is in contrast to the surgical approach used for unconstrained shoulder arthroplasty, in which the coracoacromial ligament is preserved to act as a static restraint to anterior superior migration. When we use a reverse prosthesis, the prosthetic design eliminates the need for this static restraint.

The conjoined tendon is retracted medially to expose the anterior aspect of the glenohumeral joint. The anterior humeral circumflex vessels (the "three sisters") are suture-ligated together just as in cases of unconstrained shoulder arthroplasty. The arm is then placed in forward flexion and neutral rotation, and the axillary nerve is identified by direct visualization after blunt dissection. This ensures protection of the nerve throughout the procedure.

In cases in which the subscapularis is intact, it is handled identically to cases of unconstrained shoulder

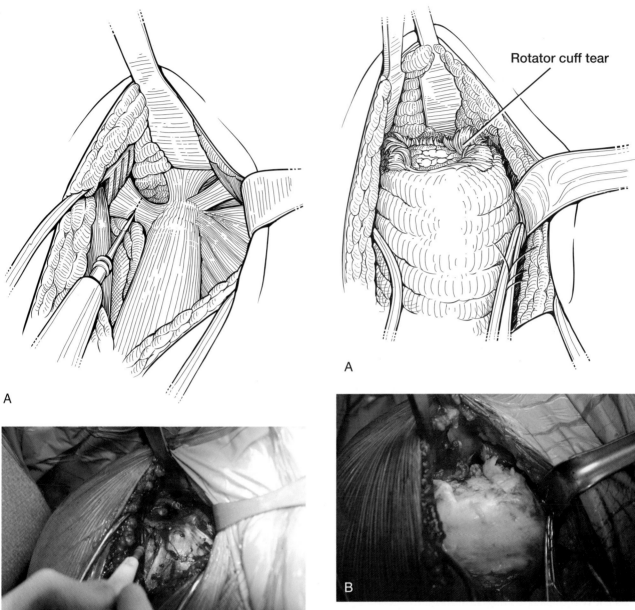

Rotator cuff tear

A

B

Figure 26-2 **A** and **B,** Release of the coracoacromial ligament with the electrocautery.

Figure 26-3 **A** and **B,** The glenohumeral joint visualized through a large rotator cuff tear.

arthroplasty. Two stay sutures of no. 2 polyester are placed in the subscapularis tendon near the musculotendinous junction. The glenohumeral joint is often already accessible through a large rotator cuff tear superiorly (Fig. 26-3). The anatomic neck of the humerus is identified, and a scalpel is used to transect the subscapularis tendon and joint capsule along the anatomic neck of the humerus. The electrocautery replaces the scalpel at the inferior portion of the sub-

scapularis to cauterize the previously ligated anterior humeral circumflex vessels. A humeral head retractor is placed in the glenohumeral joint and is used to retract the humeral head posteriorly. A circumferential release of the subscapularis tendon is performed, with release of the superior, middle, and inferior glenohumeral ligaments just as in unconstrained shoulder arthroplasty. The subscapularis is then tucked into the subscapularis fossa with forceps and held with a glenoid rim retractor. In contrast to cases of unconstrained arthroplasty, no sponge is placed in the sub-

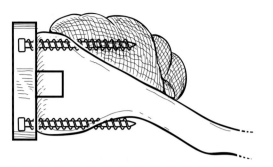

Figure 26-4   If a sponge is placed in the subscapularis fossa, screws used for base plate fixation may engage and incarcerate the sponge. When implanting a reverse prosthesis, a sponge is not used in the subscapularis fossa to avoid this situation.

scapularis fossa because insertion of screws for fixation of the glenoid base plate risks entrapment of the sponge with screws as they penetrate the anterior scapular cortex (Fig. 26-4). If the subscapularis tendon is not present, the remaining subscapularis bursa is excised to expose the glenohumeral joint, and the humeral head retractor and glenoid rim retractor are inserted. If present, the intra-articular portion of the long head of the biceps tendon is handled as described in Chapter 5 (tenotomy or tenodesis).

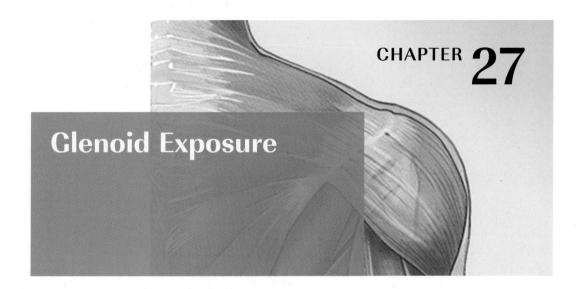

CHAPTER 27

Glenoid Exposure

The technique for glenoid exposure is no less important for implantation of a reverse prosthesis than in cases of unconstrained total shoulder arthroplasty. In fact, certain aspects of reverse prosthesis cases may make glenoid exposure more difficult than in cases of unconstrained total shoulder arthroplasty. First, static subluxation of the proximal humerus may increase the difficulty of proximal humeral retraction during glenoid exposure. Second, as detailed in Chapter 28, a smaller volume of proximal humerus is resected during humeral preparation than in cases of unconstrained shoulder arthroplasty, thus making retraction of the proximal humerus during glenoid exposure more difficult.

The steps and technique of glenoid exposure are essentially identical to that performed for unconstrained total shoulder arthroplasty. Care is taken to not release more glenohumeral joint capsule than necessary to allow adequate glenoid exposure for implantation of the reverse prosthesis glenoid exposure to avoid prosthetic dislocation. In many cases in which the reverse prosthesis is indicated, the glenohumeral joint capsule assists in providing stability to the glenohumeral joint. With the rotator cuff absent or severely compromised, stability of the prosthetic joint is provided by a combination of the inherent prosthetic biomechanics, the large muscles crossing the glenohumeral joint (deltoid, biceps), and any residual glenohumeral joint capsule. Because fibers from the large muscles crossing the glenohumeral joint are prone to elongation, which may compromise possible prosthetic tension and hence prosthetic stability over time,

every effort should be made to preserve as much joint capsule as possible to enhance prosthetic stability.

TECHNIQUE FOR GLENOID EXPOSURE

After the subscapularis, if present, is retracted medially with a small glenoid rim retractor, attention is turned to glenoid exposure. Any remaining labrum is excised from the base of the coracoid process and the exposure extended inferiorly to the 5 o'clock position in a right shoulder (7 o'clock in a left shoulder) with the needle tip electrocautery. This allows identification of the osseous anterior margin of the glenoid, as well as inspection of the superior aspect of the glenoid for evidence of erosion (Fig. 27-1). The tip of the electrocautery is used to release the inferior capsule directly off the rim of the glenoid bone, stopping initially at the 6 o'clock position (Fig. 27-2). To prevent damage to the axillary nerve, the tip of the electrocautery must be kept in contact with the glenoid bone. This release is extended sufficiently medially to completely transect the capsule and expose the muscular fibers of the triceps inserting on the inferior osseous glenoid. Adequacy of glenoid exposure is then evaluated by having an assistant provide maximal retraction on the proximal humerus and verifying complete neuromuscular paralysis with the anesthesiologist or nurse anesthetist (Fig. 27-3). An adequate release is accomplished if the surgeon believes that glenoid reaming and implantation of the reverse glenoid component would be possible after minimal humeral head resection. If exposure

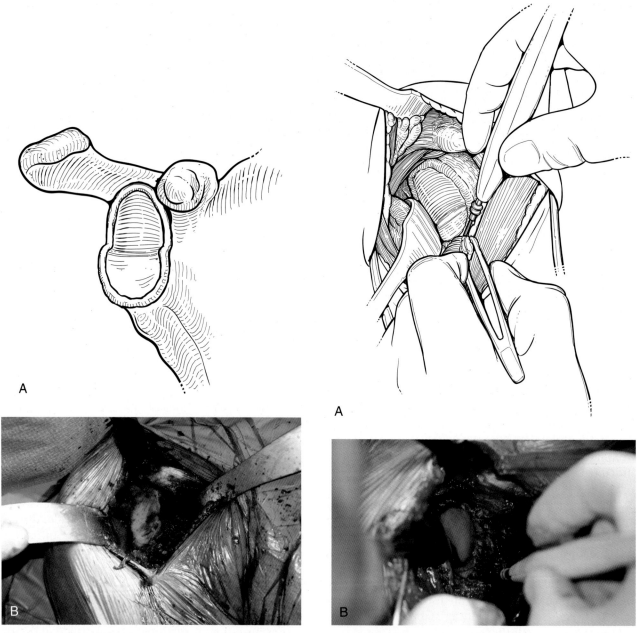

Figure 27-1   **A** and **B,** Superior erosion of the glenoid in a case of rotator cuff tear arthropathy.

Figure 27-2   **A** and **B,** Release the inferior capsule directly off the rim of the glenoid and extend it initially to the 6 o'clock position with the electrocautery.

is thought to be adequate, no further capsular release is performed. If the release is thought to be insufficient, capsular transection is continued around to the 7 o'clock position in a right shoulder (5 o'clock position in a left shoulder) and the exposure is re-evaluated. The process is repeated until the release is considered adequate. This stepwise progression helps prevent too large a release, which could potentially lead to prosthetic instability.

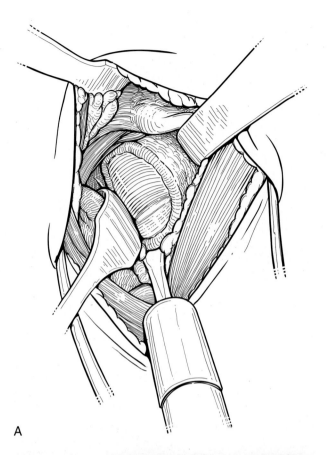

A

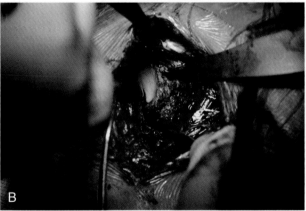

B

Figure 27-3 **A** and **B,** Evaluation of the adequacy of gleno-humeral release.

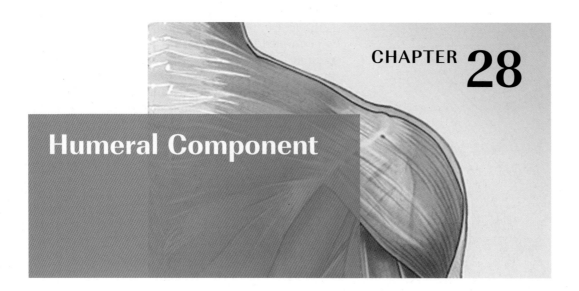

CHAPTER 28

Humeral Component

Humeral preparation and implantation of the humeral component of a reverse prosthesis are in some ways easier than with unconstrained arthroplasty. In many cases for which a reverse prosthesis is implanted, the rotator cuff is severely compromised or absent, which facilitates exposure of the proximal humerus. Additionally, because of the nonanatomic nature of the reverse prosthesis, preset resection guides are used in humeral preparation, thereby decreasing the importance of identification of the anatomic neck of the humerus, which is critical during implantation of an anatomically designed unconstrained shoulder arthroplasty.

We implant all reverse-prosthesis humeral components with polymethylmethacrylate. The forces acting on the glenohumeral joint of a reverse prosthesis combined with the proximal humeral osteopenia that is often present in candidates for implantation of a reverse prosthesis may contribute to subsidence of uncemented reverse humeral components (Fig. 28-1). Subsidence of the humeral component may cause a critical loss of soft tissue tension and lead to glenohumeral dislocation. Consequently, most manufacturers recommend the use of cement fixation of the humeral component of reverse-design prostheses.

Many different implant companies manufacture reverse-design shoulder prostheses. It is beyond the scope of this textbook to describe the specific techniques used for each of these systems. To us, the critical design feature for any reverse-prosthetic system is the Grammont-designed medialized center of rotation of the glenohumeral articulation. We believe that long-term success can be achieved if the implant

system selected adheres to this clinically tested principle. This chapter describes the technique for preparation of the proximal humerus for our preferred prosthetic system. Most of the steps, however, are applicable regardless of the system used.

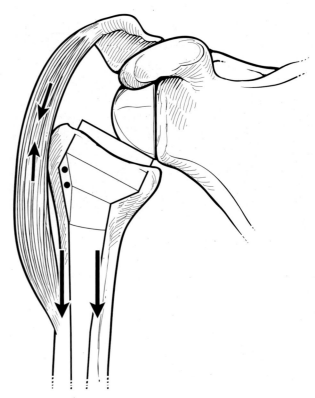

Figure 28-1 Forces acting at the glenohumeral component interface in a reverse prosthesis. These forces could contribute to subsidence of an uncemented humeral component.

TECHNIQUE FOR INSERTION OF A REVERSE-PROSTHESIS HUMERAL COMPONENT

Once the inferior capsule is released from the neck of the glenoid as described in Chapter 27, humeral preparation begins. The humeral head retractor is removed, and the humeral head is dislocated by externally rotating and extending the arm. This maneuver is typically easier than in cases of unconstrained arthroplasty because the compromised rotator cuff offers little resistance to proximal humeral dislocation. A Hohmann retractor positioned superior to the coracoid process is moved to the margin of the humeral head, which is often "bald" (devoid of any discernible rotator cuff),

and a modified Hohmann retractor is placed inferiorly and medially at the surgical neck of the humerus to complete the proximal humeral exposure (Fig. 28-2).

In most patients being treated with a reverse prosthesis, minimal if any peripheral humeral head osteophytes are present. In the uncommon situation in which large humeral osteophytes exist, they are removed with a half-inch osteotome and mallet, just as in cases of unconstrained shoulder arthroplasty (see Chapter 11). In contrast to cases of anatomic arthroplasty in which humeral osteophytes are removed to facilitate identification of the anatomic neck of the humerus to guide resection of the humeral head, osteophytes are removed in reverse-prosthesis procedures to avoid mechanical impingement between the

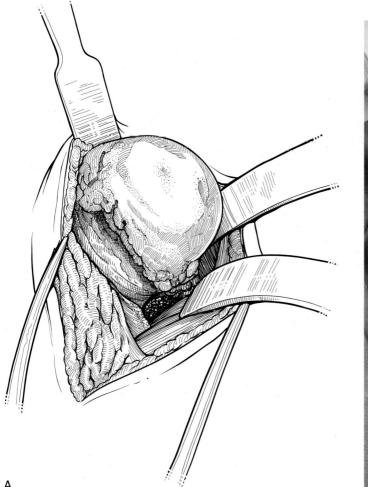
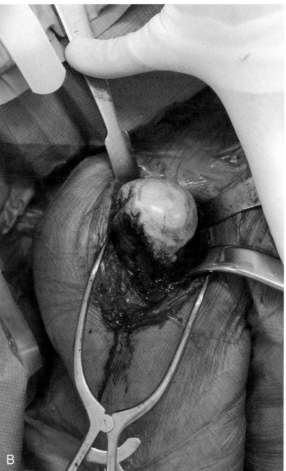

A

B

Figure 28-2   A and **B,** Completed exposure of the proximal humerus in preparation for insertion of a reverse prosthesis.

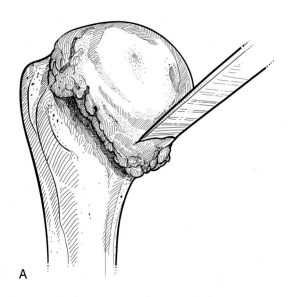

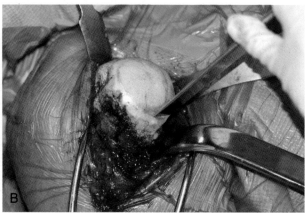

Figure 28-3 **A** and **B,** Large proximal humeral osteophytes may cause mechanical impingement after implantation of a reverse prosthesis if not removed.

osteophytes and the axillary border of the scapula (Fig. 28-3). A starter awl is used to open the humeral canal (Fig. 28-4). It is helpful to refer to preoperative radiographs to select the proper starting point for the awl, which should be in line with the humeral canal (Fig. 28-5). The humeral head can become deformed in patients with long-standing rotator cuff tears and can make identification of this starting point difficult. The humeral cutting guide, which sets resection at a 155-degree angle of inclination, is placed down the humeral canal (Fig. 28-6).

The system that we use allows selection of humeral cut version from neutral to 20 degrees of retroversion with the forearm used as a reference (Fig. 28-7). The advantage of resecting the humeral head in neutral is that less potential impingement may take place between the medial aspect of the humeral component and the lateral border of the scapula with internal rotation (Fig. 28-8). The disadvantage of resecting the humeral head in neutral is that in some cases the humeral cut may nearly miss the articular surface because the patient may normally have excessive humeral retroversion (Fig. 28-9). Conversely, the advantage of resecting the humeral head in 20 degrees of retroversion is that the humeral cut appears more nearly anatomic (Fig. 28-10). The disadvantage of

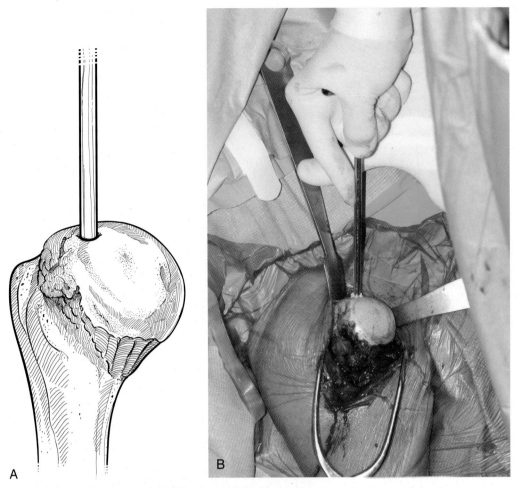

Figure 28-4   **A** and **B,** A starter awl is used to open the humeral canal.

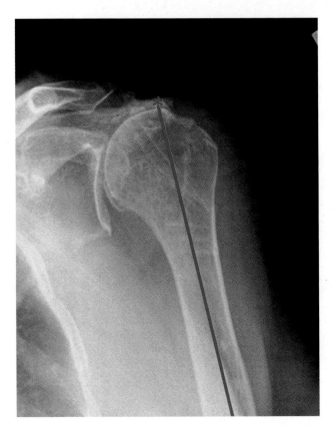

Figure 28-5   The preoperative anteroposterior radiograph is useful to approximate the position of the starting point for the awl.

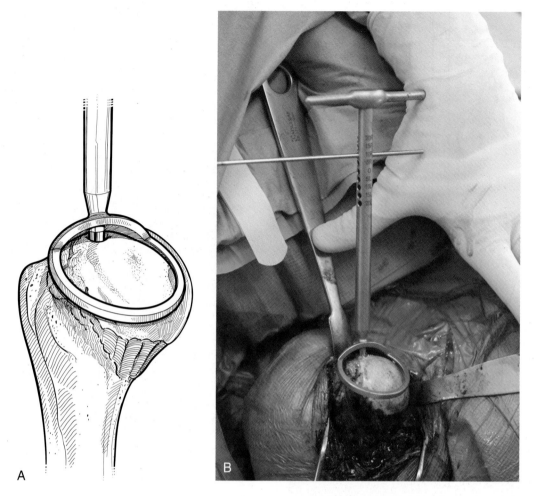

Figure 28-6   **A** and **B,** Insertion of the humeral cutting guide.

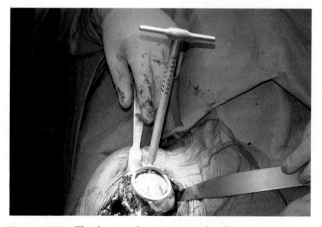

Figure 28-7   The humeral cutting guide allows resection of the humeral head from neutral to 20 degrees of retroversion with respect to the forearm.

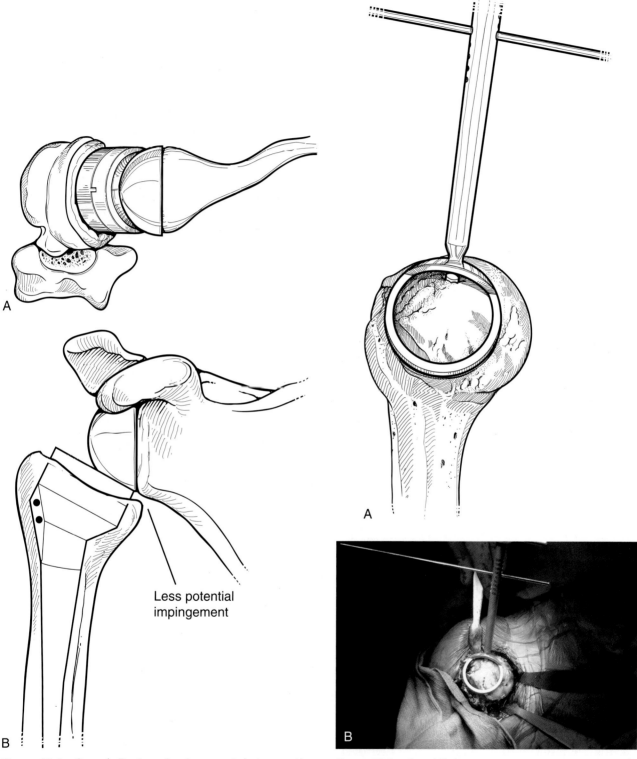

A

B

Less potential impingement

B

A

B

Figure 28-8 **A** and **B,** Less impingement between the medial aspect of the humeral component and lateral border of the scapula may occur during internal rotation with the humeral resection performed in neutral.

Figure 28-9 **A** and **B,** In some cases an attempt at resection of the humeral head in neutral may not allow resection of any humeral articular surface.

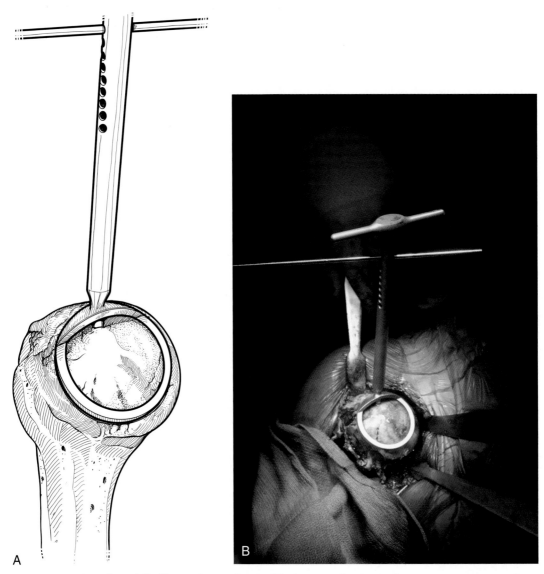

Figure 28-10   A and **B,** Humeral resection in 20 degrees of retroversion appears more nearly anatomic.

resecting the humeral head in 20 degrees of retroversion is that more inferior impingement may take place with internal rotation (Fig. 28-11). As a compromise between these two extremes, we routinely select 10-degree retroversion with the alignment guide (Fig. 28-12). Resection of the humeral head is performed by

resecting a small amount of bone by cutting just under the guide (Fig. 28-13).

With the system that we use, two epiphyseal component sizes are available, 36 and 42 mm. The advantage of the 36-mm component is that it can be used for virtually every case. The advantage of the 42-mm

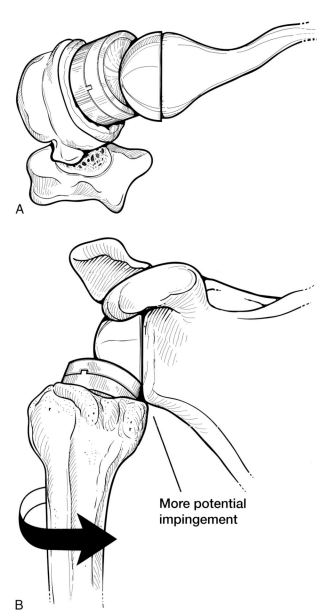

A

B

Figure 28-11 **A** and **B,** More impingement between the medial aspect of the humeral component and the lateral border of the scapula may occur during internal rotation with the humeral resection performed in 20 degrees of retroversion.

More potential impingement

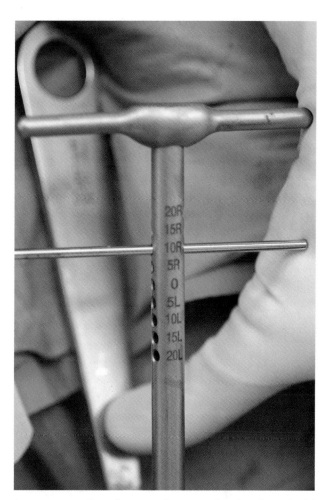

Figure 28-12 Ten degrees of retroversion is selected with the alignment guide.

component is that it may impart more stability to the prosthesis, although its large size prohibits use in many cases. Because prosthetic instability has been a rare problem in our experience, we prefer to use the 36-mm implant in nearly all cases. Epiphyseal reaming is performed with a 36-mm-diameter acetabular-type

reamer while keeping the reamer's orientation perpendicular to the cut humeral surface (Fig. 28-14). A single-size metaphyseal reamer is introduced (Fig. 28-15). Progressive diaphyseal reaming is performed until the appropriate diaphyseal diameter is attained, as evidenced by the diaphyseal reamer's reaching the inner

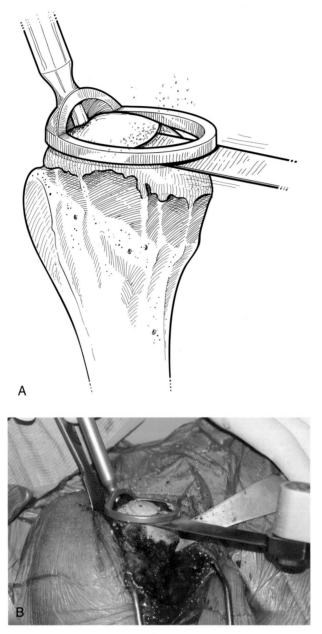

Figure 28-13   **A** and **B,** Resection of the humeral head with the cutting guide.

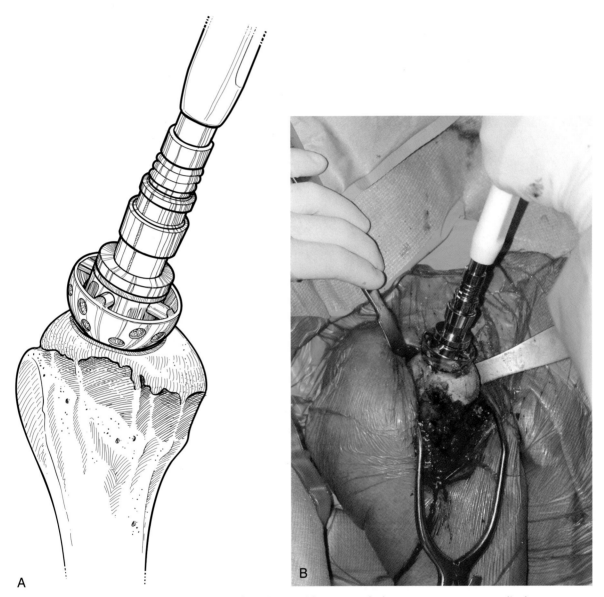

A

B

Figure 28-14 **A** and **B,** Epiphyseal reaming with an acetabular-type reamer perpendicular to the cut humeral surface.

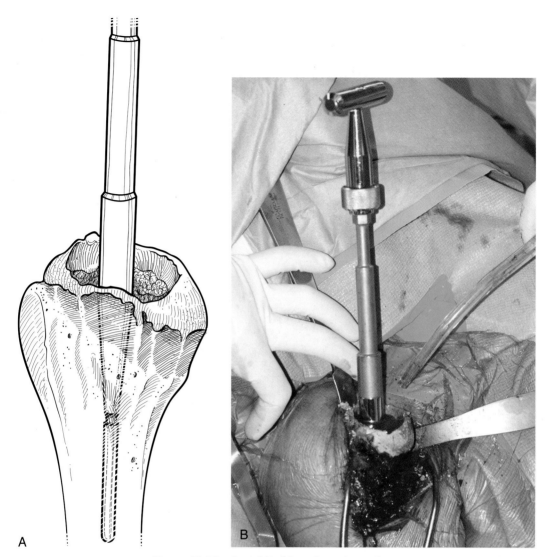

Figure 28-15 **A** and **B,** Metaphyseal reaming.

humeral cortex (Fig. 28-16). The trial stem is assembled by screwing the selected diaphyseal component onto the 36-mm metaphyseal component (Fig. 28-17). The trial is attached to the insertion guide, which is marked for humeral version with respect to the forearm (Fig. 28-18). The trial implant is inserted at 10 degrees of humeral retroversion by using the insertion guide (Fig. 28-19). The location of the lateral fin of the trial is marked with the electrocautery on the humeral metaphysis to use as a reference when later inserting the final humeral implant (Fig. 28-20). The trial implant is removed and a sponge is placed in the humeral metaphysis before retracting the humerus posteriorly for preparation of the glenoid (Fig. 28-21). Alternatively, some systems allow insertion of a

Text continued on p. 264

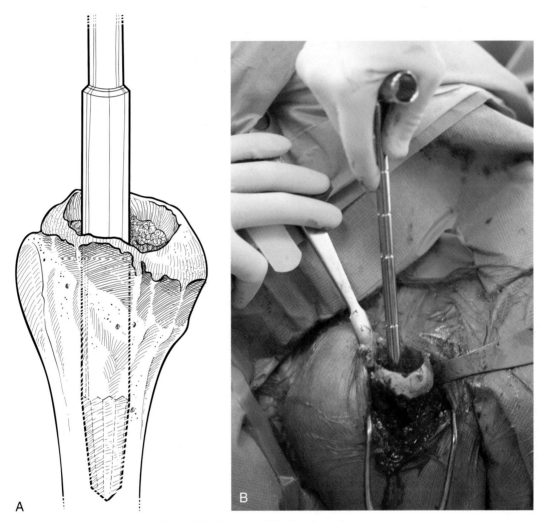

A

B

Figure 28-16   **A** and **B,** Diaphyseal reaming.

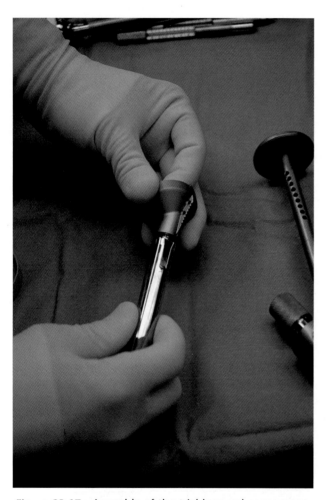

Figure 28-17   Assembly of the trial humeral component.

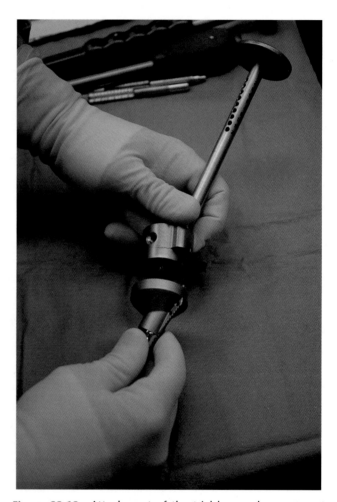

Figure 28-18   Attachment of the trial humeral component to the insertion guide.

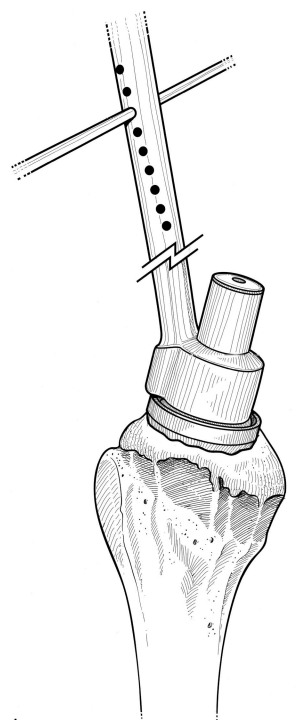

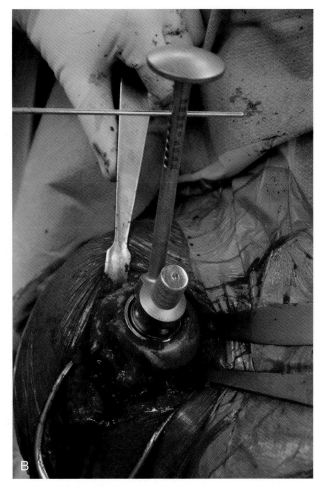

Figure 28-19 **A** and **B,** Insertion of the trial humeral component in 10 degrees of humeral retroversion.

A

B

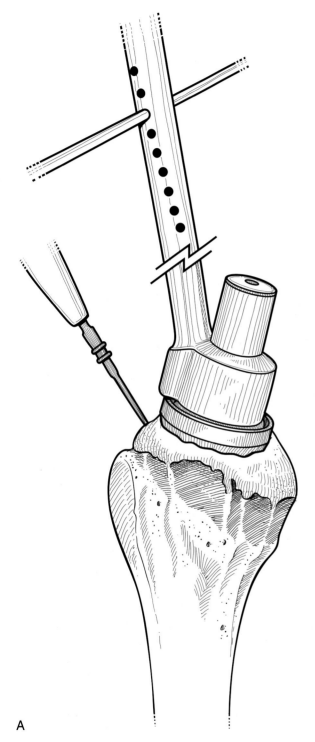

A

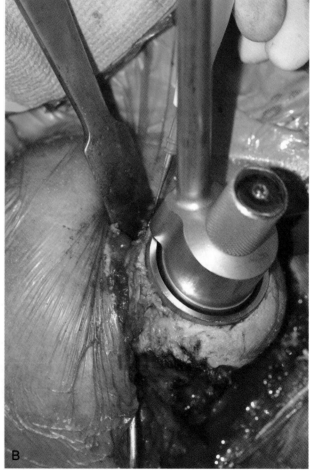

B

Figure 28-20 **A** and **B,** An electrocautery is used to mark the location of the fin of the trial implant to assist in placement of the final humeral implant in the desired version.

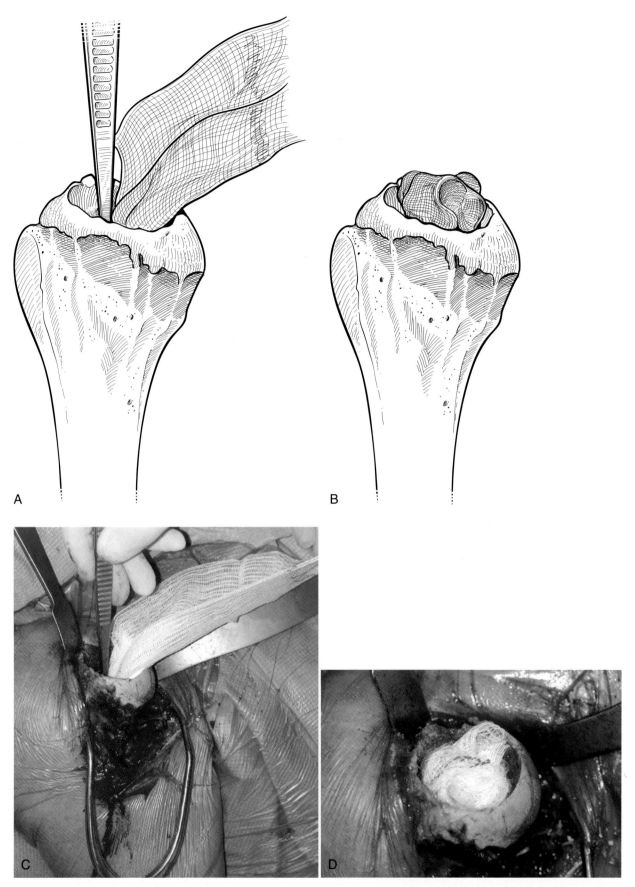

Figure 28-21 **A** to **D**, A sponge is placed in the humeral metaphysis after the trial humeral component is removed.

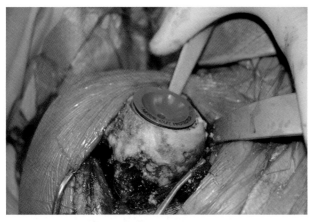

Figure 28-22 Humeral cut protector. This cut protector may prohibit glenoid exposure.

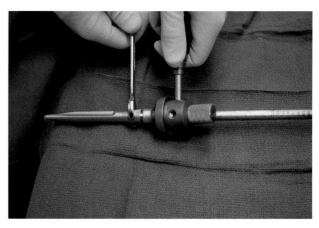

Figure 28-24 Assembly of the final humeral implant.

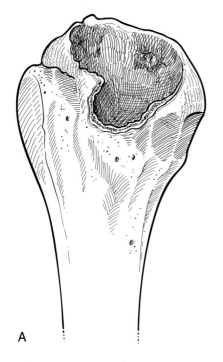

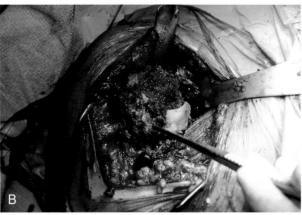

Figure 28-23 **A** and **B,** "Controlled fracture" of the anterior aspect of the proximal humerus to allow exposure of the glenoid.

humeral cut protector to avoid fracture of the anterior aspect of the humerus during posterior retraction (Fig. 28-22). We have, however, found it necessary in many cases to create a "controlled fracture" of the lesser tuberosity during posterior retraction of the humerus to obtain adequate access to the glenoid (Fig. 28-23). In our experience, this controlled fracture technique has had no detrimental consequences.

The glenoid is prepared and implanted as detailed in Chapter 29. The final humeral implant is assembled by securing the metaphyseal component to the insertion handle and screwing the diaphyseal component onto the metaphyseal portion with the wrenches provided (Fig. 28-24). The proximal humerus is dislocated anteriorly and the sponge removed from the humeral metaphysis. A cement restrictor is placed at the appropriate level to create a 1-cm cement mantle distal to the tip of the stem (Fig. 28-25). If the subscapularis is present, three transosseous no. 2 permanent braided sutures are placed through the stump of the subscapularis tendon and the lesser tuberosity for later use in reattachment of the subscapularis (Fig. 28-26). The humeral canal is irrigated and dried. Fast-curing polymethylmethacrylate cement (DePuy 2 bone cement, DePuy, Inc., Warsaw, IN) is placed in the humeral canal with a catheter tip 60-mL syringe that has been modified by cutting off the distal aspect of the plastic tip with heavy bandage scissors (Fig. 28-27). The insertion handle is used to place the prosthesis. Care is taken to ensure that the prosthesis is placed in

Text continued on p. 268

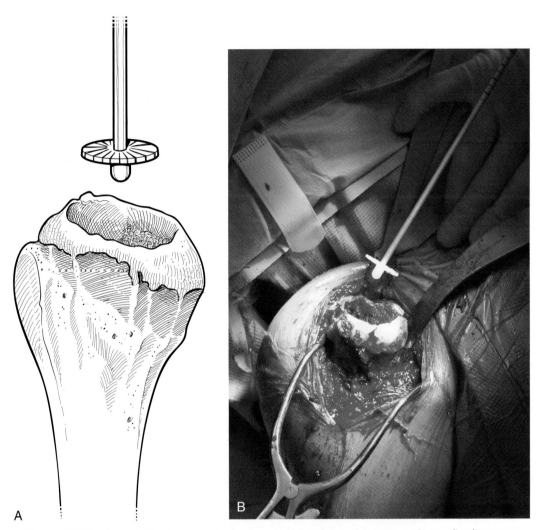

A

B

Figure 28-25 **A** and **B,** Placement of a cement restrictor to create a 1-cm distal cement mantle.

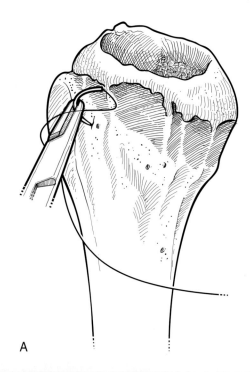

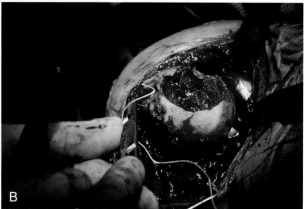

Figure 28-26 **A** and **B**, Placement of sutures for reattachment of the subscapularis.

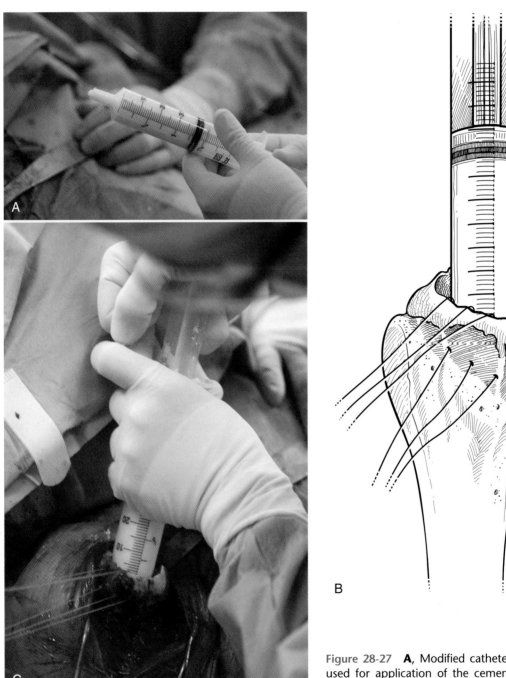

Figure 28-27 **A,** Modified catheter tip syringe used for application of the cement. **B** and **C,** Insertion of cement into the humeral canal.

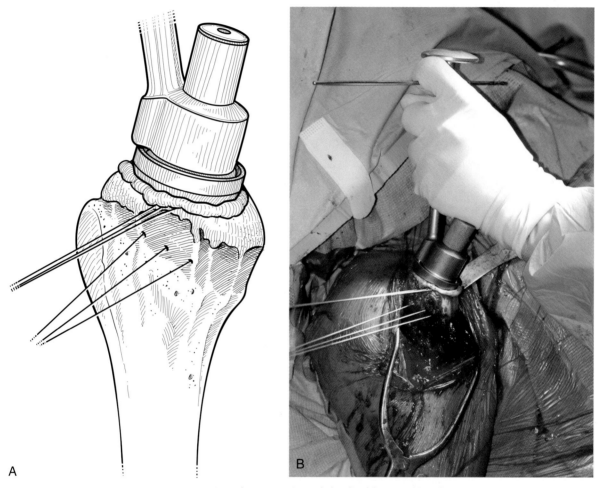

A   B

Figure 28-28   **A** and **B,** Insertion of the final humeral implant.

10 degrees of retroversion by using the previously made electrocautery mark on the humerus and the insertion guide (Fig. 28-28). In most cases the prosthesis will be rotationally stable immediately after insertion, thus allowing immediate placement of a trial spacer and reduction to check soft tissue tension (Fig. 28-29). In cases of proximal humeral bone loss, the cement should be allowed to cure completely before reduction of the prosthesis to maintain proper version (Fig. 28-30).

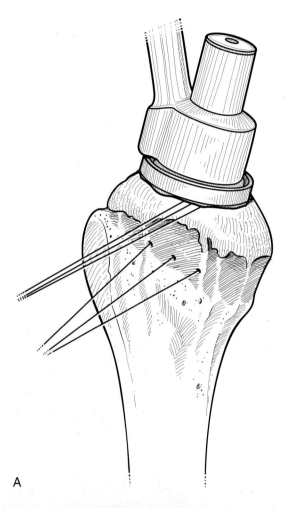

A

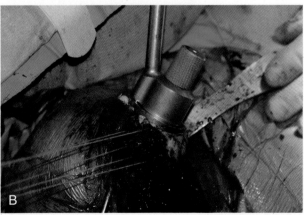

B

Figure 28-29 **A** and **B,** Case in which the humeral stem is rotationally stable. Trial reduction can be initiated before complete curing of the polymethylmethacrylate.

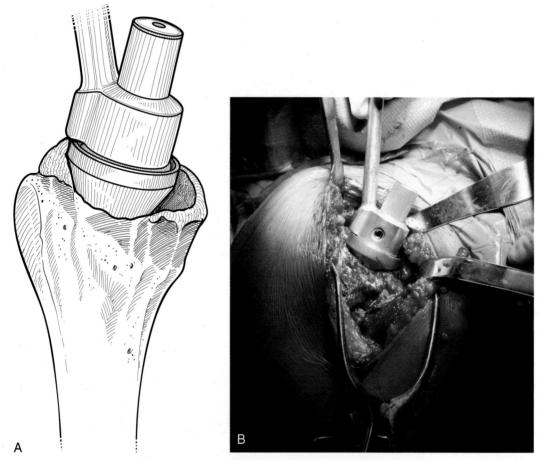

A

B

Figure 28-30 **A** and **B,** Case in which the humeral stem is rotationally unstable secondary to proximal humeral bone loss. Trial reduction should not be initiated before complete curing of the polymethylmethacrylate.

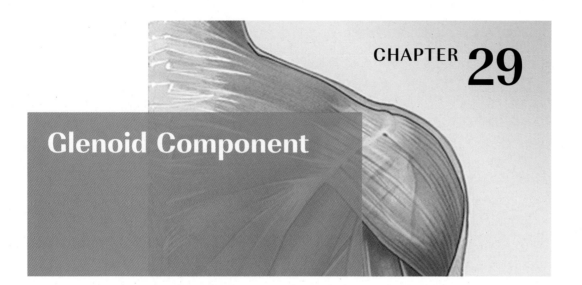

CHAPTER 29

Glenoid Component

Unlike cases of unconstrained shoulder arthroplasty, in which placement of a glenoid component is optional, the glenoid component must be placed during reverse shoulder arthroplasty. As in unconstrained arthroplasty, adequate glenoid exposure is paramount in placement of the glenoid component and is covered in Chapter 27. Many different implant companies are now manufacturing reverse-design shoulder prostheses. The glenoid components of the various brands generally consist of an uncemented metal base plate and a modular metallic glenosphere. The number and orientation of fixation screws used for the base plate and the design of the base plate (flat back versus convex back) vary among manufacturers. The specific implant with the longest and most successful follow-up is the Grammont-designed Delta (DePuy, France). Our preference is to use an implant that does not differ appreciably from this clinically tested design. The Grammont-designed Delta base plate consists of a flat back with a central peg and is fixated with four peripheral cortical screws. The glenosphere is placed over the base plate to allow a medialized center of rotation. The technique described in this chapter is applicable to this type of reverse glenoid component.

GLENOID PREPARATION AND COMPONENT IMPLANTATION

After humeral preparation is complete (see Chapter 28), the proximal humerus is retracted posteriorly with a Trillat glenohumeral retractor or a large glenoid rim retractor (see Chapter 3). We avoid using a Fukuda glenohumeral retractor during implantation of a reverse prosthesis because the base plate fixation screws may incarcerate the retractor (Fig. 29-1). After the glenoid is exposed by retracting the proximal humerus posteriorly, a drill hole is made with the inferior referencing guide provided. The guide is placed at the inferior border of the glenoid to align the inferior aspect of the glenosphere with the inferior aspect of the glenoid (Fig. 29-2). Placing the glenosphere in this position will help minimize the incidence of notching of the axillary border of the scapula as a result of the mechanical contact that occurs after implantation of the reverse prosthesis.

Reaming is performed while placing slight inferior pressure on the reamer to introduce approximately 10 degrees of inferior tilt to the surface of the glenoid. This inferior tilt serves three purposes: first, it increases stability of the prosthesis by maximizing deltoid tension through distalization of the humerus (Fig. 29-3); second, it reduces the incidence of scapular notching (Fig. 29-4); and third, it helps avoid inadvertently placing the glenoid component in a superiorly oriented position, which can lead to early glenoid failure (Fig. 29-5). Reaming is performed only to remove any remaining cartilage and flatten the glenoid surface. It is not necessary to ream to cancellous bone, and such reaming should be avoided. Additionally, many patients undergoing implantation of a reverse prosthesis have osteopenic bone that is susceptible to fracture during glenoid preparation. To help avoid fracture, the reamer is always started before contacting the bone and then gradually and gently advanced to engage the bone and ream it to a flat surface (Fig. 29-6). Once reaming is complete, the cortical aperture of the glenoid hole is opened to a slightly larger diameter (7.6 mm) to accommodate the central

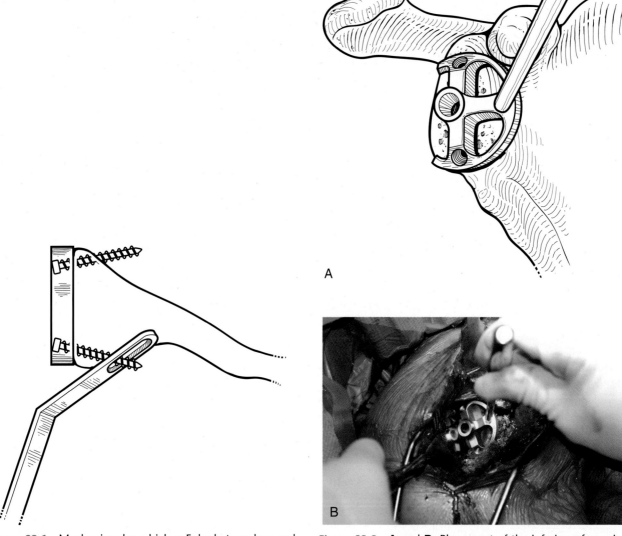

A

B

Figure 29-1 Mechanism by which a Fukuda-type humeral retractor may become incarcerated by a glenoid base plate fixation screw.

Figure 29-2 **A** and **B,** Placement of the inferior referencing guide for drilling the initial hole in the glenoid face.

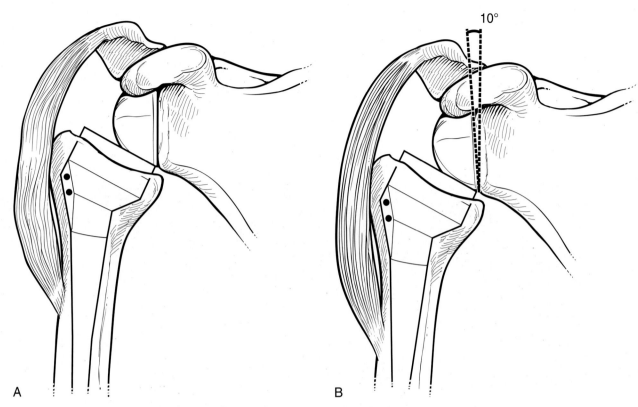

Figure 29-3   A and **B,** Mechanism by which an inferiorly tilted glenoid component maximizes deltoid tension and thereby increases prosthetic stability.

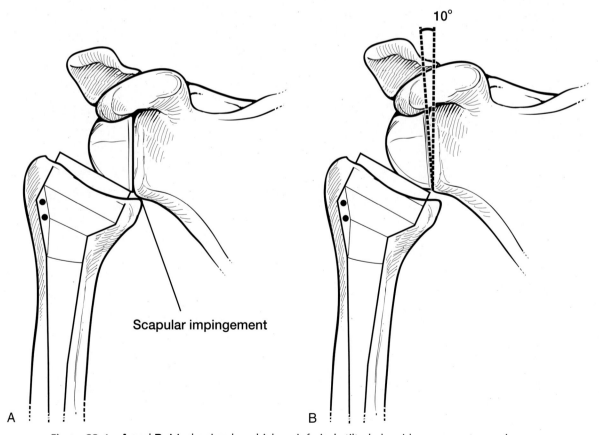

Scapular impingement

Figure 29-4   A and **B,** Mechanism by which an inferiorly tilted glenoid component may decrease the incidence of scapular notching.

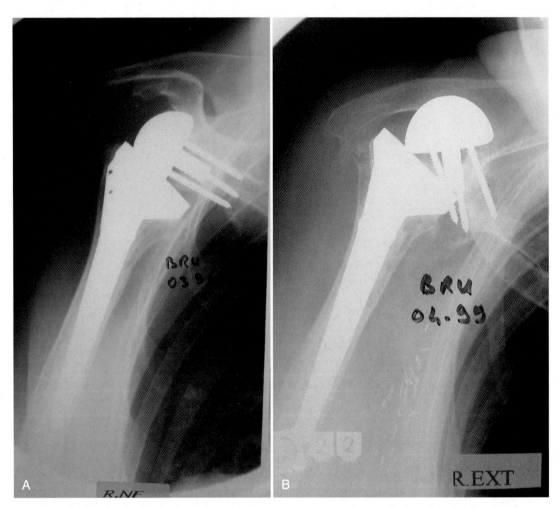

Figure 29-5 **A** and **B,** Radiographs of a glenoid component inadvertently placed with superior tilt that resulted in early glenoid failure.

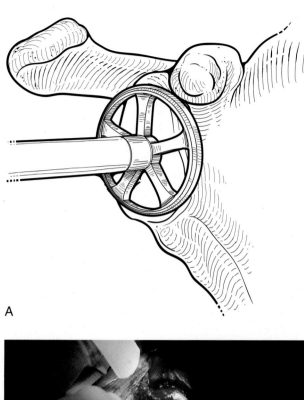

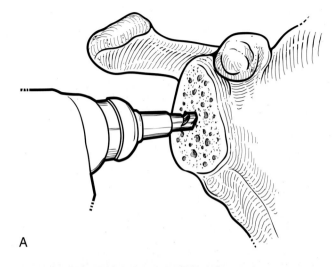

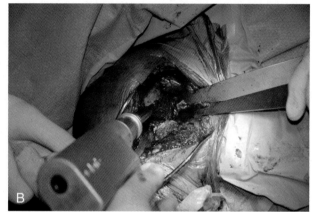

Figure 29-7   **A** and **B,** A 7.6-mm drill bit is used to enlarge the central peg hole for fixation of the base plate. This step can be omitted in patients with moderate to severe osteopenia.

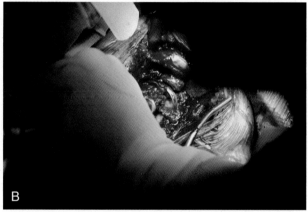

Figure 29-6   **A** and **B,** Reaming of the glenoid to a flat surface.

peg of the glenoid base plate (Fig. 29-7). In patients with moderate to severe osteopenia, this step may be omitted.

The glenoid base plate is oriented and introduced with the insertion handle (Fig. 29-8). A mallet is used to impact the base plate until it is flush with the glenoid bone circumferentially. The insertion handle is disengaged from the base plate, and the base plate is checked to ensure that it has been completely seated by inserting the tips of vascular forceps into each hole (Fig. 29-9). If any concern exists over incomplete seating of the base plate, a large smooth tamp may be used to further impact the base plate. Additionally, the peripheral inferior rim of the base plate should be confirmed to be in contact with underlying glenoid. If

the implant is not seated inferiorly, early glenoid loosening can occur. Occasionally, the base plate will be larger in anteroposterior diameter than the native glenoid, such as with bone loss or in a small patient (Fig. 29-10). This is not generally a problem as long as bone is visible in the anterior and posterior base plate holes. If the bone loss is severe, bone graft reconstruction of the glenoid may be necessary (see the following section of this chapter).

The next step involves screw insertion to complete fixation of the base plate. Fixation of the glenoid base plate in our chosen prosthetic system involves the use of two different types of screws. The inferior and superior screws lock into a mobile variable-angle washer

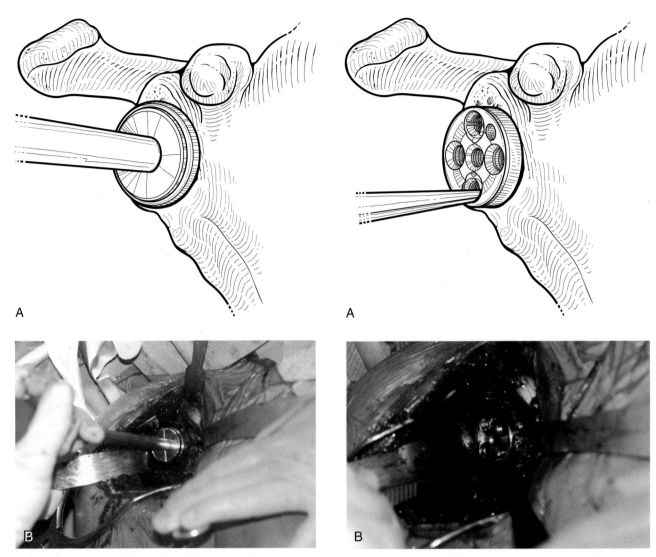

A

A

B

B

Figure 29-8 **A** and **B,** The glenoid base plate is introduced with the insertion handle.

Figure 29-9 **A** and **B,** Vascular forceps are used to ensure complete seating of the base plate.

captured in the base plate to create a fixed-angle device once the screw is tightened. The anterior and posterior screws are placed through a standard hole within the base plate that does not contain a locking mechanism (Fig. 29-11). The anterior and posterior screws can be placed at variable angles and allow compression of the base plate against the glenoid bone, whereas the inferior and superior screws "set" the distance between the implant and glenoid bone as soon as the threaded head engages the locking washer within the base plate (Fig. 29-12). Because of these special considerations, the screws are inserted and tightened in a specific order. The inferior screw is placed first to ensure maintenance of contact of the inferior aspect of the base plate with the underlying osseous glenoid. A drill guide is placed in the inferior hole of the base plate.

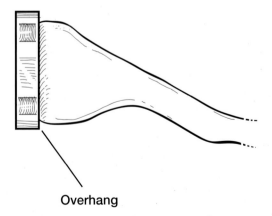

Overhang

Figure 29-10 Base plate with anterior and posterior overhang caused by a small native glenoid.

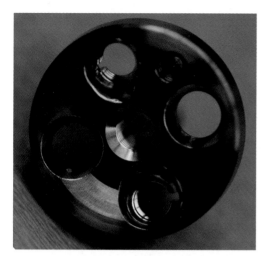

Figure 29-11 The screw holes for the base plate. The inferior and superior holes contain variable-angle locking washers that allow the screws to lock into the base plate as the screw heads are advanced into the washer, thereby fixing the angle of the screw within the base plate. The anterior and posterior screws do not lock into the base plate and serve to create compression between the base plate and the native glenoid.

A drill (3.0-mm bit) is used through the guide to create a bicortical hole (Fig. 29-13). The direction of the drill should be chosen to maximize screw length so that the strongest fixation possible is provided. Because of the inferior position of the base plate, if the drill is directed too inferiorly, it may exit the glenoid bone prematurely and result in poor fixation (Fig. 29-14). If the drill is passed perpendicular to the base plate, screw length may be shorter than desired (Fig. 29-15). We have found that directing the drill halfway between the perpendicular and the maximal inferior direction allowed by the mechanical constraints of the base plate permits consistent placement of a sufficiently long screw (Fig. 29-16).

After the second cortex is penetrated with the drill bit, a depth gauge is used to determine screw length

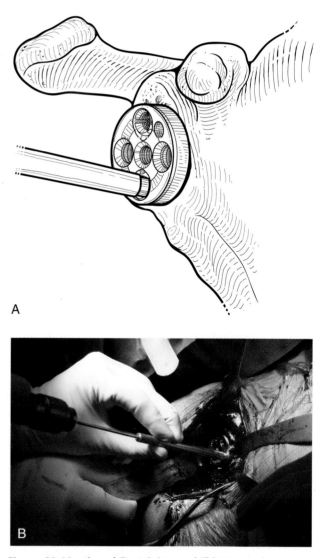

Figure 29-12 **A** and **B,** Mechanism of base plate screw fixation with anterior and posterior screws to initially compress the base plate to the native glenoid. The inferior and superior screws are then tightened to create a fixed-angle device.

Figure 29-13 **A** and **B,** A 3.0-mm drill bit is used to create the screw holes for base plate fixation.

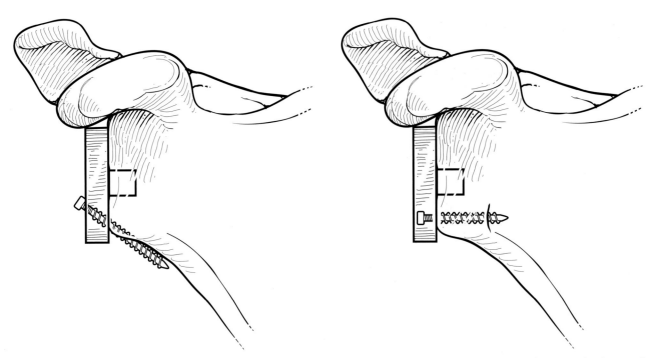

Figure 29-14   If the inferior base plate screw is directed at too steep an angle, the screw may miss the glenoid bone.

Figure 29-15   If the drill is directed perpendicular to the base plate, screw length may be shorter than desired.

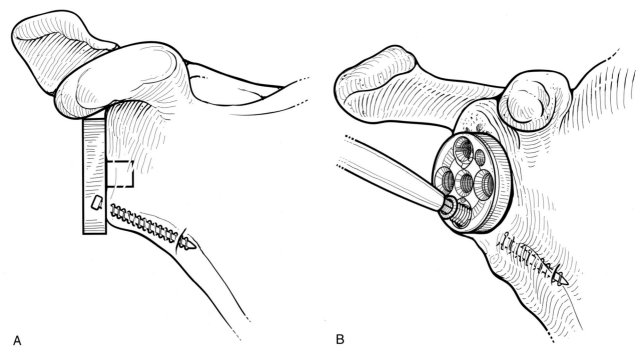

A

B

Figure 29-16   **A** and **B,** Optimal inferior screw placement.

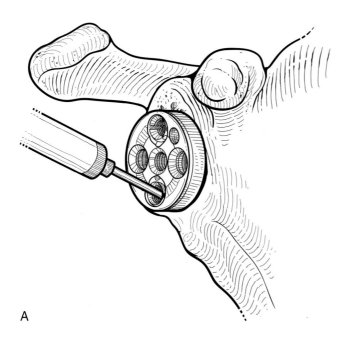

A

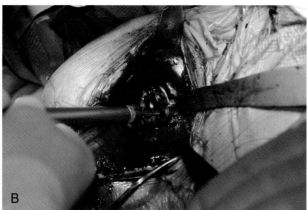

B

Figure 29-17 **A** and **B,** A depth gauge is used to determine screw length.

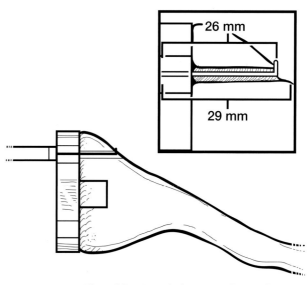

Figure 29-18 The obliquity of the scapula at the point where the screw tip exits the bone may cause too short a screw to be selected inadvertently.

(Fig. 29-17). The obliquity of the scapula may cause a screw of too short a length to be selected (Fig. 29-18). Therefore, multiple measurements are obtained with the depth gauge and the longest measurement taken. If the length measured is between two sizes, the longer size is always selected to ensure bicortical thread purchase. Muscle tissue overlies the point at which the screw tips exit the scapula; no neurovascular structures are at risk if the screw tip is slightly protruding beyond the scapular cortex. We have yet to witness symptoms caused by a screw that was radiographically too long.

A 4.5-mm screw is introduced and tightened to just before the point that the threaded screw head engages the washer of the base plate (Fig. 29-19). If the threaded head of the inferior screw engages the base plate washer, no further compression between the base plate and glenoid bone can be obtained (Fig. 29-20). The advantage of partially inserting the inferior screw first is that it assists in maintaining contact between the inferior aspect of the base plate and the native glenoid (Fig. 29-21). The drill for the superior locking screw is directed toward the base of the coracoid process (Fig. 29-22). The process of using the depth gauge is repeated for the superior locking screw. The superior screw is then inserted, once again making sure to not engage the base plate when the screw is advanced.

The anterior and posterior screws are the final phase of insertion of the base plate. These nonlocking screws are placed at insertion angles judged to be optimal for cortical purchase. Whereas the inferior and superior screws are always divergent, the anterior and posterior screws are typically convergent. The drill is typically angled toward the central peg of the glenoid base plate and passes just superior or inferior to the central peg to perforate the opposite cortex (i.e., the anterior drill hole passes just superior to the central peg and perforates the posterior cortex deep within the glenoid vault, and the posterior drill hole passes just inferior to the central peg and perforates the anterior cortex

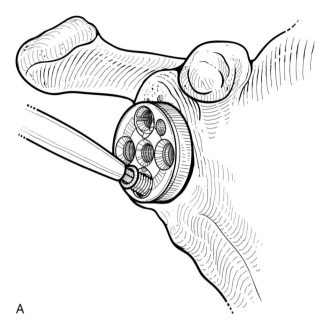

A

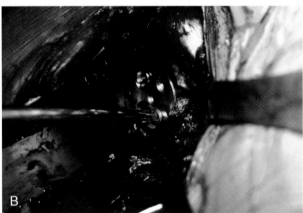

B

Figure 29-19 **A** and **B,** Partial insertion of the inferior base plate screw.

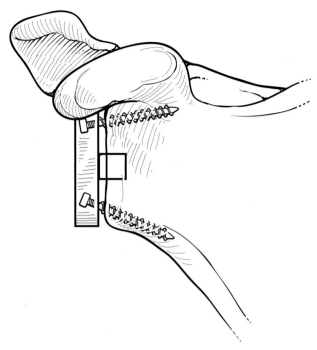

Figure 29-20 Mechanism by which compression of the base plate against the native glenoid is prohibited by completely seating the inferior or superior screw, or both screws.

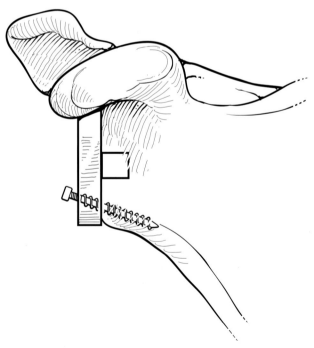

Figure 29-21 The base plate is prevented from tilting superiorly by the partially inserted inferior screw during fixation of the base plate.

deep within the glenoid vault; Fig. 29-23). The depth gauge is used for selection of screw length, and the anterior and posterior screws are inserted. In contrast to the inferior and superior screws, the anterior and posterior screws are fully tightened to provide compression between the base plate and the glenoid bone. After the anterior and posterior screws are fully seated, the inferior and then superior screws are fully tightened to engage and complete fixation of the base plate (Fig. 29-24). Occasionally, the anterior or posterior screw will not obtain satisfactory osseous purchase because of underlying osteopenia. In this case the screw is left in place to provide interference-type resistance to loosening of the glenoid component.

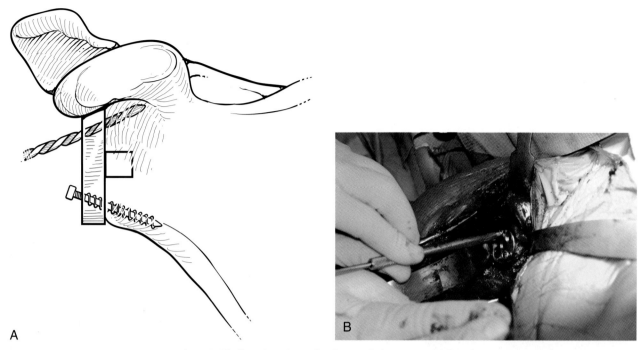

Figure 29-22 **A** and **B,** Drill direction into the base of the coracoid for the superior locking screw.

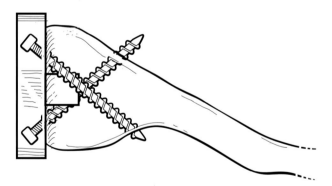

Figure 29-23 Optimal placement of the anterior and posterior compression screws.

The periphery and central hole of the base plate are cleared of soft tissue and blood, and the glenosphere component is positioned on the base plate with a screwdriver as an insertion device (Fig. 29-25). The glenosphere attaches to the base plate via a peripheral rim Morse taper and is further secured with a central safety screw (in the system that we use) (Fig. 29-26). The glenosphere is impacted into place with the impaction device (Fig. 29-27), and the safety fixation screw is advanced to complete insertion of the glenoid component (Fig. 29-28).

GLENOID BONE LOSS WITH A PRIMARY REVERSE PROSTHESIS

Glenoid bone loss is most commonly observed in two scenarios when using a reverse prosthesis as a primary shoulder arthroplasty. In patients with massive rotator cuff tears and glenohumeral arthritis, static superior migration of the humeral head may lead to nonconcentric glenoid wear and superior erosion of the osseous glenoid (Fig. 29-29). If this bone loss is not addressed, the glenoid component may inadvertently

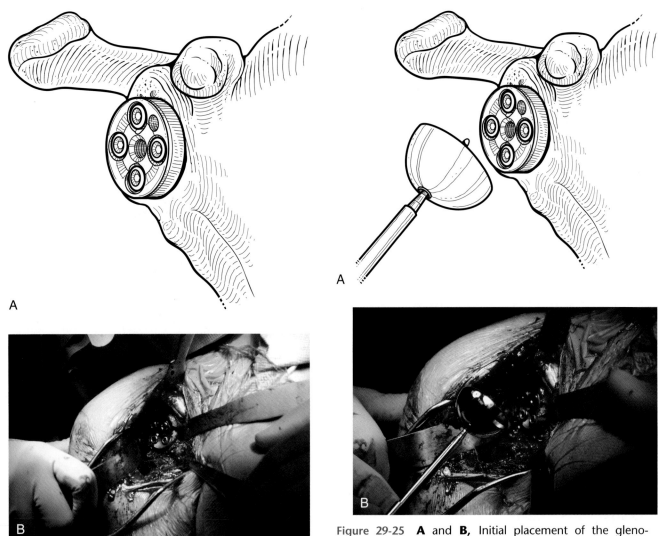

Figure 29-24 **A** and **B,** Final tightening of the inferior and superior locking screws to complete fixation of the base plate.

Figure 29-25 **A** and **B,** Initial placement of the gleno-sphere.

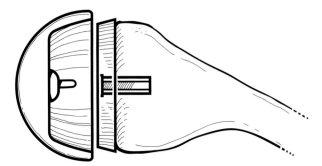

Figure 29-26 Mechanism of glenosphere fixation to the base plate.

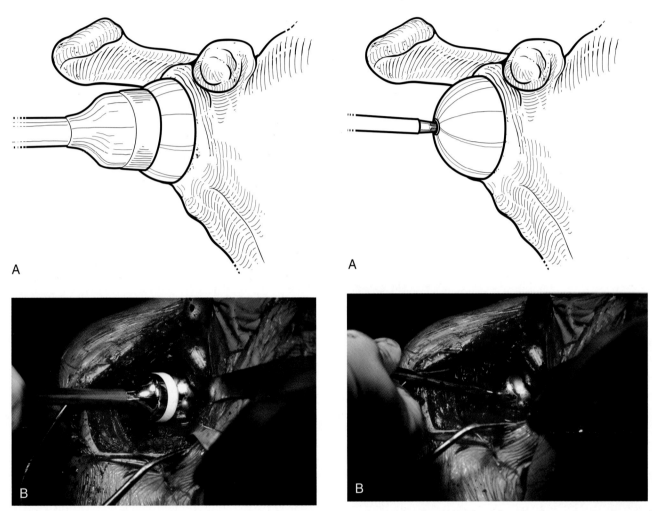

A

B

A

B

Figure 29-27 **A** and **B,** The glenosphere is impacted into place by engaging the Morse taper.

Figure 29-28 **A** and **B,** The safety fixation screw is advanced to complete insertion of the reverse-prosthesis glenoid component.

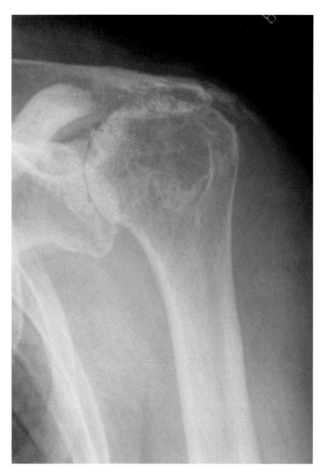

Figure 29-29 Radiograph showing superior erosion of the osseous glenoid.

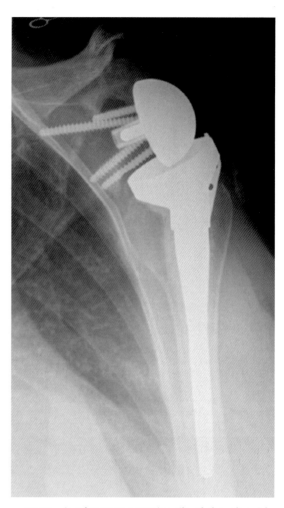

Figure 29-30 Inadvertent superior tilt of the glenoid component may be introduced by not appreciating superior glenoid erosion during glenoid preparation.

be implanted with superior tilt and risk glenoid failure (Fig. 29-30). In cases of mild superior bone loss, preferential inferior reaming alone can correct the glenoid orientation (Fig. 29-31). In moderate cases of superior glenoid bone loss, the superior orientation of the glenoid is initially corrected by preferential inferior reaming. This leaves a superior biconcave glenoid deformity. The resected humeral head can be contoured with a rongeur to fit behind the superior portion of the base plate and fill this osseous defect (Fig. 29-32). The base plate is inserted in standard fashion by placing the superior screw through the bone graft and native glenoid (Fig. 29-33). In cases of severe superior glenoid osseous deficiency the resected humeral head may be too small, and use of an autogenous iliac crest bone graft may be necessary for glenoid reconstruction. Details of this technique are provided in Chapter 40.

The less common scenario in which glenoid reconstruction may be necessary during implantation of a reverse prosthesis as a primary arthroplasty is for the treatment of fixed anterior glenohumeral dislocation.

Chronic anterior shoulder dislocations in older patients often result in erosion of the anterior glenoid. When the severity of this erosion is such that no native glenoid is seen under the anterior base plate screw hole, anterior glenoid reconstruction with iliac crest bone graft is required. The need for a bone graft is usually determined on the preoperative computed tomogram (Fig. 29-34). A tricortical segment of iliac crest bone graft is harvested as described in Chapter 40. The bone graft is shaped to fit the defect with a small oscillating saw. The bone graft is positioned anteriorly and fixated with two or three guide pins for 4.0-mm cannulated screws (Fig. 29-35). Care is taken to place the guide pins so that they will not interfere with the post of the glenoid base plate (Fig. 29-36). Partially threaded 4.0-mm cannulated screws with washers are placed after overdrilling the guide pins and measuring the appropriate length according to standard insertion technique (Fig. 29-37). After

Text continued on p. 289

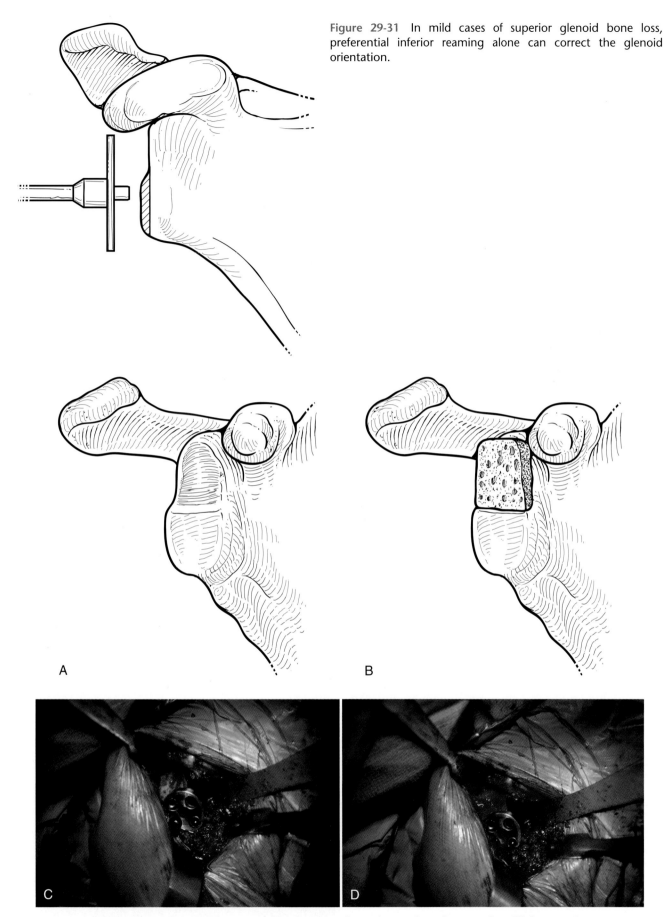

Figure 29-31 In mild cases of superior glenoid bone loss, preferential inferior reaming alone can correct the glenoid orientation.

A

B

C

D

Figure 29-32 **A** to **D,** The resected humeral head may be used as a bone graft to fill the superior glenoid defect.

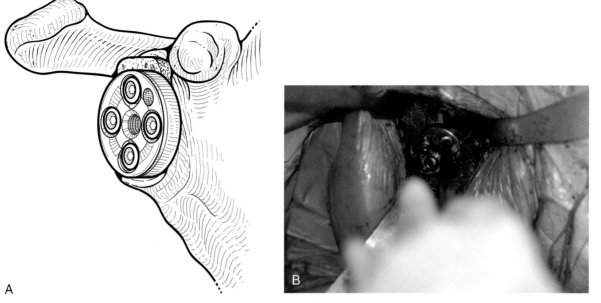

Figure 29-33 **A** and **B,** Base plate fixation after superior bone grafting of the glenoid.

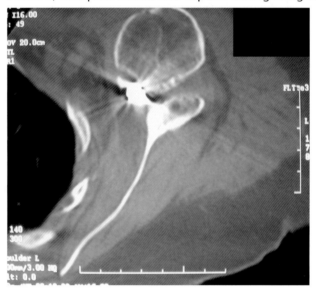

Figure 29-34 Preoperative computed tomogram in a patient with a fixed anterior dislocation showing severe anterior glenoid bone loss requiring bone grafting at the time of insertion of the reverse prosthesis.

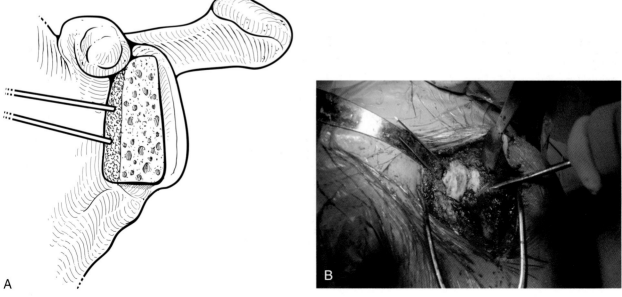

Figure 29-35 **A** and **B,** Temporary fixation of an anterior bone graft with guide wires for 4.0-mm cannulated screws.

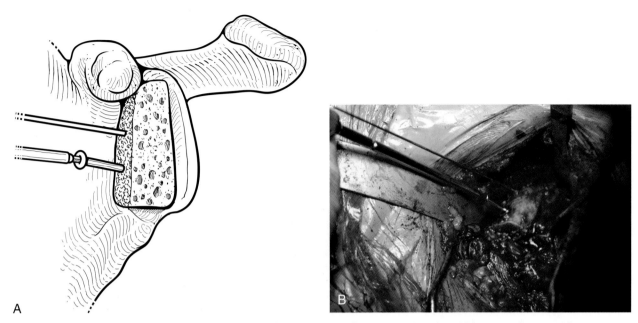

Figure 29-36 **A** and **B**, Placement of fixation screws for an anterior glenoid bone graft to avoid interference with the central peg of the base plate.

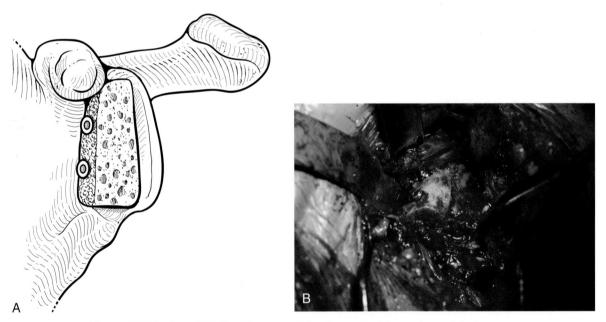

Figure 29-37 **A** and **B**, Final bone graft fixation with 4.0-mm cannulated screws.

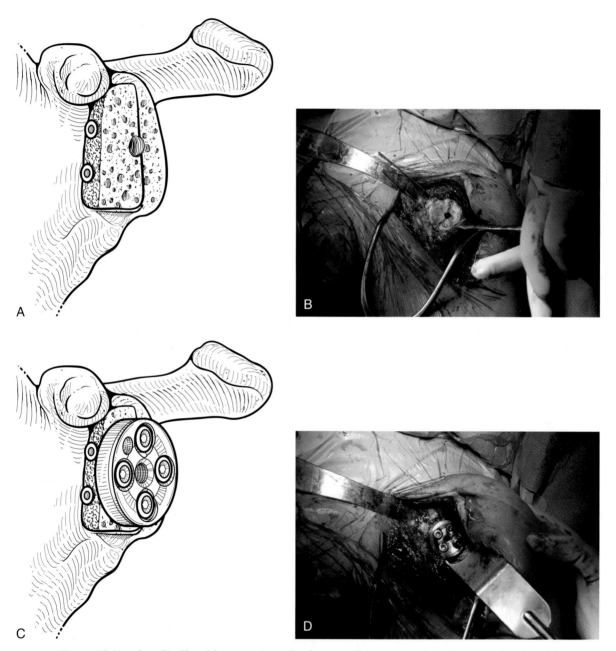

Figure 29-38   **A** to **D**, Glenoid preparation after bone graft reconstruction of an anterior glenoid defect.

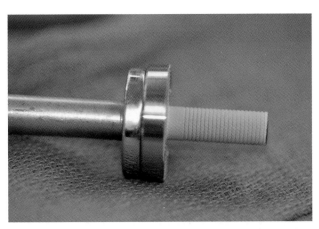

Figure 29-39 Base plate with a longer central peg to allow fixation into native glenoid bone in patients with severe glenoid osseous deficiency.

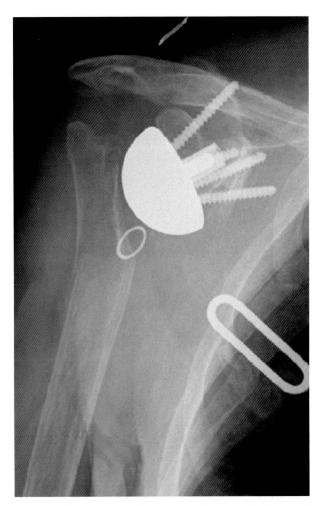

Figure 29-40 Radiograph of glenoid reconstruction with placement of the glenoid component as stage 1 of a two-stage procedure.

restoration of glenoid bone stock with the bone graft, the glenoid is prepared and the glenoid component inserted as previously described (Fig. 29-38).

If glenoid reconstruction with iliac crest bone graft is necessary before insertion of the glenoid component, every effort should be made to have a portion of the central peg of the base plate placed in native glenoid bone. Some companies manufacture base plates with a longer central peg to address this problem (Fig. 29-39). If it is not possible to place the central peg within the native glenoid bone or if the glenoid component does not seem to be securely fixed (or both), staged arthroplasty should be performed (Fig. 29-40). In staged arthroplasty, the glenoid component is inserted, and the humerus, after being prepared for the humeral component, is left without a humeral implant

for 6 months to allow the glenoid bone graft to consolidate. During this 6-month period, the patient is allowed to use the arm as tolerated, although function will be limited. After 6 months, the second stage is completed by inserting the humeral component.

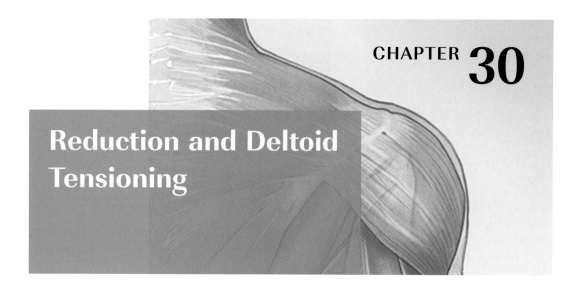

CHAPTER 30

Reduction and Deltoid Tensioning

Perhaps the most important and yet most subjective portion of the surgical technique for implantation of a reverse prosthesis is proper tensioning of the deltoid. The most frequent complication of a reverse prosthesis that requires further treatment is dislocation of the glenohumeral prosthesis. Proper tensioning of the deltoid can help minimize this complication.

HUMERAL COMPONENT TRIALING

After the humeral component has been inserted as described in Chapter 28, humeral component trialing begins. In patients with proximal humeral bone loss, component trialing should not begin before complete curing of the polymethylmethacrylate. In patients with good proximal support of the humeral component, prosthetic trialing commences immediately after insertion of the humeral component within the bone cement.

Trial reduction starts with insertion of the 6-mm polyethylene trial insert into the metaphyseal portion of the final implant (Fig. 30-1). The glenohumeral joint is reduced (this should be somewhat difficult) by applying longitudinal traction to the arm and placing a finger in the "cup" of the trial insert to guide the humeral component toward the glenosphere (Fig. 30-2). Gradually flexing the arm as traction is applied

assists in reduction. Deltoid tension is evaluated by stabilizing the scapula and applying longitudinal traction to the arm in neutral position (Fig. 30-3). We have anesthesia personnel maintain neuromuscular paralysis during this portion of the procedure, and the anterior glenoid rim retractor holding the conjoined tendon medially is relaxed. A finger is placed at the interface of the humeral and glenoid components (Fig. 30-4). Minimal (<2 mm) "pistoning" should occur with this maneuver. If tension is inadequate, the 9-mm insert is placed and reduction and testing are repeated. A 12-mm insert is available, as is a 9-mm metallic metaphyseal augment, to further increase tension if necessary (Fig. 30-5). Once appropriate tension has been obtained, it may be difficult to dislocate the implant with the trial polyethylene insert. We routinely use a bone hook on the edge of the trial insert to provide traction on the prosthesis (Fig. 30-6). As traction is applied, the arm is extended to dislocate the prosthesis.

After an insert of appropriate size is selected, the final spacer implant is impacted into the metaphyseal portion of the humeral component while taking care to align the notch in the insert appropriately (Fig. 30-7). When necessary, a metallic metaphyseal augment is placed first by impacting it into the humeral component like the polyethylene insert and then further securing it with a central screw (Fig. 30-8). The polyethylene insert is then impacted into the augment

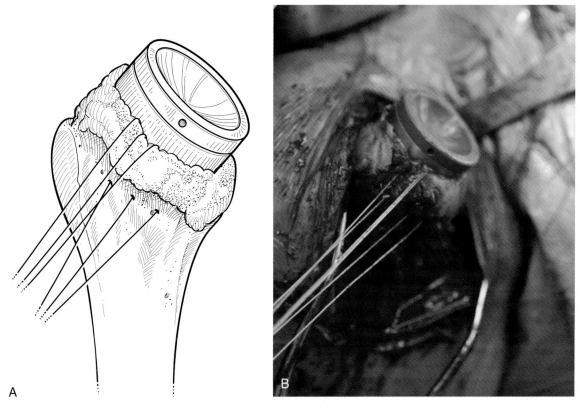

Figure 30-1 **A** and **B**, Insertion of a trial insert into the humeral stem.

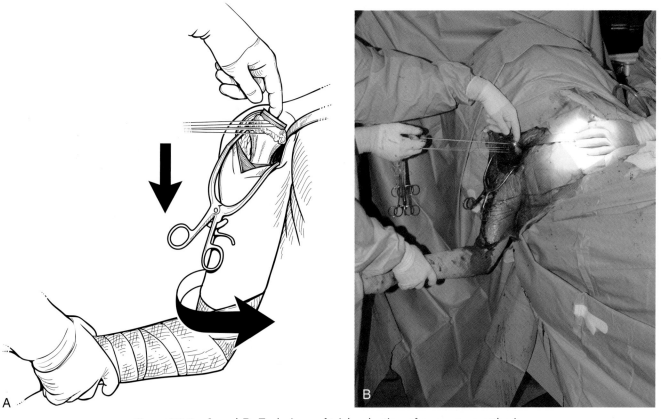

Figure 30-2 **A** and **B**, Technique of trial reduction of a reverse prosthesis.

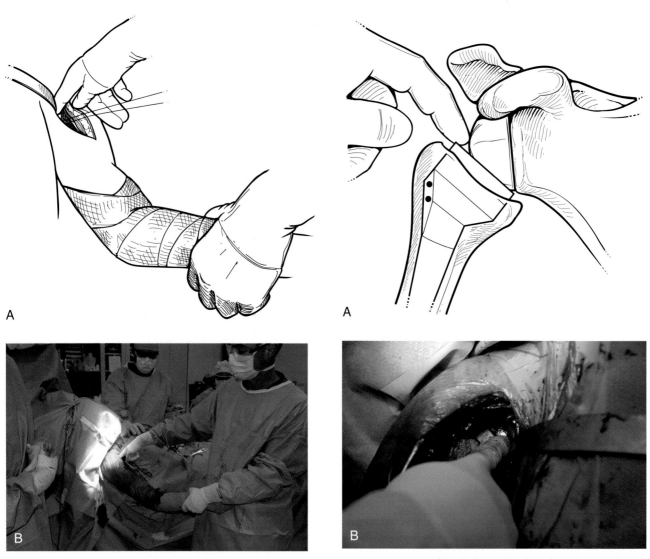

Figure 30-3 **A** and **B,** Technique for evaluating deltoid tension.

Figure 30-4 **A** and **B,** A finger is placed at the interface of the trial insert and the glenosphere to evaluate deltoid tension.

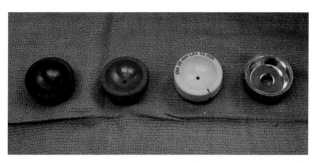

Figure 30-5 Polyethylene inserts of various sizes and a metallic metaphyseal augment used to increase deltoid tension.

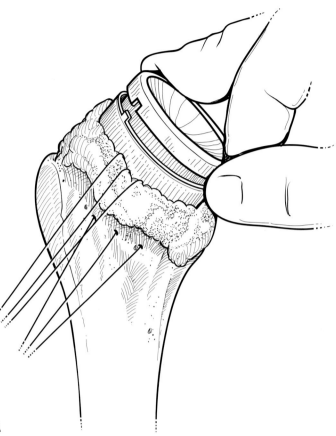

A

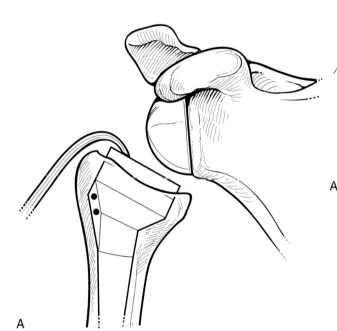

A

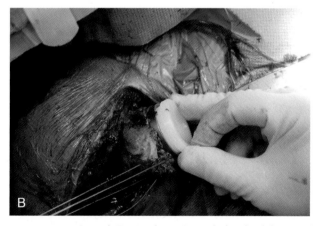

B

Figure 30-7 **A** and **B,** Implantation of the final humeral polyethylene insert.

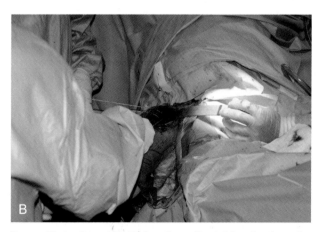

B

Figure 30-6 **A** and **B,** Dislocation after trial reduction of an adequately tensioned reverse prosthesis with a bone hook.

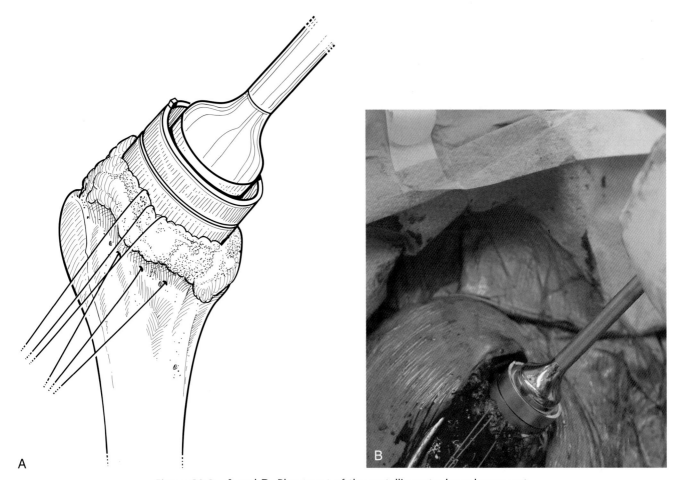

Figure 30-8   **A** and **B,** Placement of the metallic metaphyseal augment.

(Fig. 30-9). If present, the subscapularis is repaired with the previously placed transosseous sutures to further enhance prosthetic stability (Fig. 30-10).

SPECIAL CONSIDERATIONS— METAPHYSEAL BONE LOSS

Severe humeral metaphyseal bone loss merits special consideration during implantation of a reverse prosthesis. Nearly all cases of prosthetic dislocation that

we have observed have occurred in this situation. During primary arthroplasty with a reverse prosthesis, metaphyseal bone loss most commonly occurs when treating fracture sequelae (Fig. 30-11). With metaphyseal bone loss, no capsular or rotator cuff attachments exist between the scapula and humerus, thus leaving the large muscles of the shoulder girdle (deltoid, short head of the biceps, coracobrachialis) to provide nearly all the soft tissue tension and hence stability for the reverse prosthesis. Although the initial reduction of the reverse prosthesis may seem adequately tensioned,

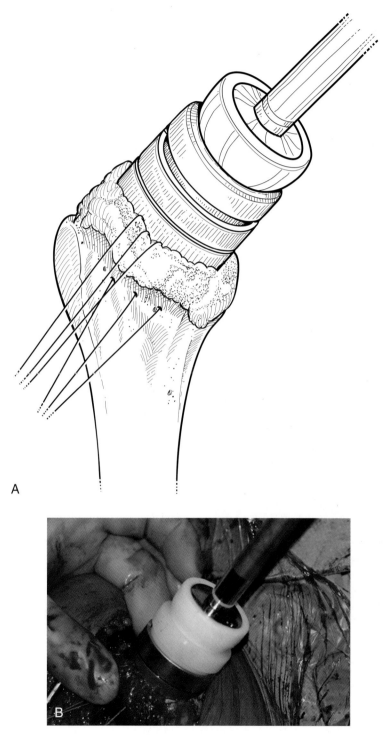

Figure 30-9 **A** and **B,** The polyethylene insert is impacted into the metallic augment.

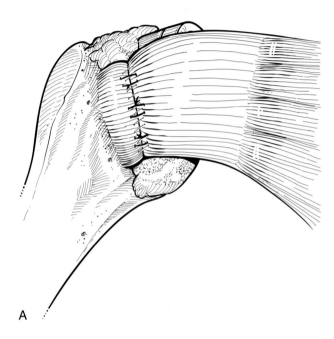

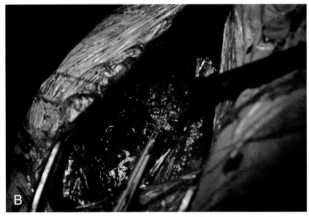

Figure 30-10 **A** and **B,** The subscapularis tendon, if present, is repaired.

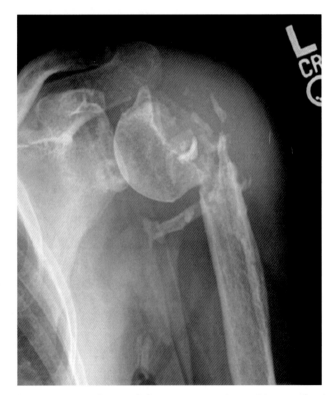

Figure 30-11 Case of fracture sequelae with proximal humeral bone loss.

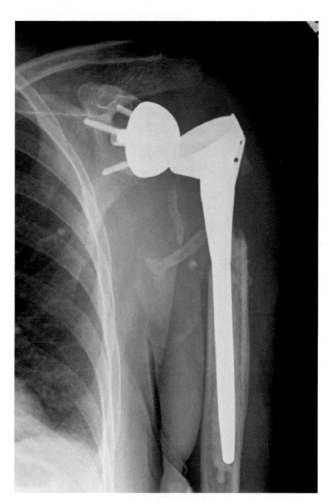

Figure 30-12 Case of prosthetic instability occurring in a patient with significant proximal humeral bone loss.

the biomechanical properties of these large muscles (compliance, stretch) allow them to lengthen over time and cause the initial tension to dissipate, thereby potentially leading to prosthetic instability (Fig. 30-12).

We address metaphyseal bone loss at the time of insertion of the reverse prosthesis by maximizing soft tissue tension during implantation and reduction of the prosthesis. In this situation, after insertion of the glenoid component, we reinsert the trial humeral stem with the 6-mm polyethylene insert and reduce the prosthetic glenohumeral joint. With longitudinal traction placed on the arm, the humeral component is manually telescoped maximally out of the humerus to the glenoid component (Fig. 30-13), and the level of the trial humeral implant with respect to the proximal humerus is marked (Fig. 30-14). The distance between the metaphyseal-diaphyseal prosthetic junction and

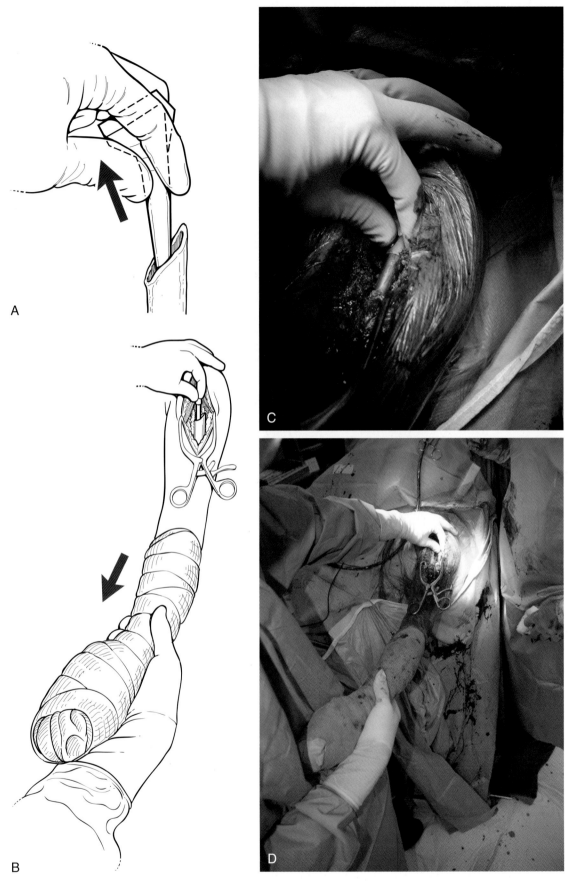

Figure 30-13 **A** to **D,** Estimation of the appropriate height for implantation of the humeral component in a patient with significant proximal humeral bone loss.

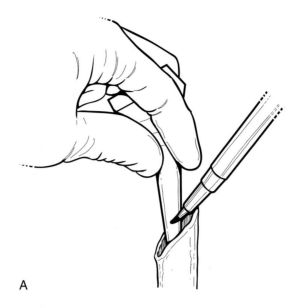

A

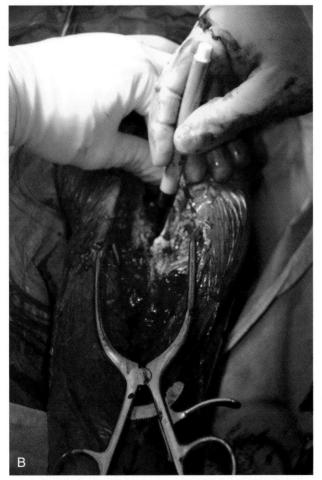

B

Figure 30-14 **A** and **B,** The implant is marked to assist in placing the humeral component at the appropriate level.

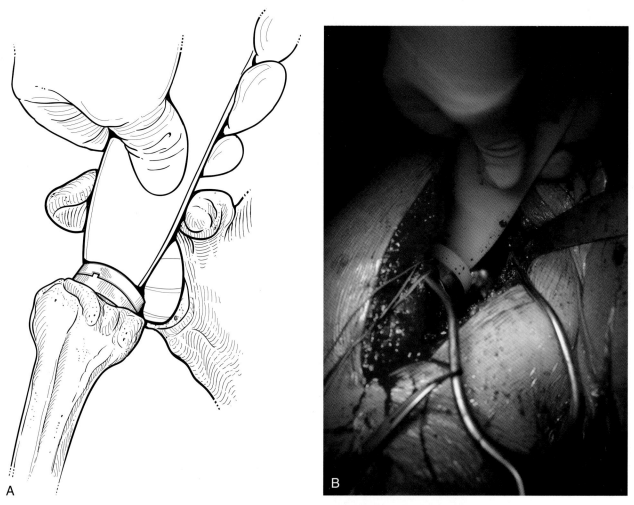

Figure 30-15   **A** and **B,** Reduction of the reverse prosthesis with the "shoe horn" technique.

the mark made with respect to the proximal humerus is compared with the distance templated preoperatively (see Chapter 25) to evaluate restoration of appropriate humeral length. This enables an estimation of the appropriate level at which to cement the humeral component. If the humeral component is cemented too distally within the humerus, adequate tension may not be obtainable. Conversely, if the humeral component is cemented too proximally within the humerus, the prosthetic joint may be irreducible.

Once the humeral component has been cemented in place within the humerus (see Chapter 28), trialing of the various inserts commences as previously described. In the scenario of metaphyseal bone loss, however, no pistoning is accepted between the components. Additionally, we often use a "shoe horn" instrument to aid in reduction by levering the humerus distally to engage the glenoid (Fig. 30-15). Once appropriate tension has been achieved, the final polyethylene insert is placed as described previously.

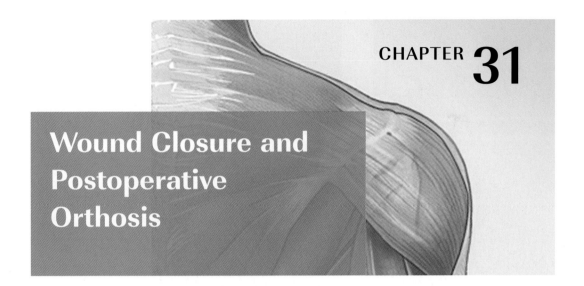

CHAPTER 31

Wound Closure and Postoperative Orthosis

The final steps in the operative procedure are wound closure and placement of the postoperative orthosis. Wound closure after implantation of a reverse prosthesis is performed similar to cases of unconstrained shoulder arthroplasty. Because of the void created by lack of a rotator cuff, wound closure becomes more important after insertion of a reverse prosthesis than in cases of unconstrained arthroplasty because postoperative hematoma has been the most commonly reported complication after this procedure.[1]

WOUND CLOSURE TECHNIQUE

After reduction of the prosthesis and closure of the subscapularis, if present, the wound is irrigated with 800 mL of antibiotic-impregnated sterile saline (50,000 units bacitracin per liter sterile normal saline) via a bulb syringe. The wound is checked to ensure that adequate hemostasis has been obtained. The electrocautery is used as necessary to minimize any residual hemorrhage. A medium-size closed suction drain is placed to help prevent postoperative hematoma formation. The trocar of the drain is used to puncture the soft tissue from inside the wound, and the skin is exited approximately 2 cm distal to the distal extent of the skin incision (Fig. 31-1). The drain is pulled through the skin until the transverse mark on the drain tube reaches the level of the skin (Fig. 31-2). The trocar is removed from the drain with scissors, and the other end of the drain is cut with scissors so that the tip of the drain rests in the void left by the absent rotator cuff (Fig. 31-3). When trimming the proximal end of the drain, care is taken to cut the drain between

holes to minimize the risk of drainage tube breakage during removal (Fig. 31-4).

Wound closure is initiated by reapproximating the deep fascial layer with no. 0 braided absorbable suture in an interrupted figure-of-eight technique (Fig. 31-5). Just as in cases of unconstrained shoulder arthroplasty, we do not close the deltopectoral interval. The subcutaneous fascia is reapproximated with 2-0 braided absorbable suture in an interrupted figure-of-eight technique (Fig. 31-6). The skin is reapproximated with 3-0 undyed absorbable monofilament suture in a subcuticular running closure technique (Fig. 31-7).

After skin closure is completed, the drain is checked to ensure that its position has been maintained. The occlusive draping is carefully removed from the site at which the drain tubing exits the skin. The skin in this area is cleaned and dried. Half-inch Steri-Strips are wrapped around the drain tubing to fix the drain to the skin and prevent inadvertent removal of the drain; we use two or three Steri-Strips (Fig. 31-8).

More of the occlusive draping is removed adjacent to the incision, and the skin is cleansed of blood with a saline-soaked sponge and then dried. Half-inch Steri-Strips are placed over the incision. Sterile gauze is then placed over the incision and a sterile absorbent pad is placed over the gauze. The dressing is secured with 3-inch foam tape. The remainder of the surgical drain is connected to the drainage tube, and the suction function of the drain is activated (Fig. 31-9). The remaining surgical drapes are then removed.

The surgical drain is removed the day after surgery regardless of the amount of drainage recorded. The dressing is maintained in place until postoperative day 3, at which time it is removed and not replaced. After removal of the dressing, the patient is allowed to

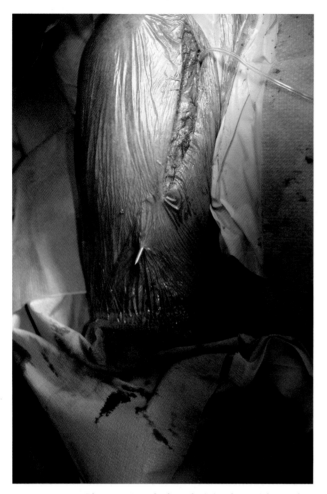

Figure 31-1 Placement of the drain tube with a sharp trocar.

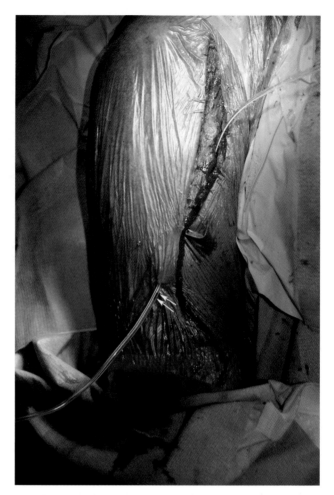

Figure 31-2 The drain is pulled through the skin until the transverse mark on the drain tube reaches the level of the skin (*arrows*).

shower, but submerging the incision in a bathtub is prohibited until 2 weeks postoperatively. The Steri-Strips are progressively removed by the patient as they lose their adhesion to the skin.

POSTOPERATIVE ORTHOSIS

The postoperative orthosis is placed in the operating room immediately after the dressing is applied. For a reverse prosthesis, we use a neutral-rotation sling (Ultrasling, Donjoy, Inc., Vista, CA; Fig. 31-10). The patient is allowed to remove the sling for performance of hand, wrist, and elbow mobility exercises and for hygiene. The duration for which the orthosis is maintained is determined by the presence or absence of humeral metaphyseal bone loss. In uncomplicated cases with sufficient metaphyseal bone, the sling is discontinued and physical therapy initiated 3 weeks after surgery. In patients with humeral metaphyseal bone loss, the sling is maintained for an additional week, and physical therapy is initiated 4 weeks after surgery. Details of the postoperative rehabilitation regimen are provided in Chapter 43.

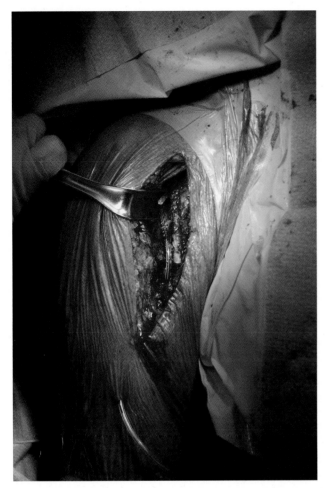

Figure 31-3 Placement of the drain in the surgical wound proximally.

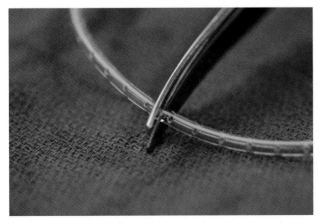

Figure 31-4 Proper trimming of the drain proximally to prevent breakage of the drain during removal.

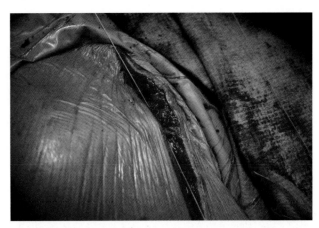

Figure 31-5 Closure of the deep fascial layer.

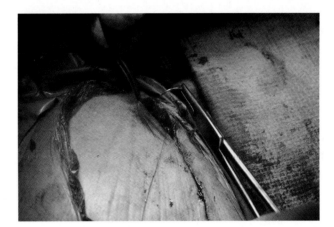

Figure 31-6 Closure of the subcutaneous fascia.

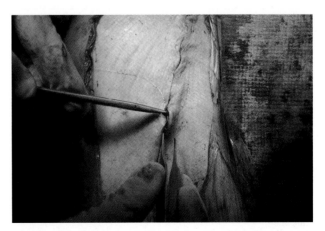

Figure 31-7 Subcuticular skin closure.

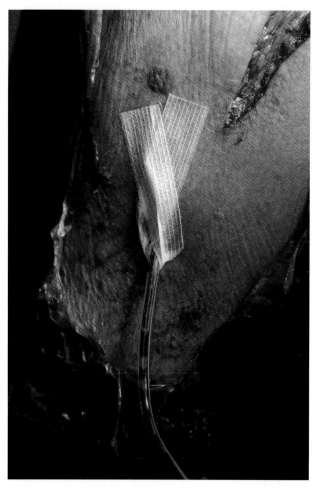

Figure 31-8   Fixation of the drainage tube with Steri-Strips.

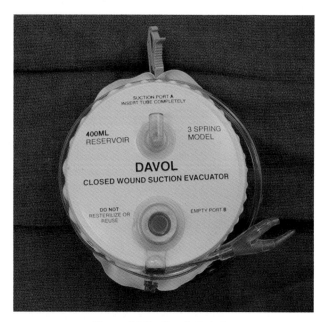

Figure 31-9   Surgical drain.

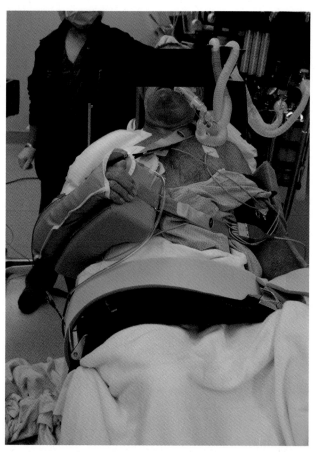

Figure 31-10   Neutral-rotation sling used after shoulder arthroplasty with a reverse prosthesis.

REFERENCE

1. Werner CM, Steinmann PA, Gilbart M, Gerber C: Treatment of painful pseudoparesis due to irreparable rotator cuff dysfunction with the Delta III reverse-ball-and-socket total shoulder prosthesis. J Bone Joint Surg Am 2005;87:1476-1486.

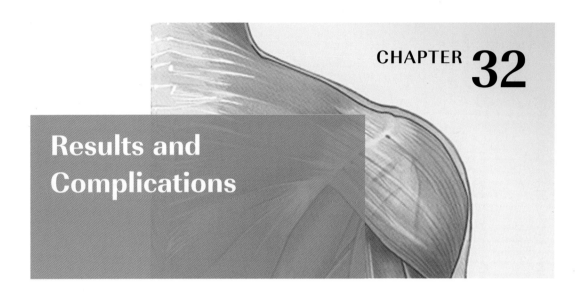

CHAPTER 32

Results and Complications

Reports on the results of reverse shoulder arthroplasty are becoming more common as implantation of this type of shoulder arthroplasty increases. The results vary predominantly by the underlying indication for which the arthroplasty was performed. We have participated in a large European-based study of the reverse prosthesis and continually enroll patients in our own database.[1] The results and complications presented in this chapter are drawn from these sources.

RESULTS

The results of reverse shoulder arthroplasty vary mainly with the etiology for which the arthroplasty was performed. The best results are obtained in the treatment of osteoarthritis with a massive rotator cuff tear (rotator cuff tear arthropathy), whereas results are least satisfactory in patients with post-traumatic arthritis. Tables 32-1 and 32-2 detail the results of reverse shoulder arthroplasty for the most common indications for which it is performed. These tables express the results in terms of active mobility; patient satisfaction; the Constant score, a shoulder-specific outcomes device incorporating pain, mobility, activity, and strength; and the age- and gender-adjusted Constant score.[2,3]

INTRAOPERATIVE COMPLICATIONS

Intraoperative complications are more common during reverse shoulder arthroplasty than during unconstrained shoulder arthroplasty performed for chronic conditions and may be divided into complications involving the humerus, glenoid, musculotendinous soft tissues (rotator cuff), and neurovascular structures.

Humerus

The most common humeral complication is iatrogenic fracture, which usually results from performing an overly aggressive dislocation maneuver without previous adequate soft tissue release. Many patients undergoing reverse shoulder arthroplasty have moderate to severe osteopenia, thus placing them at increased risk for this complication. Intraoperative tuberosity fractures during glenohumeral dislocation are less common during reverse shoulder arthroplasty than during unconstrained shoulder arthroplasty because of the lack of a rotator cuff attaching to the tuberosities, which could otherwise contribute to fracture during a dislocation maneuver. Fractures involving the humeral diaphysis should be reduced and a long-stem humeral implant placed. Allograft struts and cerclage cables may be added in patients with severe osteopenia (Fig. 32-1).

Intraoperative fractures involving the greater or lesser tuberosities (or both) are usually nondisplaced. Many of these fractures are stable or become stable once the humeral implant is inserted (Fig. 32-2). If a greater tuberosity fracture fragment that has maintained attachment of a substantial portion of the posterior rotator cuff is not satisfactorily stable, suture fixation of the tuberosity is performed and the postoperative rehabilitation adjusted accordingly to allow healing of the tuberosity. A greater tuberosity fracture fragment that is devoid of rotator cuff attachment and is unstable may simply be excised.

Table 32-1 RESULTS OF REVERSE SHOULDER ARTHROPLASTY ACCORDING TO UNDERLYING ETIOLOGY IN A LARGE EUROPEAN-BASED STUDY

Etiology	Absolute Constant Score (Points)		Active Forward Flexion (Degrees)		Active External Rotation (Degrees)		Excellent/ Good Subjective Results (%)
	Preoperative	Postoperative	Preoperative	Postoperative	Preoperative	Postoperative	
Cuff tear arthropathy (*n* = 74)	27	65	76	142	5	7	96
Massive rotator cuff tear (*n* = 41)*	28	63	89	139	11	12	96
Post-traumatic arthritis (*n* = 33)	20	53	70	113	−2	3	89
Primary osteoarthritis (*n* = 33)†	25	65	92	139	5	16	96

*Includes patients with massive rotator cuff tears and chronic pseudoparalysis but without glenohumeral arthritis.
†Includes patients with primary osteoarthritis and massive rotator cuff tears contributing to static humeral head migration.
From Wall B, Nové-Josserand L, O'Connor D, et al: Reverse total shoulder arthroplasty: A review of results according to etiology. J Bone Joint Surg Am 2007;89:1476-1485.

Table 32-2   RESULTS OF PRIMARY REVERSE SHOULDER ARTHROPLASTY ACCORDING TO UNDERLYING ETIOLOGY IN THE AUTHORS' PROSPECTIVE DATABASE FROM 2003 TO 2006

Etiology	Absolute Constant Score (Points)		Adjusted Constant Score (%)		Active Forward Flexion (Degrees)		Active External Rotation (Degrees)		Excellent/Good Subjective Results (%)
	Preoperative	Postoperative	Preoperative	Postoperative	Preoperative	Postoperative	Preoperative	Postoperative	
Cuff tear arthropathy (*n* = 63)	17	59	23	82	45	132	8	28	75
Massive rotator cuff tear (*n* = 10)*	25	72	32	94	38	161	11	29	80
Rheumatoid arthritis (*n* = 6)	13	48	18	67	32	60	3	6	50
Fixed dislocation (*n* = 8)	11	58	15	83	30	115	3	22	100
Post-traumatic arthritis (*n* = 20)	7	36	10	50	1	102	1	0	66
Acute fracture (*n* = 13)	7	60	10	82	8	142	3	15	50

*Includes patients with massive rotator cuff tears and chronic pseudoparalysis but without glenohumeral arthritis.

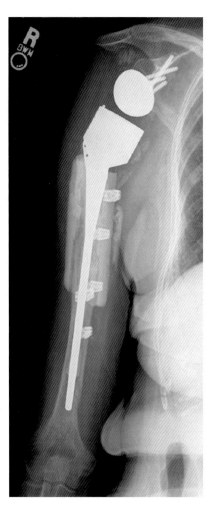

Figure 32-1   Patient with an intraoperative humeral diaphyseal fracture treated by placement of a long-stem humeral component and allograft struts fixed with cerclage cables.

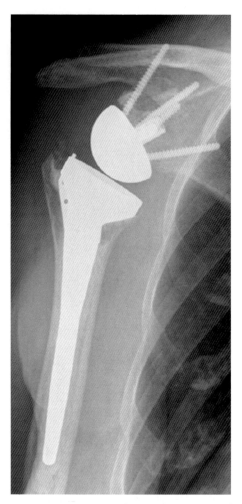

Figure 32-2   Postoperative radiograph of a patient with a nondisplaced lesser tuberosity fracture without any specific treatment.

Intraoperative lesser tuberosity fractures commonly occur during retraction of the proximal humerus in the course of glenoid preparation and insertion. The thin anterior cortex of the humeral metaphysis, including the lesser tuberosity, may be crushed by the humeral retractor (Fig. 32-3). Creation of this fracture is often necessary to obtain adequate glenoid exposure during insertion of the reverse prosthesis through a deltopectoral approach. This fracture is without clinical consequence and can largely be ignored.

Glenoid

Intraoperative glenoid fractures are more detrimental than humeral injury. Frequently, surgeons who are beginning their experience in reverse shoulder arthroplasty do not have much proficiency in glenoid preparation because they have previously performed hemiarthroplasty for most cases in which shoulder

arthroplasty is indicated. Many surgeons initially attempt to ream the glenoid as though it were an acetabulum (i.e., overaggressively), which often leads to obliteration of the glenoid bone, to glenoid fracture, or both. Patients undergoing reverse shoulder arthroplasty are at particular risk for intraoperative glenoid fracture because they tend to have more osteopenia than patients undergoing unconstrained arthroplasty for nonfracture conditions. Fractures may involve only the peripheral glenoid rim or may extend significantly into the central portion of the glenoid. Adequate capsular release helps minimize the risk for glenoid fracture. Additionally, a motorized reamer (not a drill, because the speed and torque are different) should be used for preparation of the glenoid surface. The reamer should be started before the surgeon applies force to engage the reamer onto the glenoid face. This avoids having the reamer "catch" an edge of the glenoid, which may cause a fracture.

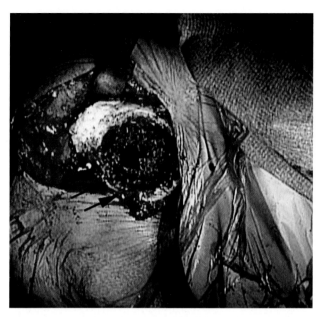

Figure 32-3 Fracture (*arrows*) of the lesser tuberosity caused by proximal humeral retraction during implantation of a reverse-prosthesis glenoid component.

Fractures that involve only a small portion of the peripheral rim generally require no treatment, and the glenoid component can be inserted as planned. Glenoid fractures that extend into the central portion of the glenoid should be bone-grafted with the humeral head. The reverse glenoid component can be inserted to help secure the bone graft and internally fix the fracture. If the central post of the reverse component is firmly seated within native glenoid bone, consideration can be given to placing the humeral component in the same surgical setting. If the glenoid component does not seem secure or the central post of the glenoid base plate is not firmly seated in unfractured native glenoid bone, the humeral component should be initially omitted for 6 months to allow the fracture to heal. After 6 months a humeral component can be placed as the second part of a two-stage procedure (Fig. 32-4). Alternatively, if an intraoperative glenoid fracture occurs, the fracture can be bone-grafted and the humeral stem plus a hemiarthroplasty adapter placed (Fig. 32-5). After the fracture has healed and remodeled (around 6 months after the index attempt at reverse shoulder arthroplasty), the second stage of the procedure, consisting of implantation of the glenoid component, may be performed (Fig. 32-6).

Rotator Cuff

With proper exposure, intraoperative injury to the rotator cuff is rare. Although patients undergoing

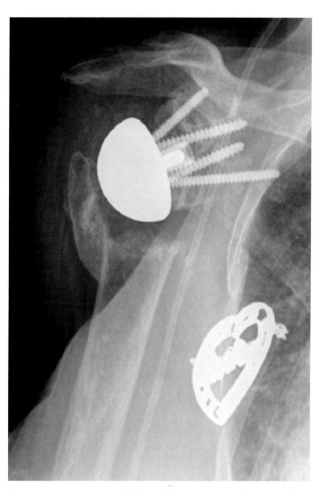

Figure 32-4 Case in which an intraoperative fracture of the glenoid was treated by bone grafting from the humeral head and placement of the glenoid component. Placement of the humeral component was delayed 6 months until the fracture had healed and remodeled.

reverse shoulder arthroplasty have a compromised rotator cuff, every effort should be made to preserve any rotator cuff function that remains, both anteriorly and posteriorly. Repair of the subscapularis tendon after reverse shoulder arthroplasty helps prevent postoperative dislocation. Preservation of the posterior rotator cuff improves outcomes by allowing active external rotation postoperatively. If the rotator cuff is adequately visualized, inadvertent damage to the rotator cuff during reverse shoulder arthroplasty can be avoided.

Neurovascular Structures

Catastrophic injury to the neurovascular structures around the shoulder is exceedingly rare during reverse shoulder arthroplasty. The neural structures most at risk during reverse shoulder arthroplasty are the axil-

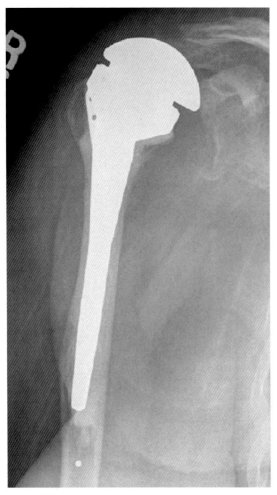

Figure 32-5   Intraoperative glenoid fracture treated by bone grafting from the humeral head and placement of the reverse stem and hemiarthroplasty adapter.

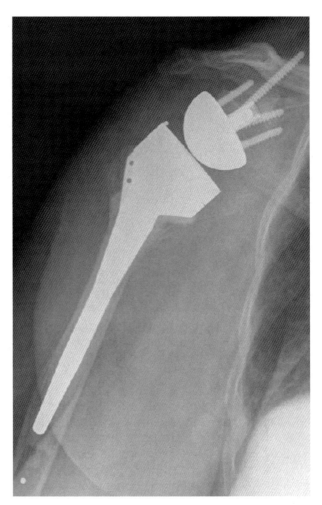

Figure 32-6   Placement of the glenoid component is performed 6 months after bone grafting of the glenoid and placement of the reverse stem and hemiarthroplasty adapter. At the time of the second stage, the hemiarthroplasty adapter is simply removed and a polyethylene insert is placed, thereby eliminating the need for exchange of the humeral stem.

lary and musculocutaneous nerves. These nerves should not be at risk for transection during primary arthroplasty using accepted operative technique. Neuropraxic injury caused by stretch most commonly involves the axillary nerve, but any nerves within the brachial plexus can be affected. Care should be taken when positioning the patient to maintain the cervical spine in neutral alignment to avoid a stretch injury to the brachial plexus. We have yet to establish risk factors for neuropraxic injury to the axillary nerve. Logic would suggest that patients with the most stiffness creating difficulty in glenoid exposure would be at the highest risk for this type of complication. Our clinical experience has not borne this out, however, and we are currently unable to predict which patients are most likely to suffer this complication. Patient education preoperatively is of paramount importance in dealing with neuropraxia inasmuch as patients are much more accepting if they have heard about the

possibility of this complication before surgery. Axillary nerve (and other nerve) neuropraxia is treated by observation, with most patients recovering by 3 to 4 months postoperatively.

Although tearing of the cephalic vein is common and largely without consequence, significant arterial and venous injuries occurring during primary reverse shoulder arthroplasty performed for nonfracture indications are exceptionally rare. Injury to the major upper extremity vessels is usually caused by overzealous medial dissection, which is not needed during shoulder arthroplasty. Should one of these injuries occur, after cross-clamping of the injured vessel, emergency intraoperative consultation with a vascular surgeon is required.

POSTOPERATIVE COMPLICATIONS

Postoperative complications are more common than intraoperative complications and occur in up to 50% of patients after reverse shoulder arthroplasty in some series.[4] The most common postoperative complications include wound problems (dehiscence, hematoma), glenoid problems, humeral problems, acromial problems, scapular notching, instability (dislocation), stiffness, and infection.

Wound Problems

Wound problems occur early after reverse shoulder arthroplasty. Hematoma is most easily avoided by extensive use of electrocautery during reverse shoulder arthroplasty and closed suction drainage for 24 hours postoperatively. The lack of a rotator cuff results in a large potential space in which a hematoma can form. Closed suction drainage minimizes hematoma formation and is highly recommended in reverse shoulder arthroplasty. Suture ligation, in addition to electrosurgical cauterization, of the anterior humeral circumflex vessels also minimizes the incidence of postoperative wound hematoma. When a hematoma occurs, it is managed by symptomatic nonoperative treatment (warm compresses, pain medication). Operative drainage is reserved for situations in which drainage persists beyond 1 week or infection is suspected (see later) and is rarely necessary.

Wound dehiscence occasionally occurs as a result of a reaction to dissolving subcutaneous sutures in susceptible patients. The presence of minimal serous drainage distinguishes this complication from the more serious deep infection. Superficial wound dehiscence is treated by local wound care, including removal of any residual dissolving suture material and chemical cauterization of any granulating tissue with silver nitrate applicators.

Glenoid Problems

Glenoid problems after reverse shoulder arthroplasty are less common than after unconstrained total shoulder arthroplasty. In all cases of which we are aware, glenoid component failure after primary reverse shoulder arthroplasty has been associated with initial placement of the glenoid component in a superiorly oriented direction (Fig. 32-7) or implantation of the prosthesis in the presence of an intraoperative glenoid fracture (Fig. 32-8). These complications are best avoided. We implant the reverse prosthesis through a deltopectoral approach to avoid inadvertent placement of the glenoid component in a superiorly oriented position,

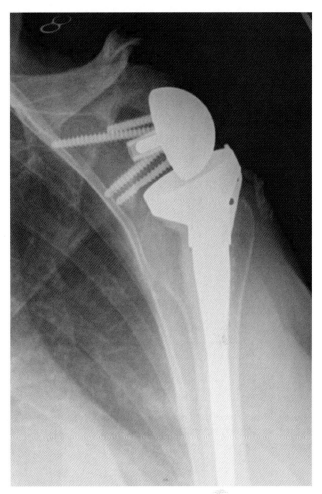

Figure 32-7 Placement of the glenoid component of a reverse prosthesis in a superiorly oriented position resulted in failure of the glenoid component.

which can occur with use of the superior lateral approach. If an intraoperative glenoid fracture occurs, we treat it as described previously in this chapter. When glenoid failure does occur, revision surgery consisting of glenoid reconstruction and conversion to a hemiarthroplasty is required (see Section Six).

Humeral Problems

Humeral problems after reverse shoulder arthroplasty are rare and can be divided into loosening of the humeral component, mechanical problems of the humeral component (polyethylene dissociation and polyethylene wear), and periprosthetic humeral fracture. Aseptic loosening of the humeral stem of a reverse prosthesis occurs in less than 1% of cases. The predominant risk factor for aseptic loosening of the humeral stem is proximal humeral bone loss (Fig. 32-9). Whenever loosening of a humeral stem occurs,

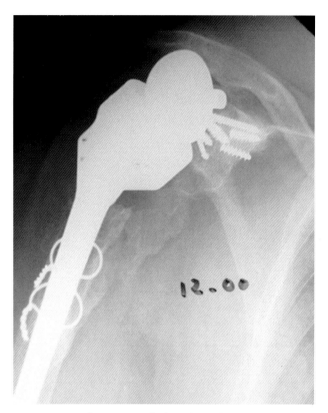

Figure 32-8 Placement of the glenoid component of a reverse prosthesis despite intraoperative glenoid fracture resulted in failure of the glenoid component.

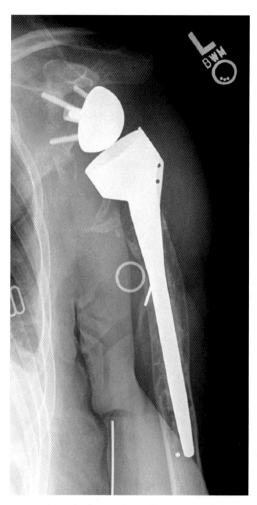

Figure 32-9 Aseptic loosening of a reverse humeral stem related to proximal humeral bone loss.

infection must be ruled out (see later). In the rare instance of symptomatic aseptic humeral component loosening, treatment consists of revision of the humeral stem, usually combined with allograft reconstruction of the proximal humerus to provide osseous support of the proximal portion of the revision stem (see Section Six).

Mechanical problems of the humeral component are exceedingly rare and are related to the polyethylene liner. We are aware of one case of dissociation of the polyethylene liner from the humeral stem that was most likely related to incomplete seating of the polyethylene component at the index arthroplasty. In this scenario, revision surgery with replacement of the polyethylene liner is indicated. Polyethylene wear occurs medially on the rim of the polyethylene liner in many patients, as noted at the time of retrieval during revision surgery (Fig. 32-10). Such wear is related to scapular notching as discussed later.

Periprosthetic humeral fractures are more common than loosening of the humeral component and are almost always the result of a fall or similar low-energy trauma (Fig. 32-11). The majority of these fractures occur just distal to the tip of the humeral stem, and

most can be treated nonoperatively. Nonoperative treatment consists of fracture bracing, activity modification, pain medication, and frequent radiographic monitoring. If the fracture has not healed within 3 months, we will incorporate the use of an external bone stimulator (OL 1000 Bone Growth Stimulator, Donjoy Orthopedics, Vista, CA). Despite these measures, periprosthetic humeral fractures treated nonoperatively may take longer than 9 months to heal.[5] Our criteria for recommending operative treatment of periprosthetic fractures (revision surgery; see Section Six) include complete displacement, angulation greater than 30 degrees, loosening or dislocation of the humeral component, or failure of nonoperative treatment (Fig. 32-12).

Acromial Problems

Occasionally, acromial stress fractures are seen after reverse shoulder arthroplasty (Fig. 32-13). These

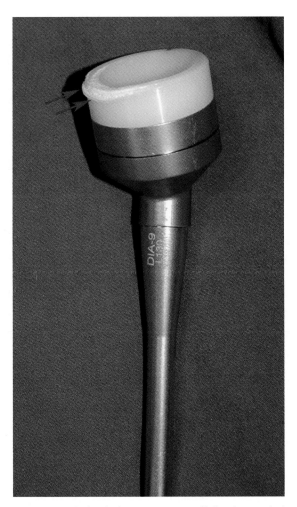

Figure 32-10 Polyethylene wear medially (*arrows*) in a retrieved reverse humeral component.

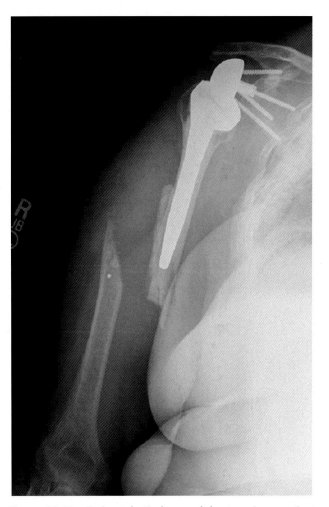

Figure 32-11 Periprosthetic humeral fracture in a patient with a reverse prosthesis occurring as a result of a fall.

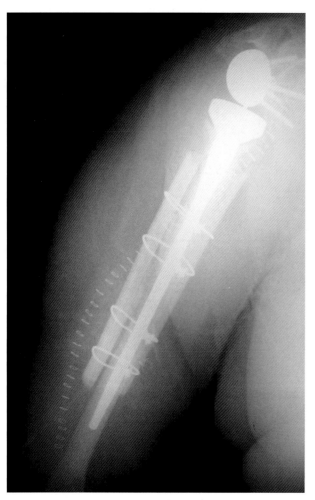

Figure 32-12   Operative treatment of a periprosthetic fracture in a patient with a reverse prosthesis.

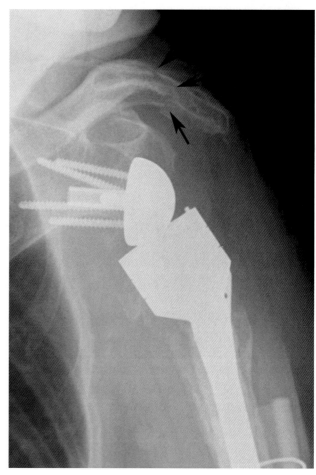

Figure 32-13   Acromial stress fracture (*arrows*) occurring after reverse shoulder arthroplasty.

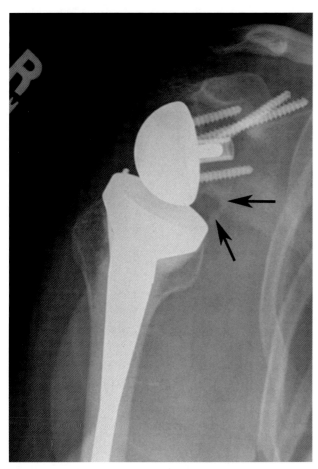

Figure 32-14 Inferior scapular notch (*arrows*), which commonly occurs in patients after reverse shoulder arthroplasty.

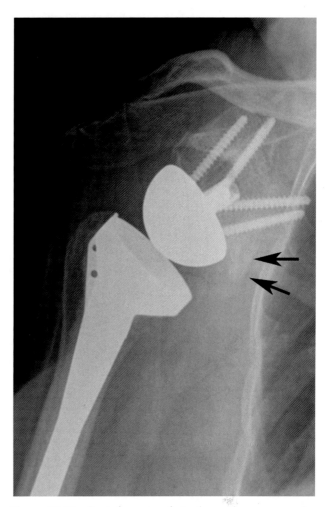

Figure 32-15 Scapular osteophyte (*arrows*) accompanying an inferior scapular notch after reverse shoulder arthroplasty.

fractures result from deltoid tension applied to osteopenic bone. Frequently, these fractures are present preoperatively as a result of chronic superior migration of the humeral head with persistent acromiohumeral articulation. Postoperatively, deltoid tension may cause the fracture fragment to tilt inferiorly. Despite these radiographic findings, no specific treatment is necessary for this complication. Additionally, patients obtain satisfactory results even with this radiographic finding.

Scapular Notching

Though whether it should be considered a complication is debatable, notching of the scapula occurs within 2 years of surgery in half the patients who undergo reverse shoulder arthroplasty (Fig. 32-14). This radiographic finding most likely occurs as a result of mechanical impingement of the medial aspect of the humeral component and the lateral aspect of the scapula just inferior to the glenoid. The impingement

is exacerbated when the patient internally rotates the shoulder. This mechanical impingement theory is further supported by the observation that patients' internal rotation seems to improve as the scapular notch progresses, thus suggesting that the prosthesis must "carve out" a portion of the scapula to maximize postoperative internal rotation. Another theory of the cause of scapular notching is polyethylene wear causing osteolysis, although this theory currently has less support than the mechanical impingement theory.

Scapular notching is commonly accompanied by a scapular osteophyte just medial to the notch (Fig. 32-15). The degree of scapular notching has also been graded by severity (Fig. 32-16).[6] The best way to avoid scapular notching seems to be by initially placing the glenoid component inferiorly on the glenoid face and introducing slight inferior tilt during glenoid reaming (Fig. 32-17). Despite the concerning appearance of

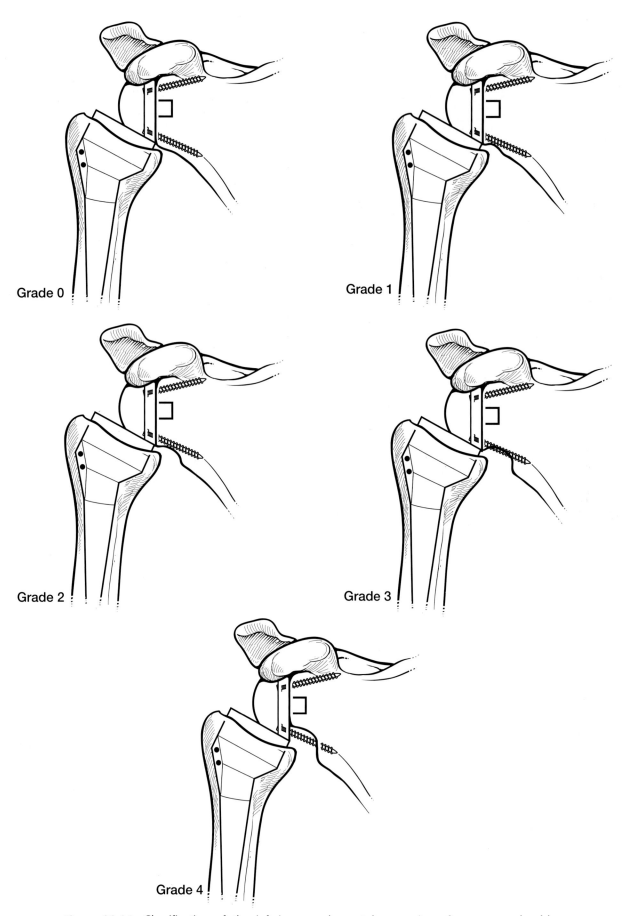

Grade 0

Grade 1

Grade 2

Grade 3

Grade 4

Figure 32-16 Classification of the inferior scapular notch occurring after reverse shoulder arthroplasty.

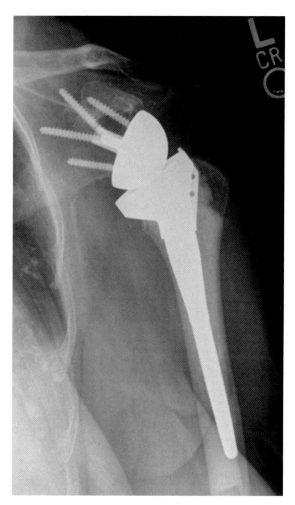

Figure 32-17 Avoidance of scapular notching by placing the glenoid component inferiorly on the glenoid face and by introducing slight inferior tilt during glenoid reaming.

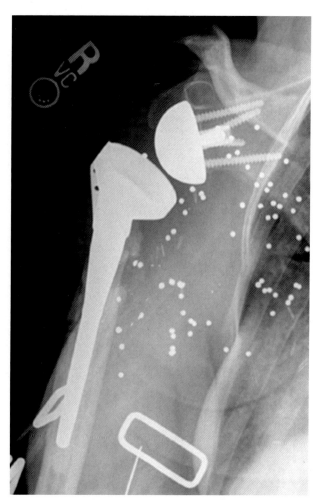

Figure 32-18 Dislocation of a reverse prosthesis.

scapular notching, its clinical implications are unclear, with most of the evidence suggesting no adverse consequence. As long as the glenoid component remains stable, no treatment of an asymptomatic scapular notch is indicated.

Instability

Instability after reverse shoulder arthroplasty is the most common complication observed in our practice,

and it occurs in approximately 5% of cases. Instability of a reverse prosthesis always occurs as a dislocation (Fig. 32-18). All dislocations that we have observed have occurred within 6 weeks of reverse shoulder arthroplasty. The majority of patients do not realize that their shoulder is dislocated, with the dislocation being detected on radiography during routine follow-up. We have observed a single case in which the patient would unintentionally dislocate his prosthesis anteriorly with arm extension but could perform a

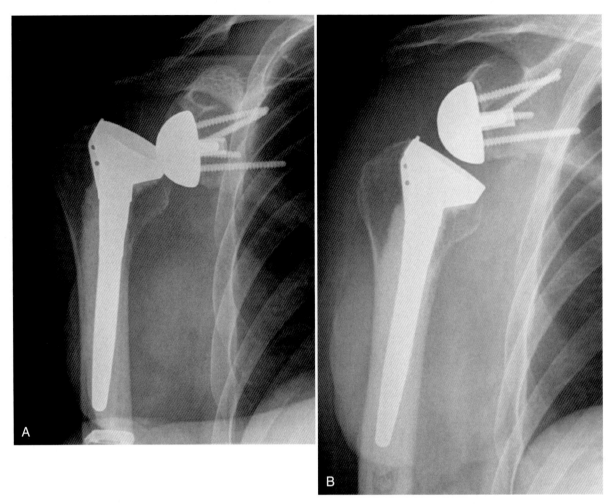

Figure 32-19   **A** and **B,** Radiographs of a patient able to dislocate and relocate his reverse prosthesis because of inadequate deltoid tension.

reduction maneuver himself to correct the dislocation (Fig. 32-19).

Instability of a reverse prosthesis can be related to various factors. In our experience, proximal humeral bone loss seems to be the greatest risk factor for dislocation of a reverse prosthesis. In this scenario, deltoid muscle tension is often solely responsible for stability of the implant because no rotator cuff or joint capsule exists to provide stability. Even if the deltoid is properly tensioned initially, it can gradually lose its tension and result in dislocation. A second major risk factor for dislocation of a reverse prosthesis is subscapularis insufficiency. All cases of dislocation that we have observed in our patients have occurred in those without a reparable subscapularis. A less common factor contributing to dislocation of a reverse prosthesis is mechanical impingement causing the prosthetic socket to be levered away from the glenoid component. This impingement usually occurs inferiorly as the arm is

adducted and is often related to positioning of the glenoid component too superior on the glenoid face (Fig. 32-20). Finally, we have observed a single case in which a patient had sustained a neuropraxic injury to the axillary nerve that resulted in prosthetic instability secondary to an inability to contract the deltoid. In most cases of dislocation, one or more of these factors are present.

In the majority of cases, treatment of a dislocated reverse prosthesis consists of closed reduction and a period of bracing. Closed reduction is performed in the operating room with the patient either heavily sedated or under general anesthesia. Under fluoroscopic guidance an attempt is made to reduce the dislocation. If the prosthesis is successfully reduced, fluoroscopic examination is performed to ensure that mechanical impingement is not responsible for the instability. If the problem is not related to mechanical impingement and the prosthesis is reduced successfully, a brace is applied to maintain the arm with the humeral component centered on the glenoid component, generally in about 90 degrees of abduction with 30 degrees of forward flexion (Fig. 32-21). The patient maintains this brace at all times for 6 weeks, with radiographs per-

formed in the brace every 7 to 10 days to confirm that the prosthesis has not dislocated (Fig. 32-22). After 6 weeks, the brace is discontinued and a normal rehabilitation regimen ensues.

If the prosthesis is not reducible by closed means, mechanical impingement is causing the dislocation, or closed reduction with bracing has failed, open reduction with insertion of a thicker polyethylene spacer or metallic augment (or both) ensues (Fig. 32-23). Any mechanical impingement can simultaneously be addressed by careful removal of bone at the lateral aspect of the scapula just inferior to the glenoid component if necessary. Postoperatively, the patient is treated with the same bracing protocol used after closed reduction of a dislocated reverse prosthesis.

Stiffness

Glenohumeral stiffness after reverse shoulder arthroplasty is rare. Limitation of mobility after implantation of a reverse prosthesis is usually related to mechanical limitation of the prosthetic design and not capsular contracture. We personally have no experience in dealing with postoperative capsulitis after implantation of a reverse prosthesis.

Infection

Infection after reverse shoulder arthroplasty occurs at the same frequency as after unconstrained shoulder arthroplasty (<1% of cases). Patients most at risk for infection are those with systemic illness (diabetes mellitus), those with compromised soft tissues (radiation-induced osteonecrosis, post-traumatic arthritis), and those with inflammatory arthropathy (rheumatoid

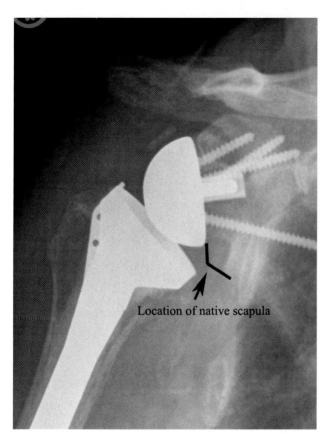

Figure 32-20   Positioning of the reverse glenoid component too superior on the glenoid face resulted in mechanical impingement.

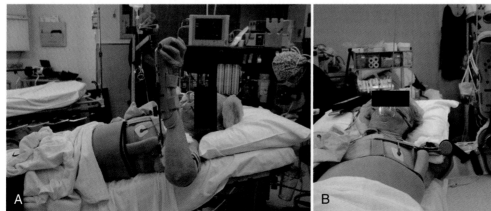

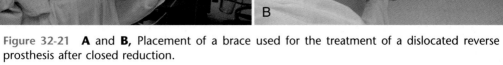

Figure 32-21   A and **B,** Placement of a brace used for the treatment of a dislocated reverse prosthesis after closed reduction.

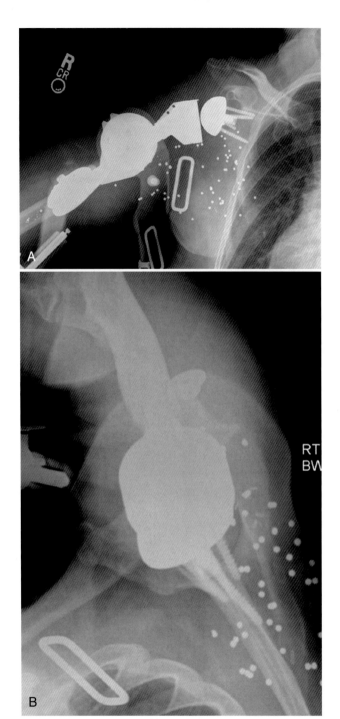

Figure 32-22 **A** and **B,** Radiograph obtained in the brace confirming maintenance of prosthetic reduction.

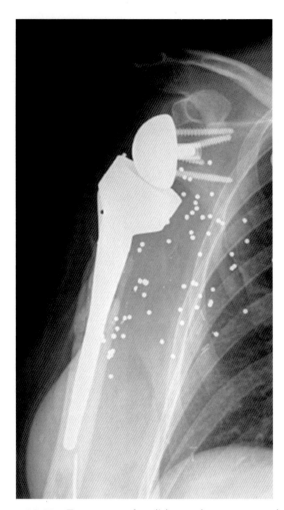

Figure 32-23 Treatment of a dislocated reverse prosthesis with the addition of an augment to increase deltoid tension.

arthritis). These infections are most commonly caused by *Staphylococcus aureus* or *Propionibacterium acnes.* Infections after shoulder arthroplasty can be divided into perioperative (within 6 weeks of surgery) and late (hematogenous) infections.

Early perioperative infections are initially treated with two or three irrigation and débridement proce-

dures and retention of the fixed components. With each irrigation and débridement procedure, the polyethylene liner of the humeral component is removed and the prosthesis is thoroughly cleaned. The original polyethylene liner is replaced after being cleaned during the initial one or two irrigation and débridement procedures. At the last planned irrigation and débridement procedure, absorbable antibiotic-impregnated beads (Stimulan, Biocomposites, Inc., Staffordshire, England) are placed in the soft tissues around the shoulder, and the polyethylene liner is replaced. Consultation with an infectious disease specialist is obtained, and a minimum of 6 weeks of intravenous antibiotics tailored to the specific organism causing the infection (or covering the most likely offending organisms, if cultures remain negative despite obvious infection) is usually recommended. If this regimen fails, prosthetic removal ensues as detailed in Section Six.

Late-appearing infections are treated by removal of the prosthesis and intravenous administration of antibiotics as detailed in Section Six. The decision whether to place a revision shoulder arthroplasty or continue with a resection arthroplasty is patient specific.

REFERENCES

1. Wall B, Nové-Josserand L, O'Connor D, et al: Reverse total shoulder arthroplasty: A review of results by etiology. J Bone Joint Surg Am 2007;89:1476-1485.
2. Constant CR, Murley AH: A clinical method of functional assessment of the shoulder. Clin Orthop Relat Res 1987;214:160-164.
3. Constant CR: Assessment of shoulder function. In Gazielly D, Gleyze P, Thomas T (eds): The Cuff. New York, Elsevier, 1997, pp 39-44.
4. Werner CML, Steinmann PA, Gilbart M, Gerber C: Treatment of painful pseudoparesis due to irreparable rotator cuff dysfunction with the Delta III reverse-ball-and-socket total shoulder prosthesis. J Bone Joint Surg Am 2005;87:1476-1486.
5. Kumar S, Sperling JW, Haidukewych GH, Cofield RH: Periprosthetic humeral fractures after shoulder arthroplasty. J Bone Joint Surg Am 2004;86:680-689.
6. Valenti P, Boutens D, Nerot C: Delta 3 reversed prosthesis for osteoarthritis with massive rotator cuff tear: Long term results (>5 years). In Walch G, Boileau P, Molé D (eds): 2000 Prothèses d'Epaule . . . Recul de 2 à 10 Ans. Paris, Sauramps Medical, 2001, pp 253-259.

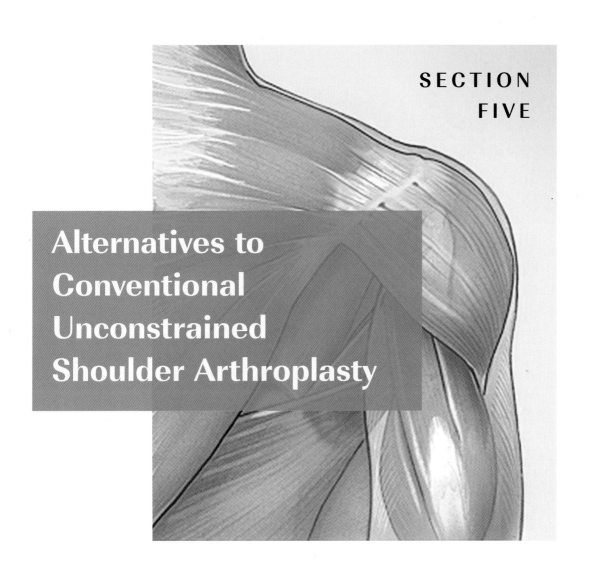

Alternatives to Conventional Unconstrained Shoulder Arthroplasty

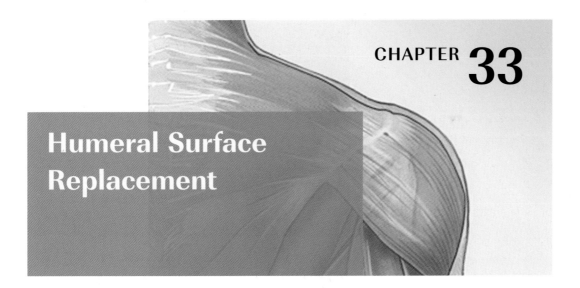

CHAPTER 33

Humeral Surface Replacement

The advantage of complete surface replacement of the humeral head lies mainly in preservation of subchondral bone.[1] In our practice, few situations exist in which complete surface replacement of the humeral head is more advantageous than conventional humeral head replacement with a stemmed implant. Additionally, use of these surface replacement implants hinders glenoid exposure and thus prevents implantation of a prosthetic glenoid implant in many cases.

Alternatively, some devices and biologic implants offer subtotal resurfacing of the humeral head for focal loss of humeral head articular cartilage. Situations in which subtotal resurfacing of the humeral head is indicated are rare, but these devices and biologic implants prove useful in certain scenarios. This chapter outlines our preferred use of humeral surface replacement.

INDICATIONS AND CONTRAINDICATIONS

Complete Surface Replacement

We rarely perform complete surface replacement of the humeral head in our practice. As detailed in Chapter 6, we perform glenoid resurfacing in most shoulder arthroplasty candidates with an indication other than acute fracture. The most common indication for which we will use a complete humeral surface replacement is early-stage humeral head osteonecrosis in an active patient younger than 50 years in whom the segment of necrotic bone is sufficiently small that it will not jeopardize implant fixation, typically less than 25% of the humeral head. An additional indication is an exceptionally young, otherwise healthy patient who is a candidate for shoulder arthroplasty.

Most of our patients falling into this category have chondrolysis of the glenohumeral joint after an arthroscopic instability procedure. In these cases we will consider use of a complete humeral head surface replacement combined with biologic resurfacing of the glenoid (see Chapter 34).

In addition to the standard contraindications to unconstrained shoulder arthroplasty (see Chapter 6), any condition jeopardizing implant fixation is a contraindication to humeral head surface replacement (i.e., proximal humeral fracture, extensive proximal humeral osteonecrosis). Moreover, insertion of a standard polyethylene glenoid component is a relative contraindication to use of a humeral head surface replacement, and in the vast majority of cases a conventional stemmed humeral implant should be used instead. As detailed in Chapter 10, glenoid exposure is the most important portion of prosthetic glenoid resurfacing, and preservation of a portion of the humeral head should never be favored over optimal glenoid exposure. Conversely, biologic resurfacing typically does not involve correction of glenoid deformity and does not entail the use of a pegged or keeled glenoid component. These concessions usually make biologic glenoid resurfacing possible with the more limited glenoid exposure available during humeral head resurfacing.

Partial Surface Replacement

Partial surface replacement is indicated in patients with localized full-thickness defects of the articular cartilage of the humeral head who have failed other treatments. When patients with full-thickness articular cartilage lesions of the humeral head are seen in

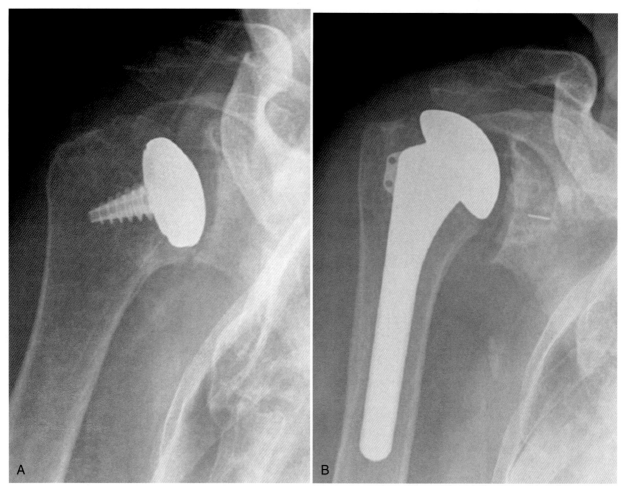

Figure 33-1 **A** and **B,** Radiographs of a patient who had undergone partial resurfacing of the humeral head for primary osteoarthritis. The patient never improved after surgery, and revision to a standard unconstrained total shoulder arthroplasty was eventually performed.

our practice, we initially treat them nonoperatively with nonsteroidal anti-inflammatory medications, selective rest, and activity modification for a period of 6 to 12 weeks. If such treatment proves unsuccessful, we offer arthroscopic treatment of the lesion with débridement and drilling of subchondral bone to stimulate the formation of fibrocartilage. If patients remain symptomatic 6 months after arthroscopic treatment, we will offer them partial surface replacement. In patients older than 30 years, we opt for prosthetic replacement with a metallic device (Hemicap, Arthrosurface, Inc., Franklin, MA). In younger patients, we opt for matched osteochondral allograft replacement. In our experience, it is rare for a patient to fail arthroscopic treatment of these localized articular cartilage lesions, thus minimizing the indications for partial surface replacement.

Contraindications specific to partial surface replacement include cartilaginous lesions larger than 35 mm in diameter (the diameter of the largest implant available), the presence of nonlocalized disease (Fig. 33-1), and the absence of sufficient bone quality to support the implant.

TECHNIQUE FOR PROSTHETIC RESURFACING

The operating room setup, anesthesia, patient positioning, skin preparation, surgical draping, and surgical approach are identical to that for humeral surface replacement and other shoulder arthroplasties (see Chapters 3, 4, and 8). The first difference in the technique involves handling of the anterior humeral circumflex vessels and subscapularis. When performing humeral surface replacement, we prefer to leave the anterior humeral circumflex vessels intact to maintain optimal blood flow to the humeral head. Consequently, after placing stay sutures in the subscapularis

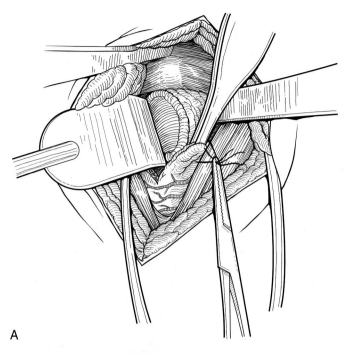

A

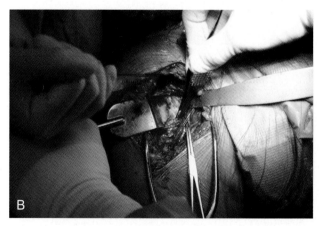

B

Figure 33-2 **A** and **B,** Distal extent of the subscapularis tenotomy used during humeral head resurfacing. The anterior humeral circumflex vessels are left intact.

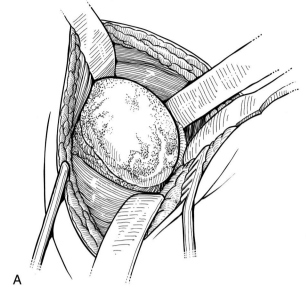

A

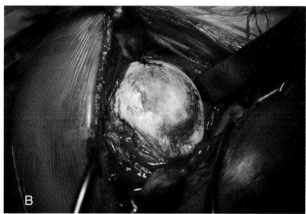

B

Figure 33-3 **A** and **B,** Completed proximal humeral exposure for surface replacement of the humeral head.

tendon as for unconstrained shoulder arthroplasty, we end our subscapularis tenotomy just superior to the anterior humeral circumflex vessels (Fig. 33-2). Subscapularis and capsular release is rarely necessary in patients undergoing humeral surface replacement. Next, the humeral head is dislocated by externally rotating and extending the arm. Hohmann retractors are placed circumferentially around the humeral head to complete the proximal humeral exposure (Fig. 33-3).

Complete Surface Replacement

For complete surface replacement, we use a system (Tornier, Inc., Stafford, TX) that allows the same 12

different humeral head sizes available for stemmed unconstrained arthroplasty. We believe that selection of the appropriate humeral head size is no less important in humeral surface replacement than in stemmed humeral arthroplasty. After exposure of the humeral head is complete and peripheral humeral osteophytes are removed, the size of the humeral head is determined with the sizing guides (Fig. 33-4). If the native humeral head is between two sizes, the smaller size is selected. The pin guide corresponding to the selected humeral head size is centered over the humeral articular surface (Fig. 33-5). The guide pin is drilled into the proximal humerus through the cannulated pin guide until it engages the lateral humeral cortex (Fig. 33-6). The pin guide is removed and the guide pin left in place (Fig. 33-7). A reamer of the appropriate size is advanced over the guide pin, and the humerus is

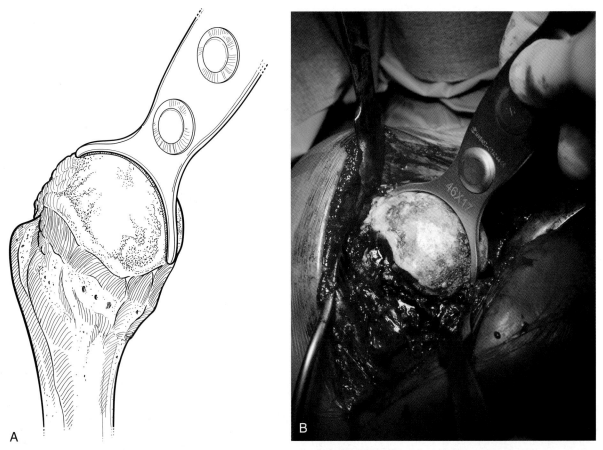

Figure 33-4 **A** and **B,** Determination of the proper humeral head implant diameter.

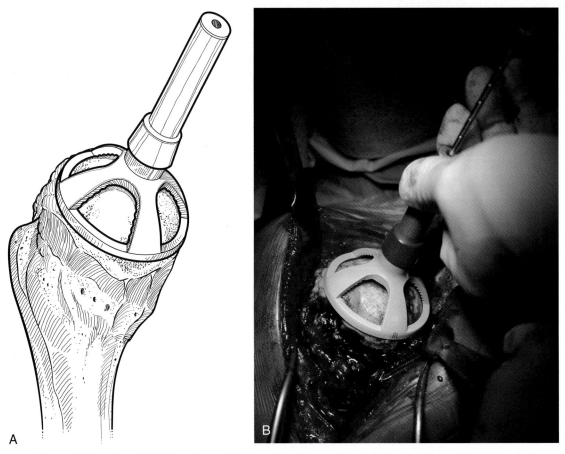

Figure 33-5 **A** and **B,** The pin guide is centered over the articular surface of the humeral head.

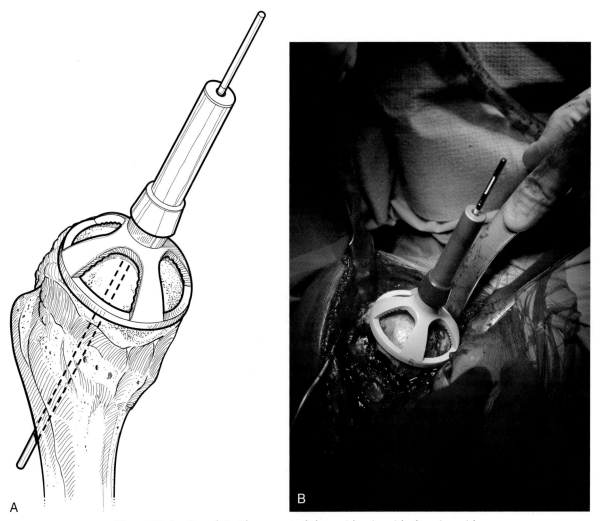

A

B

Figure 33-6   **A** and **B,** Placement of the guide pin with the pin guide.

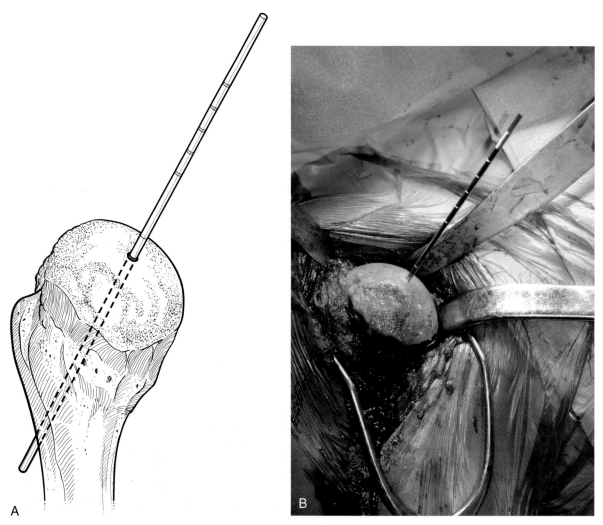

Figure 33-7 **A** and **B,** Final position of the guide pin.

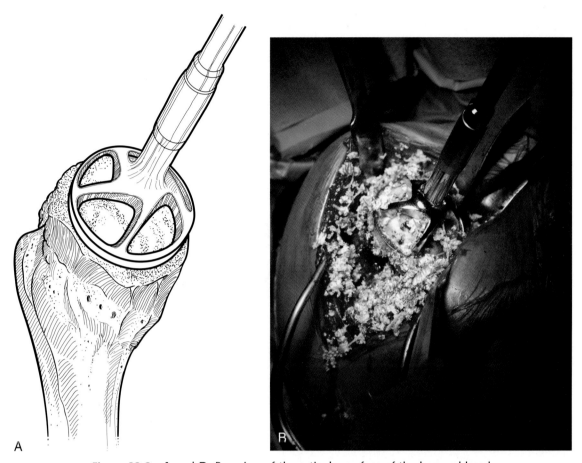

Figure 33-8 **A** and **B,** Reaming of the articular surface of the humeral head.

reamed until the leading edge of the reamer is in contact with the humeral anatomic neck (Fig. 33-8). The reamer is removed and a trial head gauge is inserted over the guide pin to ensure that the reamed humeral surface conforms to the back surface of the implant by looking through fenestrations in the trial head gauge (Fig. 33-9). The trial head gauge is removed, and a cannulated stem compactor of appropriate size is advanced over the guide pin until the collar is flush with the humeral surface (Fig. 33-10). The cannulated

stem compactor is removed with the guide pin. The final humeral implant is oriented in the stem hole and impacted into place with the smooth compactor (Fig. 33-11). The glenohumeral joint is reduced.

The subscapularis is closed with interrupted no. 2 braided permanent tendon-to-tendon suture. The closure is reinforced with a running no. 1 braided absorbable suture. The wound is then closed as for other cases of shoulder arthroplasty.

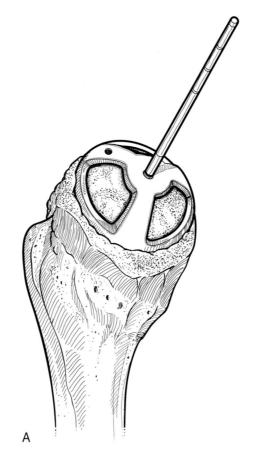

A

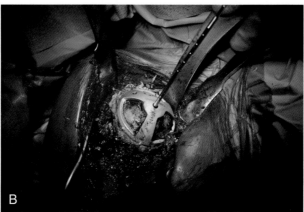

B

Figure 33-9 **A** and **B,** Placement of the trial head gauge to ensure that the implant will fully seat.

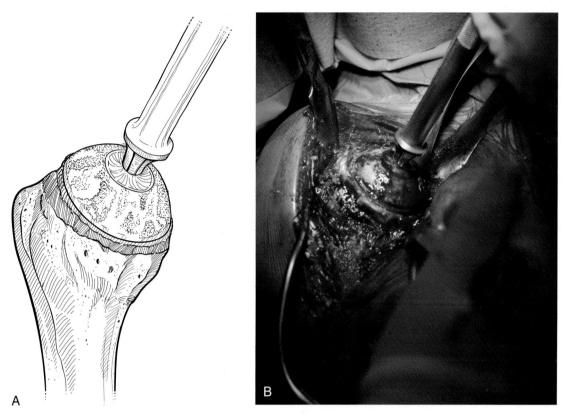

Figure 33-10   **A** and **B,** Insertion of the cannulated stem impactor.

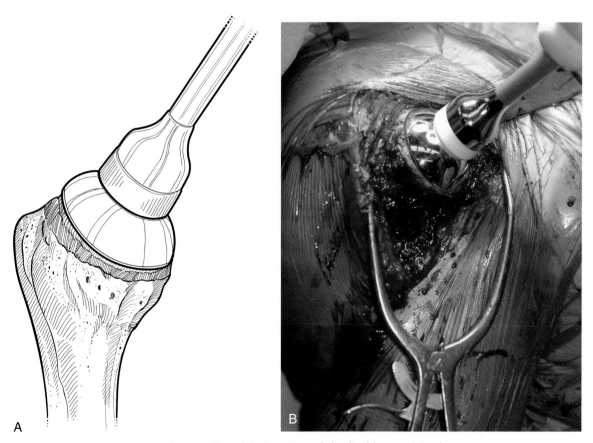

Figure 33-11   **A** and **B,** Insertion of the final humeral implant.

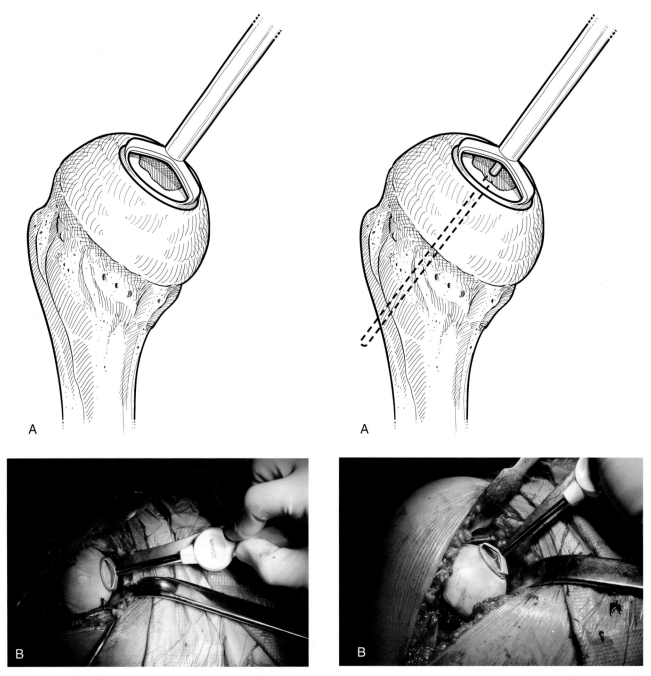

Figure 33-12 **A** and **B,** Drill guide used for partial humeral head resurfacing.

Figure 33-13 **A** and **B,** Insertion of the guide pin used in partial humeral head resurfacing.

Partial Surface Replacement

A drill guide just large enough to circumscribe the articular cartilage lesion is selected (Fig. 33-12). Available sizes are 25, 30, and 35 mm. A guide pin is inserted to the level of the laser mark by using the drill guide centered in the articular cartilage defect (Fig. 33-13). The drill guide is removed and a cannulated drill is passed over the guide pin until it is flush with the humeral head articular surface (Fig. 33-14). A tap is advanced over the guide pin and removed (Fig. 33-15). The central screw is advanced over the guide pin until the laser mark on the screw driver is flush with the articular surface of the humeral head (Fig. 33-16). The guide pin is removed and the central hole of the screw is cleaned with the taper cleaner (Fig. 33-17). A trial cap is inserted and should be at or below the level of the articular cartilage (Fig. 33-18). If the trial cap is

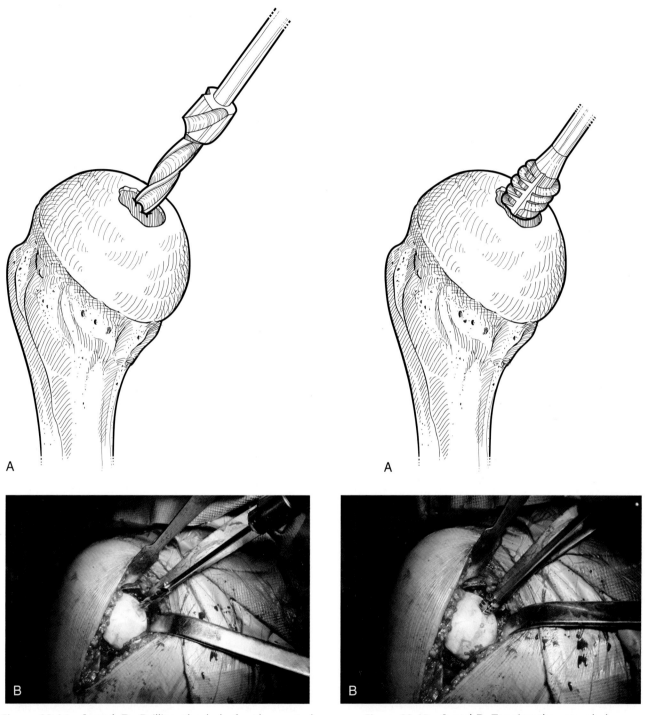

A

B

A

B

Figure 33-14 **A** and **B,** Drilling the hole for the central screw used in partial humeral head resurfacing.

Figure 33-15 **A** and **B,** Tapping the screw hole.

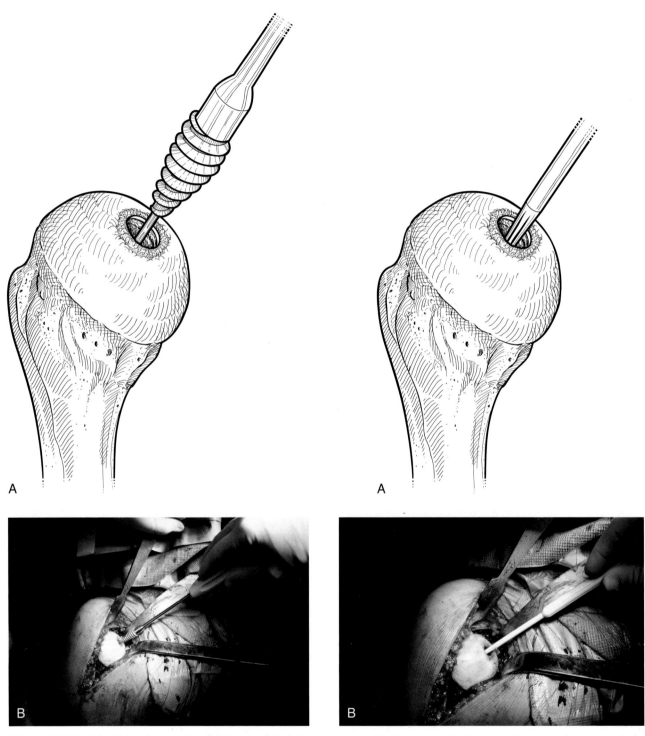

Figure 33-16 **A** and **B,** Placement of the central screw.

Figure 33-17 **A** and **B,** Cleaning the central screw with the taper cleaner.

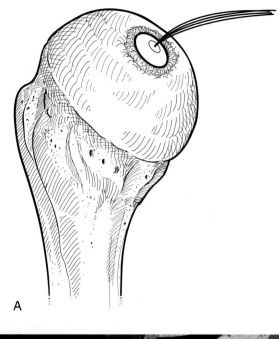

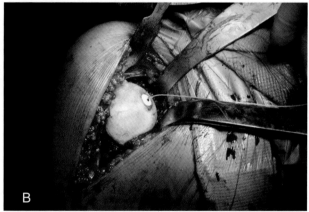

Figure 33-18 A and **B,** The trial cap is inserted to ensure that the central screw has been advanced sufficiently.

prominent, it is removed, the screw is advanced half a revolution, and the position of the trial cap is rechecked. The centering shaft is placed in the central hole of the screw, and measurements are made with the specially designed measurement contact probe at the superior, inferior, medial, and lateral margins (Fig. 33-19) and recorded on the sizing card (Fig. 33-20). Selection of implant diameter is based on the measurements recorded on the sizing card, and the maximal measurement recorded is used. An example is shown in Figure 33-21. The centering shaft is removed and a guide pin is replaced in the central hole of the screw.

A surface reamer appropriate for the implant chosen is selected and used for reaming until it contacts the screw (Fig. 33-22). The reamer and guide pin are removed, and the central screw hole is cleaned with

the taper cleaner. The appropriate sizing trial is placed in the central screw hole to ensure that the final implant will not be prominent (Fig. 33-23). The edges of the trial implant should be flush or slightly recessed with respect to the surrounding intact articular surface. The trial is removed and the central screw hole cleaned with the taper cleaner. The final implant is placed onto the central screw with the suction inserter (Fig. 33-24). The inserter is removed by disconnecting the suction, and the implant is impacted into place with the impactor provided (Fig. 33-25). The glenohumeral joint is reduced.

The subscapularis is closed with interrupted no. 2 braided permanent tendon-to-tendon suture. The closure is reinforced with running no. 1 braided absorbable suture. The wound is then closed as for other cases of shoulder arthroplasty.

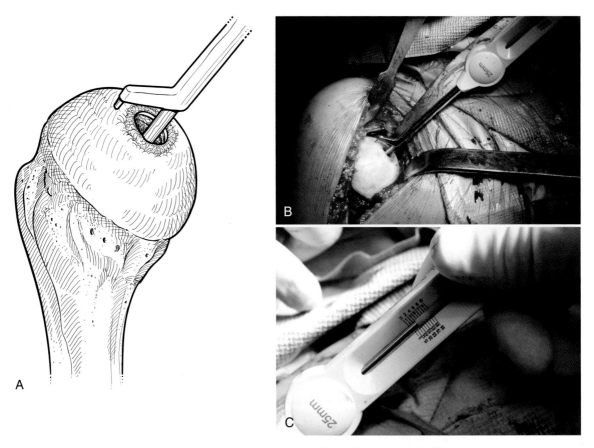

Figure 33-19 **A** to **C,** Each quadrant of the humeral head is measured with the contact probe placed over the centering shaft.

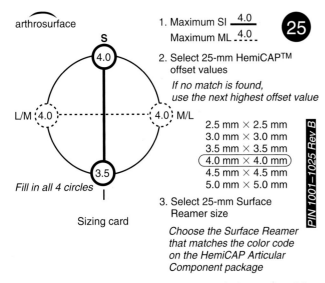

arthrosurface

S

4.0

L/M 4.0 - - - - - - - - - - 4.0 M/L

3.5

Fill in all 4 circles

Sizing card

1. Maximum SI __4.0__
   Maximum ML __4.0__   **25**

2. Select 25-mm HemiCAP™ offset values
   If no match is found, use the next highest offset value

   2.5 mm × 2.5 mm
   3.0 mm × 3.0 mm
   3.5 mm × 3.5 mm
   (4.0 mm × 4.0 mm)
   4.5 mm × 4.5 mm
   5.0 mm × 5.0 mm

3. Select 25-mm Surface Reamer size

   Choose the Surface Reamer that matches the color code on the HemiCAP Articular Component package

P/N 1001–1025 Rev B

Figure 33-20 Measurements are recorded on the sizing card.

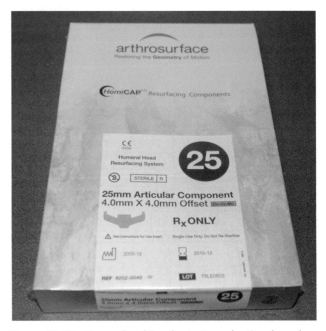

Figure 33-21 Example of implant size selection based on information recorded on the sizing card.

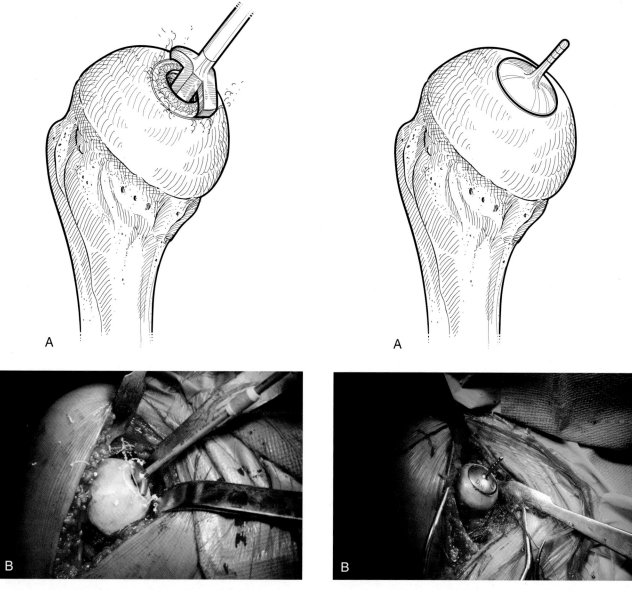

Figure 33-22 **A** and **B,** Reaming with a surface reamer corresponding to the selected implant size.

Figure 33-23 **A** and **B,** Placement of the sizing trial to ensure that the final implant will not be prominent.

TECHNIQUE FOR BIOLOGIC RESURFACING

The operating room setup, anesthesia, patient positioning, skin preparation, surgical draping, and surgical approach are identical to that for humeral surface replacement and other shoulder arthroplasties (see Chapters 3, 4, and 8). Handling of the subscapularis is the same as for prosthetic surface replacement, as described previously in this chapter. Biologic resurfacing necessitates greater preoperative planning in that

it is necessary for the company supplying the proximal humeral allograft to locate an appropriately sized specimen (we use the Musculoskeletal Transplant Foundation). Magnification-controlled radiographs and computed tomography scans of the proximal humerus are provided to the allograft supplier to allow appropriate specimen selection. Our supplier has usually been able to provide specimens within 6 weeks of receiving the preoperative imaging studies. Once the specimen has been obtained, surgery is scheduled.

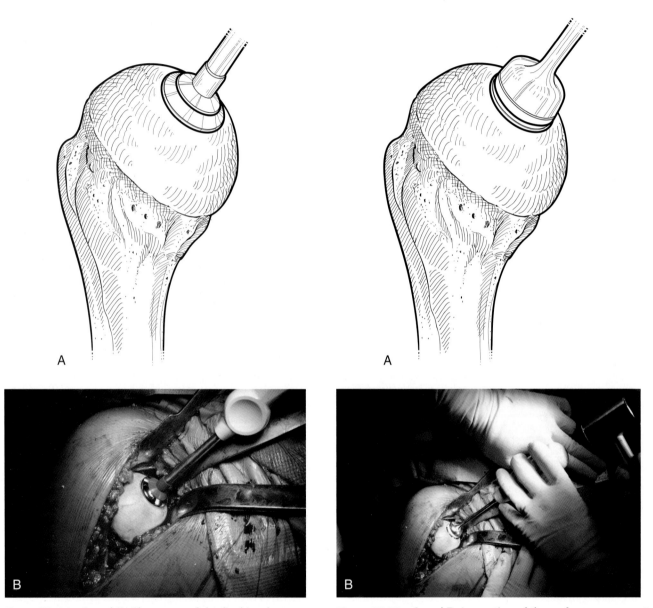

Figure 33-24   **A** and **B,** Placement of the final implant onto the central screw with the suction inserter.

Figure 33-25   **A** and **B,** Impaction of the surface component of the final implant.

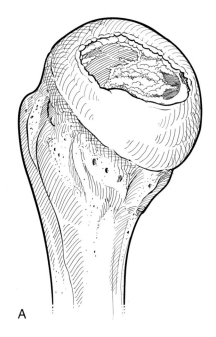

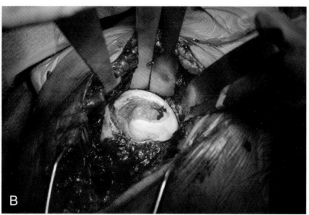

Figure 33-26   A and **B,** Completed exposure of the humeral head.

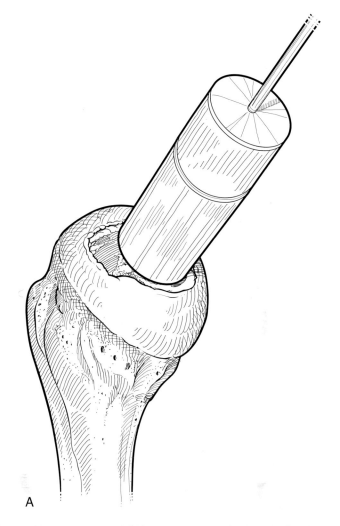

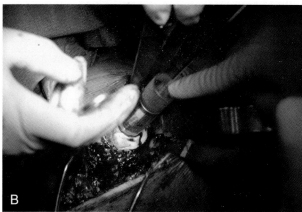

Figure 33-27   A and **B,** The size of the humeral head articular cartilage lesion is measured.

The humeral head is dislocated to expose the articular cartilage lesion (Fig. 33-26). The size of the lesion is measured with a templating device from the instrumentation set (Arthrex, Inc., Naples, FL) (Fig. 33-27), and a guide pin is placed in the humeral head at the center of the articular cartilage lesion with the templating device used as a guide (Fig. 33-28). A specialized cannulated drill is used to score the periphery of the lesion (Fig. 33-29), and a cannulated triflange reamer is used to create an osseous defect in which to place the osteochondral allograft (Fig. 33-30). If associated osteonecrosis is present in addition to the articular cartilage lesion, the reamer is advanced to a depth sufficient to eliminate the necrotic bone as determined on preoperative imaging studies. If no or minimal osteonecrosis is present, the reamer is advanced a

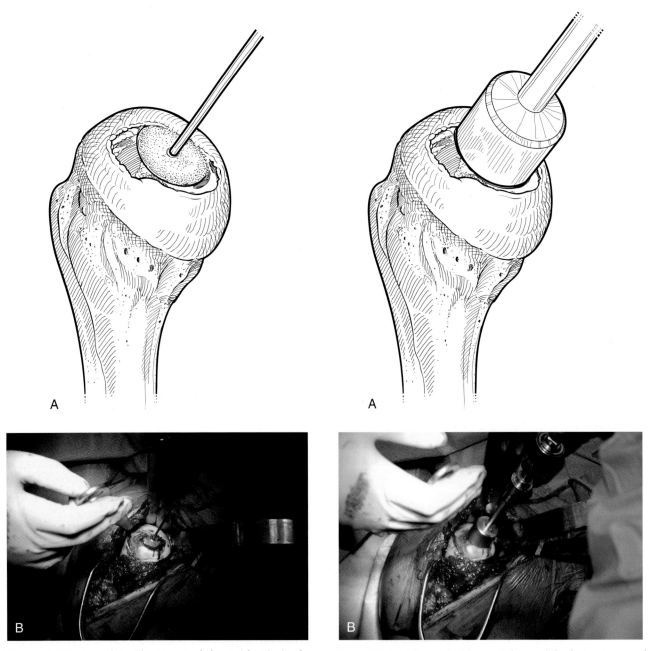

Figure 33-28   **A** and **B,** Placement of the guide pin in the center of the lesion.

Figure 33-29   **A** and **B,** The periphery of the lesion is scored with a special instrument.

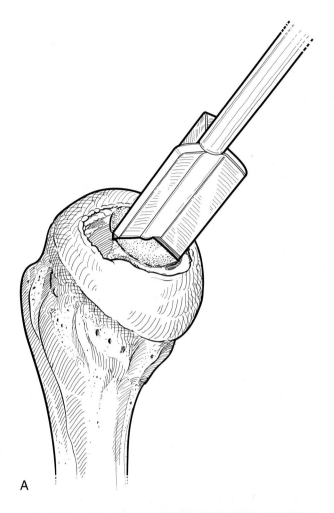

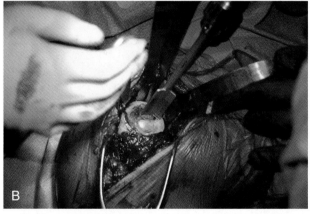

Figure 33-30 **A** and **B,** Reaming of the humeral head with a triflange reamer.

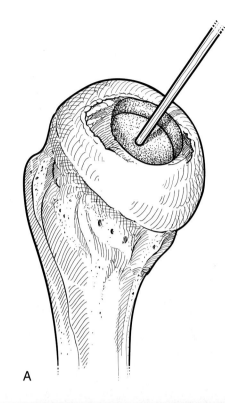

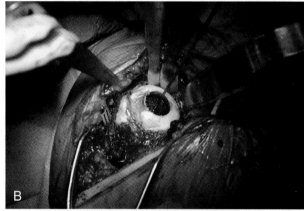

Figure 33-31 **A** and **B,** Completed humeral preparation.

minimum of 10 mm deep to provide an adequate interference fit for the osteochondral allograft. Figure 33-31 shows the humerus after reaming has been completed.

The proximal humeral allograft is positioned in the cutting jig, and the selected donor site is marked with a surgical marker (Fig. 33-32). A cutting guide of appropriate diameter is assembled onto the cutting jig, and a coring drill is used to harvest the osteochondral allograft plug (Fig. 33-33). The allograft plug is placed in a specialized clamp, and a saw is used to trim the deep surface of the allograft to match the depth penetrated by the triflange reamer (Fig. 33-34). The bone plug is progressively impacted into the prepared humeral defect until it is fully seated (Fig. 33-35).

The subscapularis is closed with interrupted no. 2 braided permanent tendon-to-tendon suture. The closure is reinforced with running no. 1 braided absorbable suture. The wound is then closed as for other cases of shoulder arthroplasty.

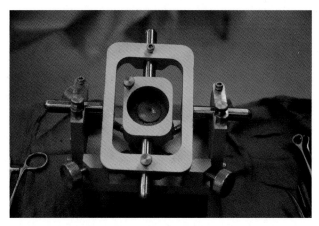

Figure 33-32   Placement of the proximal humeral allograft in the cutting jig.

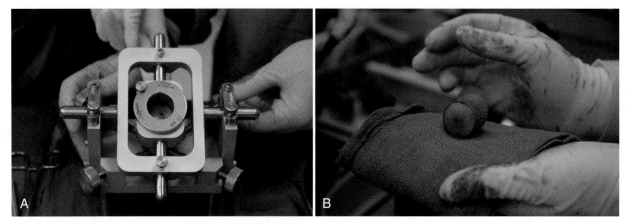

Figure 33-33   **A** and **B**, A coring drill is used to harvest the osteocartilaginous allograft plug.

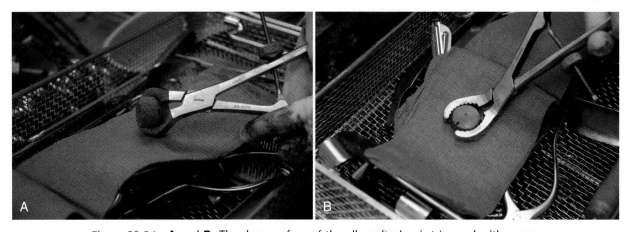

Figure 33-34   **A** and **B**, The deep surface of the allograft plug is trimmed with a saw.

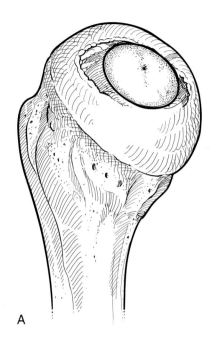

REFERENCE

1. Levy O, Copeland SA: Cementless surface replacement arthroplasty of the shoulder. 5- to 10-year results with the Copeland Mark-2 prosthesis. J Bone Joint Surg Br 2001;83:213-221.

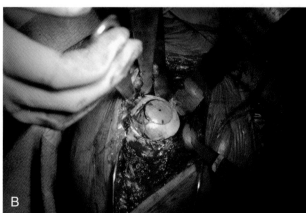

Figure 33-35 **A** and **B,** The allograft plug is seated into the prepared humerus.

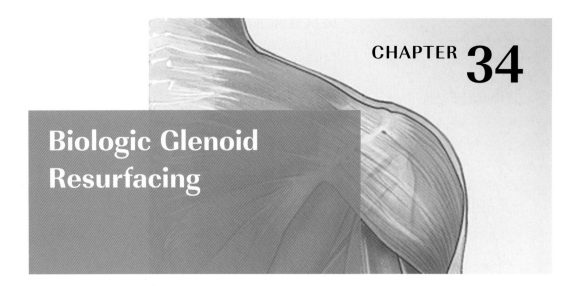

CHAPTER 34

Biologic Glenoid Resurfacing

Biologic resurfacing of the glenoid has been performed with various materials, including fascia lata autograft, fascia lata allograft, meniscal allograft, and Achilles tendon allograft.[1] The main advantage of biologic glenoid resurfacing lies in providing a new articulating surface for the glenoid while avoiding potential late-term complications associated with polyethylene wear and failure. Consequently, consideration of biologic glenoid resurfacing is most reasonable in younger patients. Biologic glenoid resurfacing also allows resurfacing of localized glenoid articular cartilage lesions that may result from trauma in young patients. In our practice, we almost always combine biologic glenoid resurfacing with humeral head arthroplasty (hemiarthroplasty or surface replacement) because our patients with glenoid articular cartilage disease almost always have associated humeral head articular cartilage disease.

Of the available tissues for use in biologic glenoid resurfacing, we prefer autogenous fascia lata. Use of the patient's own tissue minimizes the risk of graft rejection, a phenomenon that we have observed with allografts. Additionally, the morbidity associated with harvest of a fascia lata autograft is minimal.

INDICATIONS AND CONTRAINDICATIONS

Indications in our practice for biologic glenoid resurfacing are limited to a young patient (<40 years old) with glenoid disease; in an older patient, the use of a prosthetic glenoid component would be indicated. We have performed biologic resurfacing most commonly in patients with a generalized arthritic condition (i.e., glenohumeral chondrolysis; Fig. 34-1) but have also

used it for localized traumatic glenoid articular cartilage lesions. One situation in which we opt for a prosthetic glenoid component in a young patient is a diagnosis of juvenile rheumatoid arthritis.

A rare situation in which we use biologic glenoid resurfacing is a revision case with a competent rotator cuff in which hemiarthroplasty has resulted in symptomatic glenoid erosion and insufficient bone exists to permit prosthetic resurfacing (Fig. 34-2). In these scenarios, biologic resurfacing represents an alternative to resection arthroplasty (see Chapter 35 for more on indications for revision shoulder arthroplasty). In most primary cases in older patients in whom unconstrained arthroplasty is indicated yet insufficient glenoid bone exists for prosthetic resurfacing, we generally perform isolated hemiarthroplasty because most of these patients obtain satisfactory pain relief and function (although these results are inferior to those obtained with total shoulder arthroplasty) without prosthetic or biologic glenoid resurfacing.

Contraindications to biologic glenoid resurfacing include the standard contraindications to unconstrained shoulder arthroplasty. Additionally, any situation in which the native glenoid is insufficient to allow anchorage of the biologic tissue is a contraindication to biologic resurfacing (Fig. 34-3).

TECHNIQUE FOR BIOLOGIC GLENOID RESURFACING

Autogenous Fascia Lata Harvest

The operating room setup, anesthesia, patient positioning, skin preparation, surgical draping, and surgi-

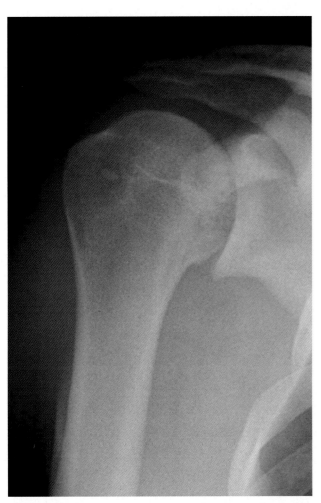

Figure 34-1 Radiograph of a young patient with glenohumeral joint chondrolysis after shoulder arthroscopy.

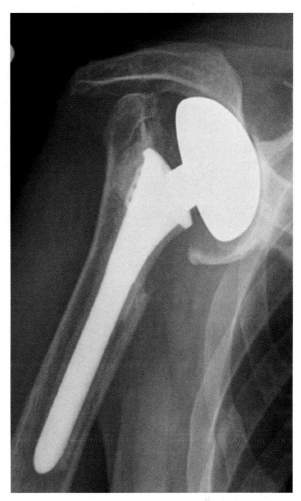

Figure 34-2 Glenoid erosion after hemiarthroplasty. The residual glenoid bone is insufficient to permit insertion of a prosthetic glenoid component.

cal approach are identical to that for other shoulder arthroplasties. Additionally, the contralateral lower extremity and hip region are prepared and draped (Fig. 34-4). Using the contralateral lower extremity permits an assistant to close the fascia lata harvest wound while the approach is made to the shoulder. An 8-cm incision is started 3 cm distal to the greater trochanter of the femur and extended distally along the longitudinal axis of the femur (Fig. 34-5). A needle tip electrocautery is used to obtain hemostasis and aids in dissection through the subcutaneous layer down to the fascia lata. The fascia lata is cleared of the overlying subcutaneous fat to complete the exposure (Fig. 34-6). A scalpel is used to harvest an 8-cm-long by 3-cm-wide segment of fascia lata (Fig. 34-7). The wound is irrigated; it is not necessary to close the residual defect in the fascia lata (Fig. 34-8). The subcutaneous tissue is

closed with 2-0 absorbable braided suture in an interrupted technique. The skin is closed with 3-0 absorbable monofilament suture in a continuous running subcuticular technique. Steri-Strips and sterile dressings are applied. The fascia lata is folded to double its thickness. Braided 2-0 absorbable suture is used to suture the perimeter of the autograft (Fig. 34-9).

Implantation of the Fascia Lata Autograft

A standard deltopectoral approach is performed as described in Chapter 8. The subscapularis is treated as described in Chapter 9 if hemiarthroplasty is planned. If humeral head resurfacing is planned, the anterior humeral circumflex vessels are preserved as detailed in Chapter 33. The glenoid is exposed by releasing the inferior glenohumeral joint capsule from the glenoid

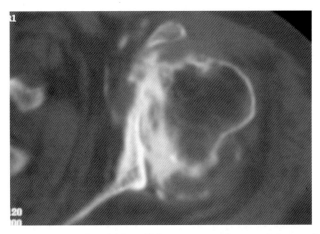

Figure 34-3 Glenoid insufficiency preventing anchorage of a biologic resurfacing graft.

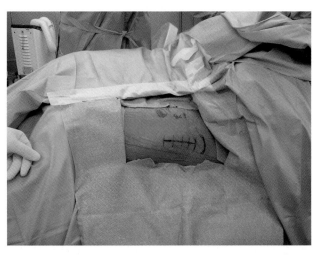

Figure 34-4 Preparation and draping for harvest of an autogenous fascia lata graft.

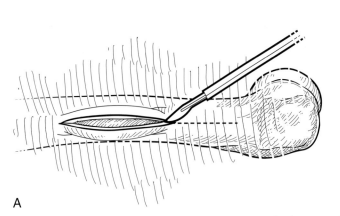

A

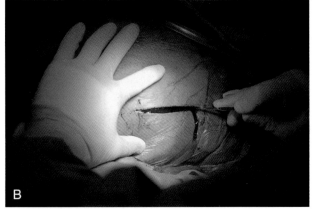

B

Figure 34-5 Incision for harvest of an autogenous fascia lata graft.

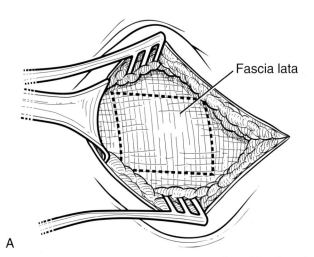

A

Fascia lata

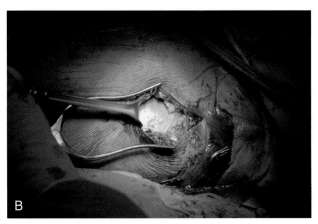

B

Figure 34-6 **A** and **B,** Completed exposure of the fascia lata graft.

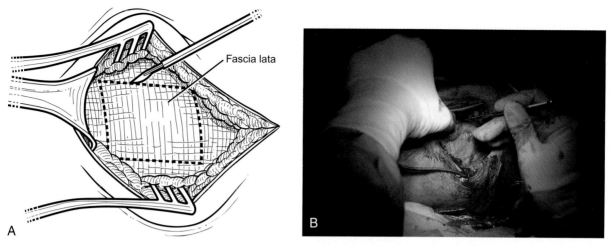

Figure 34-7   **A** and **B,** Harvesting of the fascia lata graft with a scalpel.

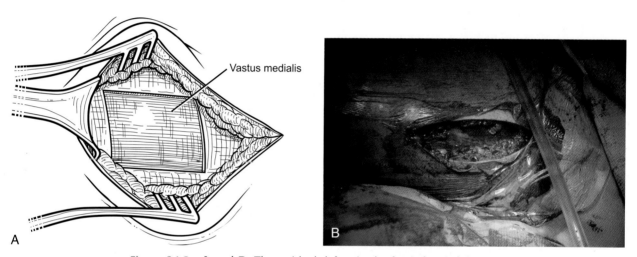

Figure 34-8   **A** and **B,** The residual defect in the fascia lata is left open.

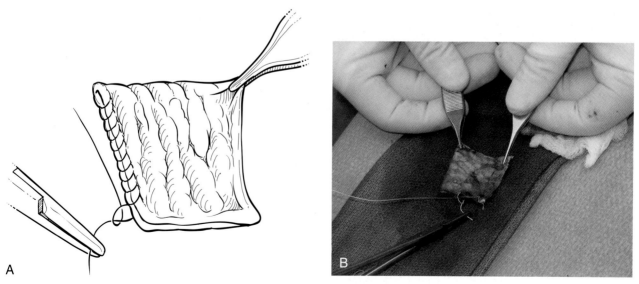

Figure 34-9   **A** and **B,** Preparation of the fascia lata graft by doubling it and suturing the three "free" sides.

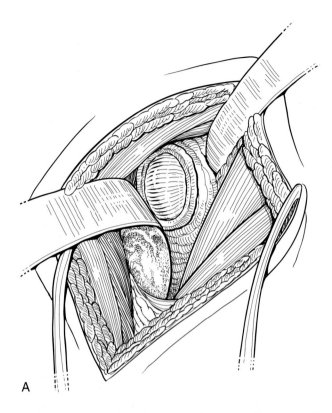

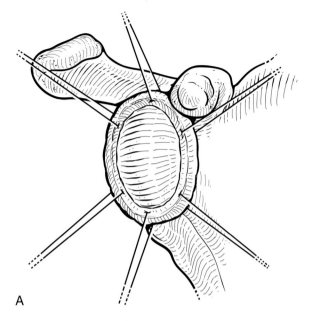

A

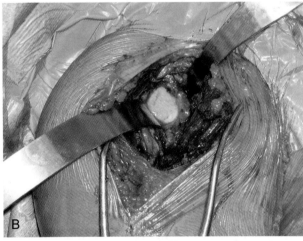

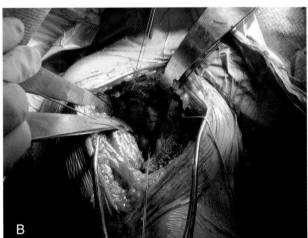

Figure 34-11 **A** and **B,** Sutures placed circumferentially around the labrum for use in fixation of the autogenous fascia lata.

Figure 34-10 **A** and **B,** Exposure of the glenoid before biologic resurfacing.

neck (Fig. 34-10). The glenoid joint surface is prepared by removing any residual articular cartilage with a Cobb elevator or motorized burr, if necessary. Any nonconcentric wear is corrected with the burr or a reamer (see Chapter 12), if needed. Two options exist for graft fixation. If the glenoid labrum is intact circumferentially, the autograft can be sutured directly to the intact glenoid labrum. If the glenoid labrum is absent or diseased to the extent that graft fixation would be compromised, bioabsorbable suture anchor fixation is used to secure the graft (we use a 2.9-mm

Bioraptor anchor, Smith Nephew, Inc., Andover, MA).

In patients with an intact glenoid labrum, no. 2 braided permanent sutures are placed through the labrum at the 12, 2, 4, 6, 8, and 10 o'clock positions (Fig. 34-11). These sutures are kept separate by tagging them with hemostats. The autograft is oriented so that the nonsutured side of the graft is superior. The glenoid side suture at each location is passed through the perimeter of the graft at each position (12, 2, 4, 6, 8, and 10 o'clock; Fig. 34-12). The graft is then passed down the sutures until it rests on the glenoid surface (Fig. 34-13). The sutures are tied sequentially to complete the resurfacing (Fig. 34-14). Alternatively, in patients with an insufficient labrum, a doubly loaded

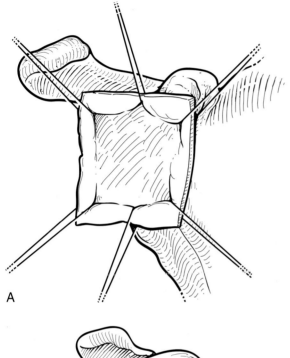

Figure 34-12 **A** to **C,** Sutures are passed through the autograft outside the wound to facilitate graft placement and fixation.

A

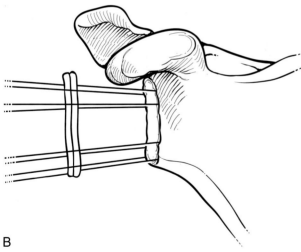

B

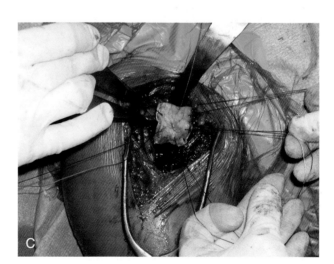

C

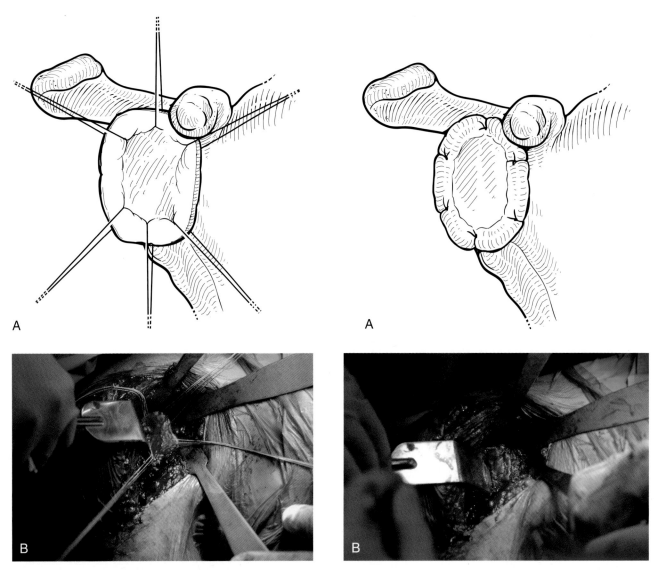

Figure 34-13 **A** and **B,** The graft is shuttled down the sutures to the glenoid face.

Figure 31-14 **A** and **B,** Final glenoid resurfacing after all sutures are tied.

bioabsorbable suture anchor can be placed on the glenoid margin in each quadrant of the glenoid (a total of four anchors), and the same suturing process used (Fig. 34-15). When using anchor fixation, a 3.0-mm hole is predrilled at each location and the anchors placed via standard insertion technique.

We have also performed biologic glenoid resurfacing for incomplete defects of glenoid articular cartilage. In this circumstance, only the area of full-thickness cartilage loss is prepared with the Cobb elevator or motorized burr. The fascia lata autograft is prepared as previously described, except that it is trimmed to fit

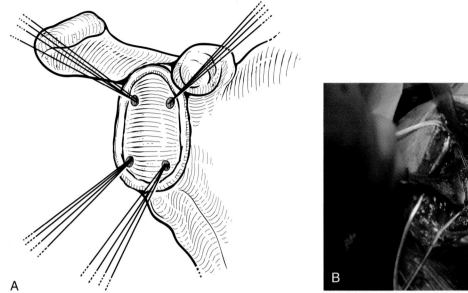

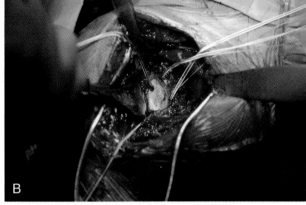

Figure 34-15 **A** and **B,** Suture anchor placement for biologic glenoid resurfacing in a patient with a deficient labrum.

the glenoid articular cartilage defect (Fig. 34-16). In this circumstance it is often helpful to use suture anchors to fix the graft at the location immediately adjacent to the remaining intact glenoid articular cartilage (Fig. 34-17). Figure 34-18 shows the final

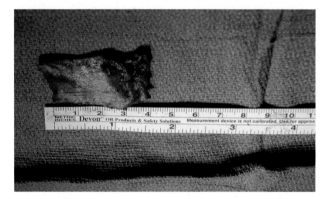

Figure 34-16 Fascia lata autograft used for resurfacing the superior half of the glenoid in a young patient in whom the inferior half of the glenoid articular cartilage is intact.

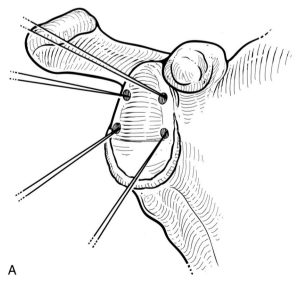

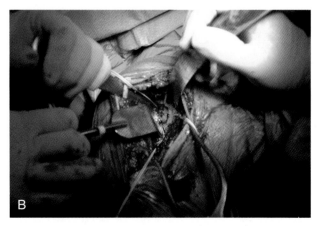

Figure 34-17 **A** and **B,** Suture anchor placement for fixation of a fascia lata autograft used for resurfacing the superior half of the glenoid.

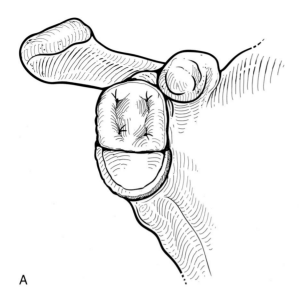

A

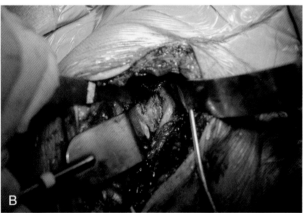

B

Figure 34-18 **A** and **B,** Final construct after resurfacing of the superior half of the glenoid.

construct after resurfacing of the superior half of the glenoid.

After biologic glenoid resurfacing is complete, the humeral portion of the surgery is performed and the subscapularis and wound are closed as for unconstrained shoulder arthroplasty.

REFERENCE

1. Burkhead WZ Jr, Hutton KS: Biologic resurfacing of the glenoid with hemiarthroplasty of the shoulder. J Shoulder Elbow Surg 1995;4:263-270.

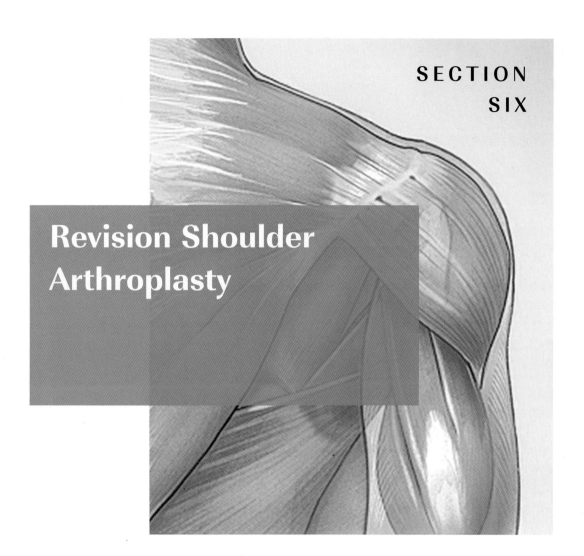

SECTION SIX

Revision Shoulder Arthroplasty

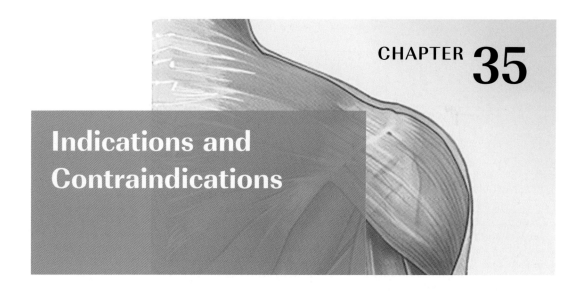

CHAPTER 35

Indications and Contraindications

Just as with hip and knee arthroplasty, as the volume of shoulder arthroplasties performed each year increases, so will the number of patients requiring revision shoulder arthroplasty. Indications for performing revision shoulder arthroplasty are variable and numerous and can include problems related to the glenoid, problems related to the humerus, and problems related to the soft tissues (rotator cuff, instability). Rarely, infection, either early postoperative or late-appearing hematogenous, is an indication for revision arthroplasty. Complications related to healing of the greater and lesser tuberosities can be observed after unconstrained shoulder arthroplasty performed for proximal humeral fractures. Finally, certain periprosthetic humeral fractures are an indication for revision shoulder arthroplasty. This chapter details our specific indications and contraindications for revision shoulder arthroplasty.

PROBLEMS RELATED TO THE GLENOID

Problems related to the glenoid are the most common indications for revision shoulder arthroplasty in our practice. One category consists of patients with problems of their native glenoid (glenoid erosion), and a second category includes patients who have problems with a previously placed glenoid component.

Glenoid Erosion

Glenoid erosion after hemiarthroplasty is a multifactorial problem.[1] It may occur early or late and does not seem to be related to any readily identifiable risk factor. This problem occurs when the metallic prosthetic humeral head erodes into the softer glenoid bone (Fig. 35-1). Initially, pain may be the sole manifestation of this problem. As the erosion progresses medially, the normal length-tension relationships of the rotator cuff may become compromised and result in substantial weakness (Fig. 35-2).

Glenoid erosion may be central or peripheral. If the rotator cuff is intact, as in primary osteoarthritis, the erosion is usually central or, less commonly, posterior (Fig. 35-3). If the rotator cuff is deficient, the erosion is generally superior (Fig. 35-4) or, less commonly, anterior (if the subscapularis is deficient; Fig. 35-5).

Glenoid erosion is best treated by resurfacing of the glenoid if sufficient native glenoid bone is available for implantation of a glenoid component (see Chapter 36). Frequently, the humeral component will require revision for glenoid exposure, and two options are available to the surgeon. We may exchange the component for a smaller head size in an unconstrained arthroplasty (Fig. 35-6) or change to a reverse-design arthroplasty. In general, with a functioning rotator

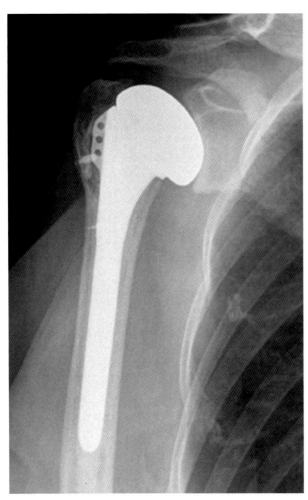

Figure 35-1 Radiograph demonstrating osseous glenoid erosion after hemiarthroplasty.

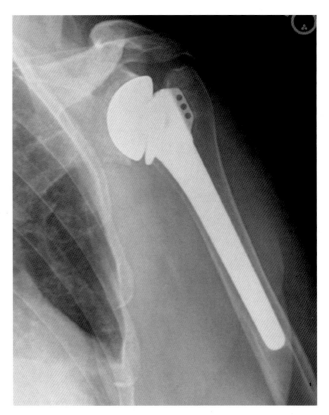

Figure 35-2 Severe medialization of the humeral head caused by progressive glenoid erosion.

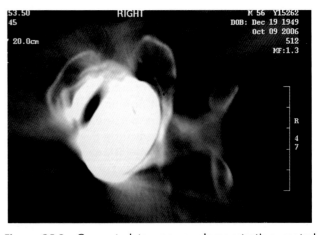

Figure 35-3 Computed tomogram demonstrating central glenoid erosion after hemiarthroplasty for primary osteoarthritis.

cuff, an unconstrained arthroplasty is performed for revision arthroplasty. If rotator cuff function is significantly compromised, revision to a reverse prosthesis is performed.

Glenoid Component Failure

Glenoid component failure can vary from subtle loosening to migration of the component with severe glenoid bone loss (Fig. 35-7). Additionally, mechanical failure of the implant can necessitate revision surgery (Fig. 35-8). When considering revision surgery for failure of a glenoid component, the surgeon must first decide whether to simply remove the failed glenoid component or to remove the failed glenoid component and reconstruct the osseous glenoid. In debilitated patients seeking mainly pain relief without significant concern for function, isolated removal of

Text continued on p. 363

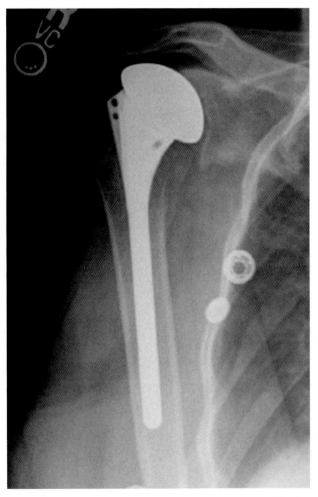

Figure 35-4 Superior glenoid erosion in a patient who has undergone hemiarthroplasty for rotator cuff tear arthropathy.

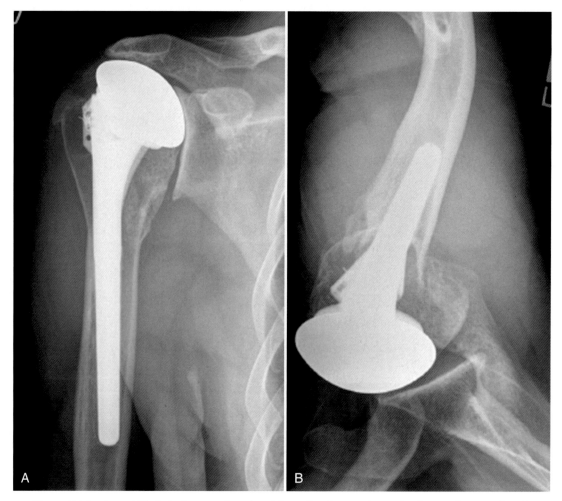

Figure 35-5   A and **B,** Anterior superior glenoid erosion in a patient who has undergone hemi-arthroplasty for anterior superior rotator cuff insufficiency.

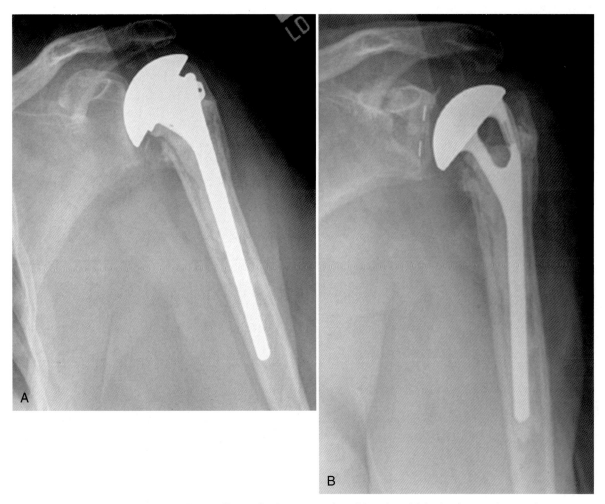

Figure 35-6 **A,** Pre-revision radiograph. **B,** Humeral revision in which the humeral stem has been exchanged and the humeral head exchanged for a smaller size.

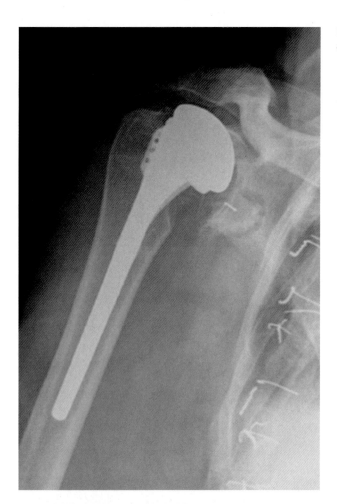

Figure 35-7 Radiograph showing loosening of a glenoid component.

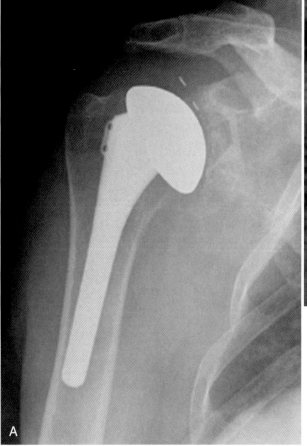

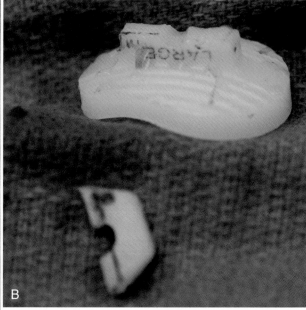

Figure 35-8 **A** and **B,** Mechanical failure of a glenoid implant.

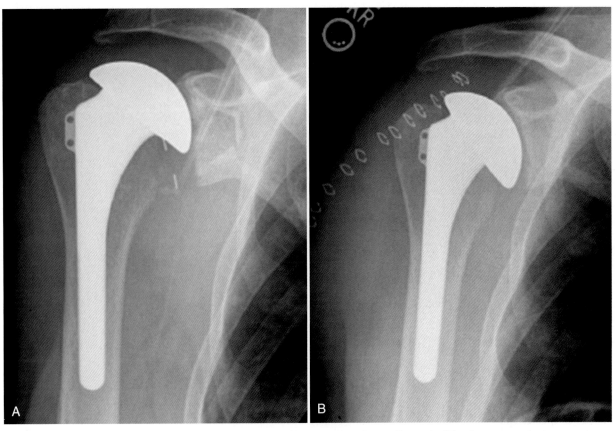

Figure 35-9   Preoperative radiograph (**A**) and postoperative radiograph (**B**) after removal of a loose glenoid component and bone grafting of the residual osseous defect in the glenoid.

the glenoid component is usually the best treatment option. In other patients, glenoid reconstruction with iliac crest bone graft is indicated. For patients undergoing revision with an unconstrained prosthesis, we reconstruct the glenoid with an iliac crest bone graft as the first stage. Six months later, after complete incorporation of the bone graft, if the shoulder is still painful, we perform the second stage, which consists of placement of a new glenoid component (Fig. 35-9). When performing revision surgery with a reverse-design prosthesis, glenoid reconstruction and revision can often be performed as a single stage, provided that the central post of the revision glenoid component can be firmly seated in native glenoid bone (Fig. 35-10).

Just as in cases of glenoid erosion, patients requiring revision surgery for a problem with the glenoid component often require revision of the humeral component for glenoid exposure, and the surgeon can exchange the component for a smaller head size in an unconstrained arthroplasty or change to a reverse-design arthroplasty. As previously mentioned, in a

patient with a functioning rotator cuff, an unconstrained arthroplasty is used for revision arthroplasty. If rotator cuff function is significantly compromised, revision to a reverse prosthesis is performed.

Reverse Glenoid Component

In our experience, failure of the glenoid component of a reverse prosthesis is less common than failure of the glenoid component of an unconstrained shoulder arthroplasty. The most common problem that we observe is inadvertent placement of the glenoid component in a superiorly oriented position (Fig. 35-11). This usually occurs when a superior surgical approach has been used to place the reverse prosthesis. Although this radiographic finding does not merit revision surgery in and of itself, revision is indicated if this problem evolves into early glenoid loosening (Fig. 35-12).

Another radiographic finding related to a reverse glenoid component is inferior scapular notching. This finding can be related to excessive superior placement

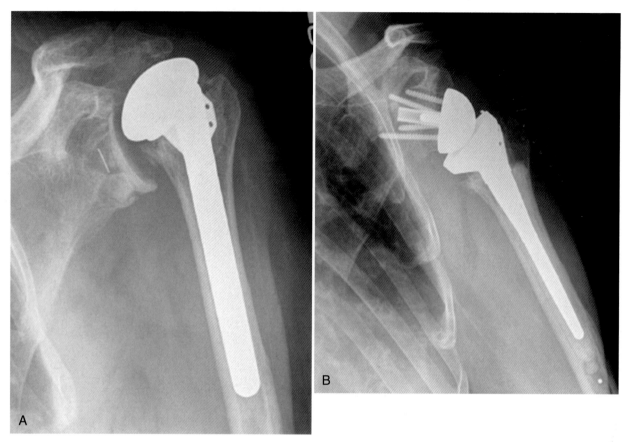

Figure 35-10   **A,** Preoperative radiograph. **B,** Postoperative radiograph after revision of a failed unconstrained shoulder arthroplasty to a reverse shoulder arthroplasty with bone grafting of the glenoid.

of the reverse glenoid component (Fig. 35-13). Notching, even when it is severe, has not been shown to cause loosening of the glenoid component, and revision surgery is unnecessary in the absence of glenoid loosening.

PROBLEMS RELATED TO THE HUMERUS

Humeral component problems requiring revision surgery are much less common than glenoid problems. Specifically, aseptic loosening of both unconstrained and reverse humeral components is rare. More commonly, revision surgery for a humeral component problem results from positioning or size of the humeral component.

Unconstrained Humeral Components

The main problem that leads us to revise an unconstrained humeral component is placement of a humeral head prosthesis that is too large (Fig. 35-14). This can lead to stiffness, glenoid problems, and rotator cuff problems. If the stem of the humeral implant is acceptably positioned, the humeral head is simply exchanged for a smaller size.

Less frequently, a humeral implant will be improperly positioned, generally with respect to humeral version. Problems with humeral component version can lead to instability of the component; nonconcentric glenoid loading, wear, and loosening; and failure of subscapularis repair. These scenarios are indications for revision of the humeral component.

Reverse Humeral Components

Even in cases in which a reverse humeral component is properly positioned, the deltoid muscle can "stretch out" and result in loss of prosthetic stability and, ultimately, dislocation. Patients most at risk for this complication are those with proximal humeral bone loss (Fig. 35-15). In such cases it is sometimes necessary to add more length to the humeral component to restore

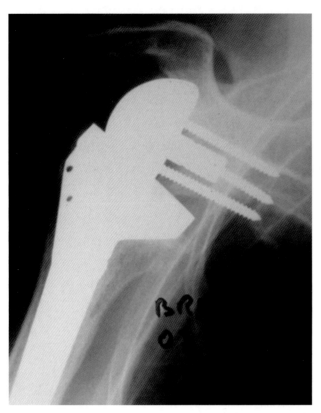

Figure 35-11 Superiorly oriented glenoid component after reverse shoulder arthroplasty performed through a superior approach.

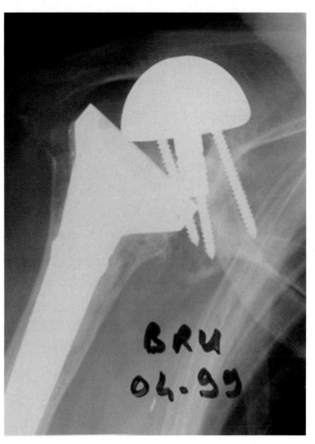

Figure 35-12 Failure of the glenoid component in reverse shoulder arthroplasty. The glenoid component was initially placed in a superiorly directed orientation.

prosthetic stability via restoration of deltoid tension. This can usually be accomplished by exchanging the primarily placed polyethylene liner for a thicker liner or adding a metallic augment, or both (Fig. 35-16). Tensioning the deltoid by adding length to the prosthesis almost never requires removal of the humeral stem. In cases in which use of a metallic augment and the thickest polyethylene liner fails to stabilize the prosthesis, multiple metallic augments can be stacked together and secured with a custom-manufactured screw (Fig. 35-17).

PROBLEMS RELATED TO SOFT TISSUE

Soft tissue problems necessitating revision shoulder arthroplasty can be divided into those related to instability and those related to the rotator cuff. These problems often occur concomitantly because rotator cuff insufficiency can lead to glenohumeral prosthetic instability.

Subscapularis Problems

Occasionally, subscapularis dehiscence will develop after unconstrained shoulder arthroplasty. In many circumstances, postoperative failure of a subscapularis repair will be asymptomatic or minimally symptomatic and is a contraindication to revision surgery. If the patient has early (<6 weeks postoperatively) subscapularis failure without instability, subscapularis repair with retention of all components can be considered, provided that they are appropriately sized and positioned. If the patient complains only of weakness and pain without instability and has chronic subscapularis insufficiency, a subcoracoid pectoralis major transfer with retention of all components can be considered, provided that they are appropriately sized and positioned.

If subscapularis insufficiency is coupled with either dynamic or static anterior instability after unconstrained shoulder arthroplasty, our experience has been that revision to a reverse-design prosthesis is the

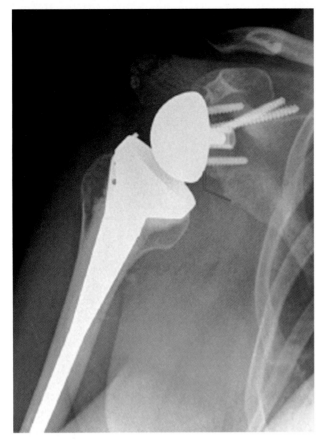

Figure 35-13 Scapular notching after reverse shoulder arthroplasty in which the glenoid component was placed superiorly on the glenoid face. The red line indicates the original border of the glenoid.

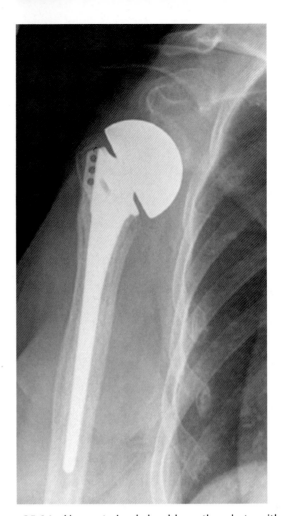

Figure 35-14 Unconstrained shoulder arthroplasty with an excessively large humeral head component.

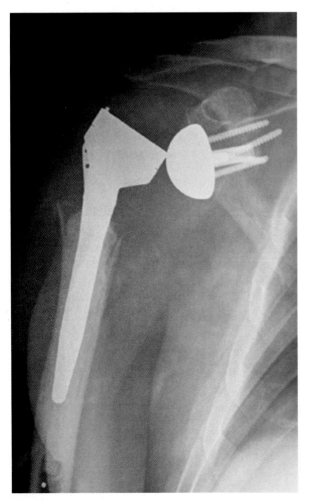

Figure 35-15 Patient with severe proximal humeral bone loss resulting in dislocation of the reverse prosthesis.

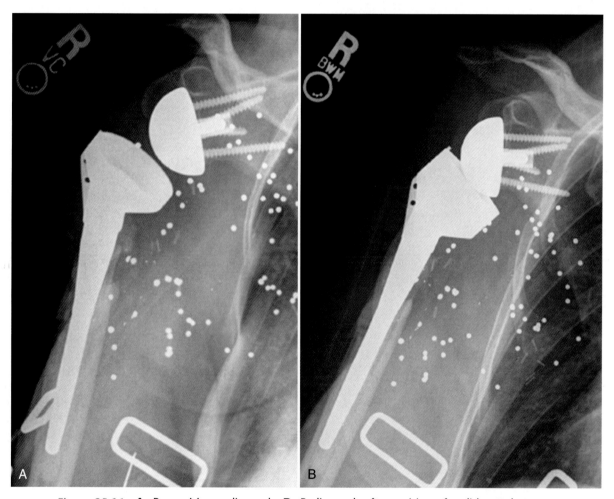

Figure 35-16 **A,** Pre-revision radiograph. **B,** Radiograph after revision of a dislocated reverse prosthesis by adding a metallic augment with a thicker polyethylene spacer to increase deltoid tension and prosthetic stability.

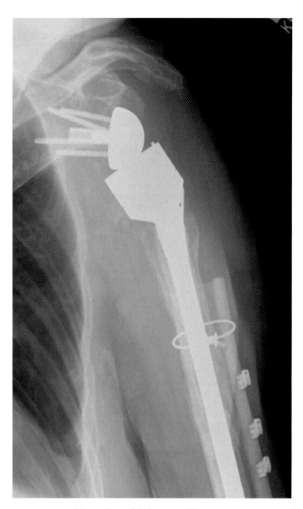

Figure 35-17 Use of multiple metallic augments to stabilize a dislocated reverse prosthesis. This requires the use of a custom-manufactured screw to hold the augments together.

only reliable way of restoring glenohumeral stability (Fig. 35-18).

Other Rotator Cuff Problems

The development of rotator cuff insufficiency after unconstrained shoulder arthroplasty is very rare. In cases in which a patient has sustained a massive (two or more tendons) rotator cuff tear after unconstrained shoulder arthroplasty that has resulted in severe dysfunction and static or dynamic glenohumeral prosthetic instability, revision to a reverse-design prosthesis can be considered (Fig. 35-19).

Instability

Glenohumeral instability after unconstrained shoulder arthroplasty usually occurs in one of two scenarios. First, instability can occur with rotator cuff insuffi-

ciency, as previously mentioned. Second, instability can occur in patients who have undergone unconstrained shoulder arthroplasty for primary osteoarthritis with posterior glenoid wear and posterior capsular distention (Fig. 35-20). In these cases we have found soft tissue procedures unpredictable in restoration of glenohumeral stability. We opt for revision to a reverse-design prosthesis (Fig. 35-21).

A less common problem causing instability is an unconstrained humeral implant positioned in incorrect version (Fig. 35-22). This is an indication for revision of the humeral component and placement of the revision component in correct humeral version.

INFECTION

Fortunately, infections are rare after shoulder arthroplasty. When infections do occur, surgery is indicated. Early postoperative infections (<2 weeks after surgery) can be treated initially with multiple irrigation and débridement sessions, exchange of any nonfixed modular components (i.e., humeral head), and retention of the remainder of the components. Late infections and early infections failing component-retaining procedures should be treated with component removal. Revision arthroplasty can be considered as a second stage after appropriate treatment of the infection (Fig. 35-23).

SPECIAL SITUATION—TUBEROSITY PROBLEMS AFTER UNCONSTRAINED ARTHROPLASTY FOR FRACTURE

Tuberosity malunion and nonunion after unconstrained shoulder arthroplasty for proximal humeral fracture are an indication for revision shoulder arthroplasty with a reverse-design prosthesis (Fig. 35-24). Our experience in achieving reliable tuberosity union once tuberosity migration has occurred has not been favorable.

PERIPROSTHETIC FRACTURE

Displaced periprosthetic fractures not amenable to nonoperative treatment or treatment by open reduction and internal fixation because of inability to achieve adequate fixation proximally are an indication for revision shoulder arthroplasty (Fig. 35-25). In this scenario, we believe it best to remove the existing humeral stem and revise to a long-stem humeral component to act as an intramedullary fixation device.

Text continued on p. 374

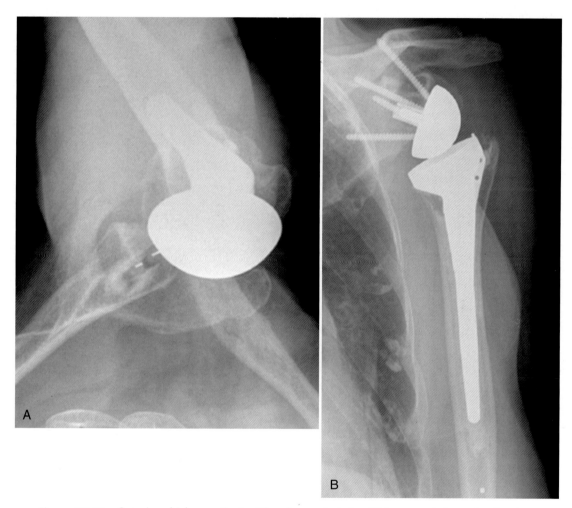

Figure 35-18 Case in which a patient with subscapularis insufficiency and dynamic glenohumeral prosthetic instability (**A**) underwent revision with a reverse prosthesis (**B**).

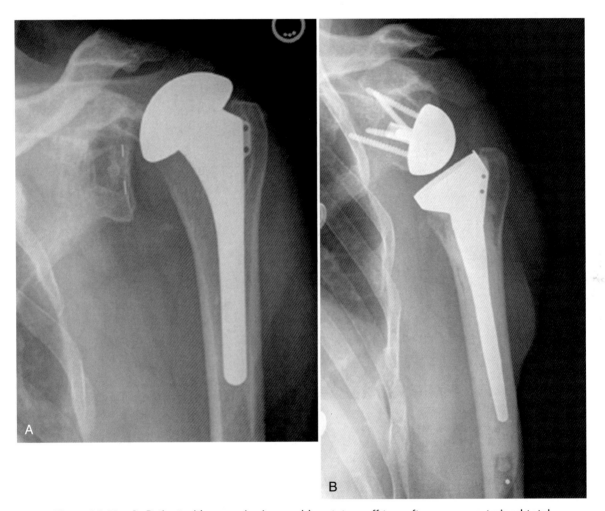

Figure 35-19   **A,** Patient with a massive irreparable rotator cuff tear after an unconstrained total shoulder arthroplasty. **B,** Static superior migration of the humerus required revision to a reverse prosthesis.

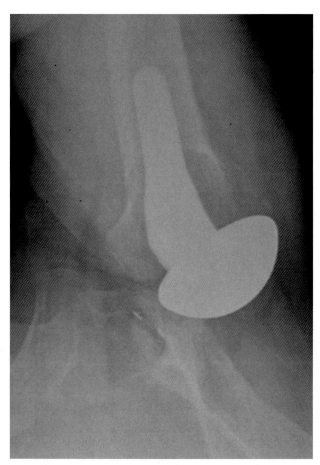

Figure 35-20   Posterior dislocation of a total shoulder arthroplasty performed for primary osteoarthritis in a patient with severe posterior glenoid wear.

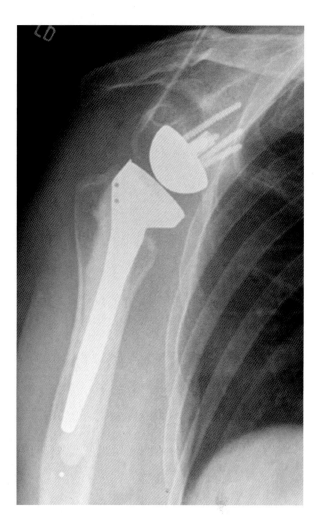

Figure 35-21   Revision of a posteriorly dislocated unconstrained total shoulder arthroplasty to a reverse prosthesis.

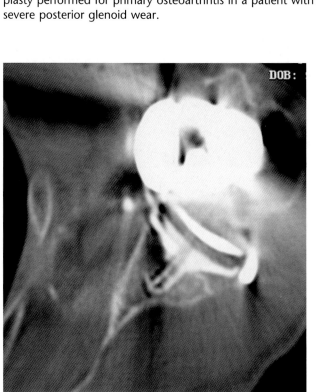

Figure 35-22   Computed tomogram of a patient with a humeral component placed in excessive anteversion that resulted in anterior instability.

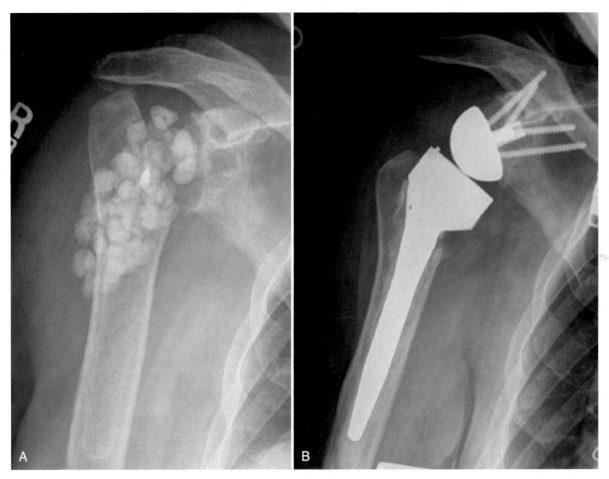

Figure 35-23 Infection of the primary arthroplasty (**A**) required revision shoulder arthroplasty (**B**).

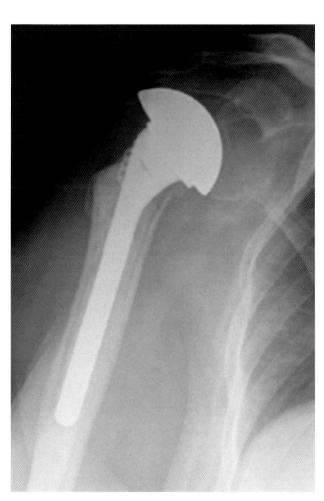

Figure 35-24 Tuberosity nonunion after hemiarthroplasty for the treatment of a proximal humeral fracture.

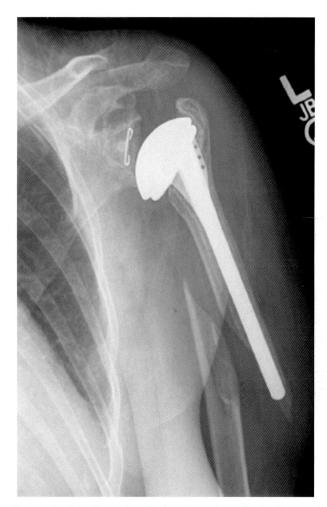

Figure 35-25 Severely displaced periprosthetic humeral fracture.

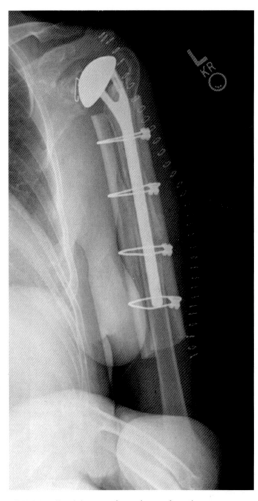

Figure 35-26   Revision arthroplasty for the treatment of a periprosthetic fracture.

Table 35-1	**CONTRAINDICATIONS TO REVISION SHOULDER ARTHROPLASTY**	
Contraindication	**Absolute or Relative**	**Comments**
Poor generalized health	Relative	Appropriate perioperative medical treatment required
Active infection	Absolute	Must clear infection first. May be candidate for revision as a second stage
Axillary nerve palsy	Absolute	Better suited for resection arthroplasty
Deltoid insufficiency	Absolute	Better suited for resection arthroplasty
Insufficient humeral bone stock	Relative	May be able to restore bone stock with a proximal humeral reconstruction
Insufficient glenoid bone stock	Relative	May be able to restore bone stock with a staged procedure
Poor patient motivation	Absolute	

This is combined with allograft struts placed peripherally at the fracture site and fixated with cerclage cables (Fig. 35-26). In addition to this scenario, any periprosthetic fracture in which the humeral stem is loose is an indication for revision of the humeral component via the same technique.

CONTRAINDICATIONS TO REVISION SHOULDER ARTHROPLASTY

Contraindications to revision shoulder arthroplasty are listed in Table 35-1. Some of these contraindications are absolute, whereas others are relative.

REFERENCE

1. Hertel R, Lehmann O: Glenoid erosion after hemiarthroplasty of the shoulder. In Walch G, Boileau P, Molé D (eds): 2000 Prothèses d'Epaule . . . Recul de 2 à 10 Ans. Paris, Sauramps Medical, 2001, pp 417-423.

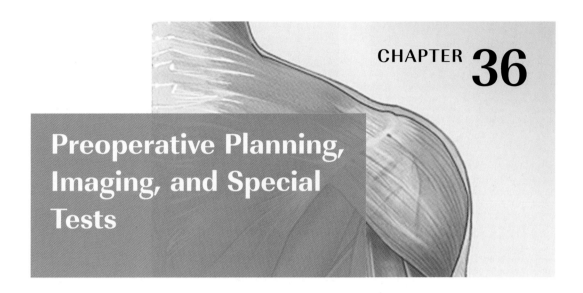

CHAPTER 36

Preoperative Planning, Imaging, and Special Tests

Revision shoulder arthroplasty is more challenging overall than primary shoulder arthroplasty. Preoperative planning for a revision arthroplasty case is critically important and is initiated as soon as revision arthroplasty is being considered; it should never be an afterthought the morning of surgery. Preoperative planning for revision shoulder arthroplasty is similar to, albeit more complex than, planning for primary shoulder arthroplasty and consists of reviewing the patient's clinical history and physical examination, radiographs, and secondary imaging studies, as well as any special tests obtained. This chapter reviews our approach to preoperative planning for revision shoulder arthroplasty.

CLINICAL HISTORY AND EXAMINATION

Although description of a detailed shoulder history and examination are beyond the scope of this textbook, certain aspects of the history and physical examination are important in preoperative planning for revision shoulder arthroplasty. The patient's complaints are reviewed, such as the type of symptoms (pain, stiffness, weakness), duration of symptoms (weeks, months, years), indication for the primary arthroplasty, initial results of the primary arthroplasty (relief of all symptoms, relief of some symptoms, no improvement from surgery), and the presence of any symptoms of infection (previous history of infection, fevers, wound redness, wound drainage). These shoulder-specific complaints help the surgeon decide which

patients are candidates for revision shoulder arthroplasty. A patient with complaints of only mild pain, mild weakness, or mild stiffness may initially best be treated with nonoperative modalities even if radiographs demonstrate positive findings such as glenoid erosion after hemiarthroplasty. Similarly, a patient with a sudden onset of symptoms of a short duration to date may be experiencing a transient acute rotator cuff tendinitis not directly related to the shoulder replacement. In this situation, a period of nonoperative treatment would certainly be indicated. Special attention is given to factors that could make the operative procedure more difficult. The number and type of all previous shoulder surgeries, arthroplasty and nonarthroplasty, should be recorded in the patient's history. Chronic use of nonsteroidal anti-inflammatory medications can result in excessive operative blood loss, so they should be discontinued the week before surgery.

Any medical history of systemic illness (diabetes mellitus, cardiac problems) should be considered in preoperative planning. Although these factors may not affect the actual surgical procedure, they may necessitate special considerations in the patient's postoperative care. Appropriate medical consultations should be obtained well in advance of the surgery date. The availability of appropriate care of these systemic illnesses, including the availability of consultants, should be confirmed before surgery.

All of our patients undergo a thorough shoulder examination, much of which is detailed in Chapter 7. The visual appearance of the shoulder yields useful

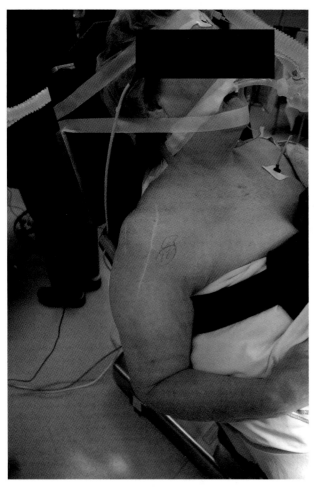

Figure 36-1   Previous skin incision used in primary shoulder arthroplasty.

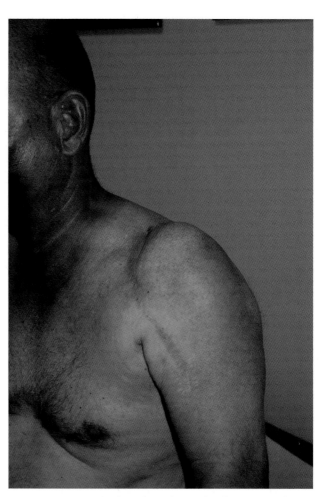

Figure 36-2   Hemiarthroplasty located subcutaneously secondary to anterior superior escape.

information in candidates for revision shoulder arthroplasty. The presence and location of surgical scars are noted. The preoperative plan should include whether all or part of a previous skin incision site is to be used or whether a completely new incision is to be created (Fig. 36-1). In thin patients, anterior superior escape of a prosthetic humeral head caused by anterior superior rotator cuff deficiency may be obvious (Fig. 36-2). Special attention should be paid to the condition of the deltoid, especially if it has previously been surgically violated (Fig. 36-3). Atrophy of the supraspinatus and infraspinatus should be noted as well (Fig. 36-4).

Both active and passive mobility is recorded, as detailed in Chapter 7. Special attention should be paid to evaluation of the deltoid muscle. If deltoid contractility appears to be compromised, further evaluation with electromyography and nerve conduction studies should be performed before revision shoulder arthroplasty.

The integrity of the rotator cuff is tested (see Chapter 7). Details of this examination are of paramount importance in preoperative planning for revision surgery. Although a minor rotator cuff deficiency such as an isolated supraspinatus tendon tear may have little influence on preoperative planning, larger rotator cuff tears (two-, three-, and four-tendon tears), especially when coupled with static or dynamic glenohumeral instability, may change the type of revision prosthesis to be inserted (reverse instead of unconstrained).

The results of the clinical history and examination are documented in the patient's chart and reviewed well in advance of surgery as part of preoperative planning.

RADIOGRAPHY

Recent (within 3 months) magnification- and fluoroscopy-controlled radiographs are obtained in all patients

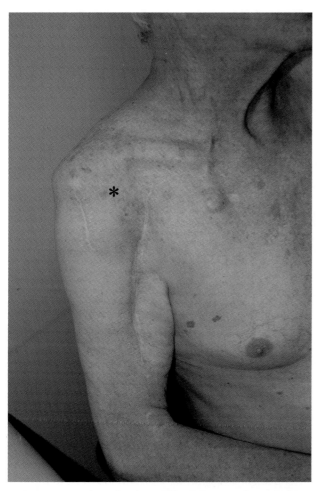

Figure 36-3 Atrophy (*asterisk*) of the anterior deltoid.

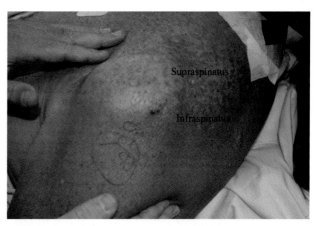

Figure 36-4 Atrophy of the supraspinatus and infra-spinatus.

who are candidates for revision shoulder arthroplasty. The same views obtained for primary arthroplasty, including an anteroposterior view of the glenohumeral joint with the arm in neutral rotation, an axillary view, and a scapular outlet view, are obtained in the revision scenario. Additionally, full-length orthogonal views of the humerus (anteroposterior and lateral) are obtained to evaluate diaphyseal cortical bone quality (Fig. 36-5). The previous arthroplasty is inspected on these radiographs for signs of loosening of the glenoid and humeral components, signs of mechanical failure of components (Fig. 36-6), appropriateness of compo-

nent size and position, signs of static or dynamic instability (Fig. 36-7), and signs of infection (Fig. 36-8).

Preoperative radiographic templating can be useful in planning revision shoulder arthroplasty, especially in cases of proximal humeral deficiency. In most of these cases, the proximal humeral deficiency with resultant rotator cuff compromise constitutes an indication for revision with a reverse-design prosthesis. In patients demonstrating proximal humeral bone loss, bilateral full-length magnification-controlled antero-posterior humeral radiographs are obtained. These radiographs are used to help select the height at which to implant the humeral stem. Using the full-length humeral radiographs, the desired position of the reverse prosthesis is templated on the radiograph of the unaffected humerus, and the level of the metaphy-seal-diaphyseal junction of the humeral component is marked (Fig. 36-9). The distance from the transepicon-dylar axis at the elbow to this point is measured (Fig. 36-10). A mark is made at the same distance from the transepicondylar axis on the affected radiograph. A second mark is made at the most proximal extent of the humeral shaft (Fig. 36-11). The distance between the desired prosthetic level at the metaphy-

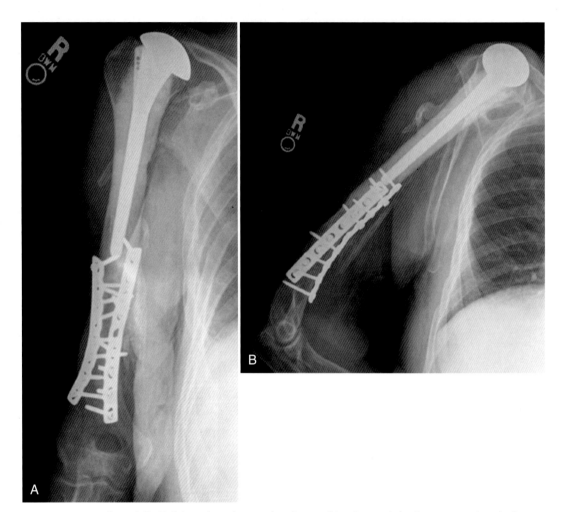

Figure 36-5 **A** and **B,** Full-length orthogonal radiographic views of the humerus taken before revision shoulder arthroplasty.

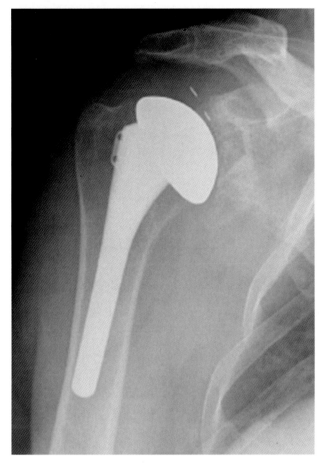

Figure 36-6   Mechanical failure of a keeled glenoid component detected on anteroposterior radiography.

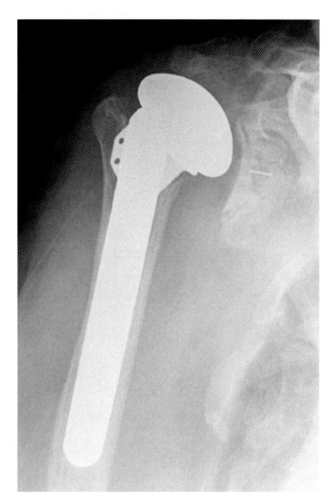

Figure 36-7   Static superior migration after total shoulder arthroplasty.

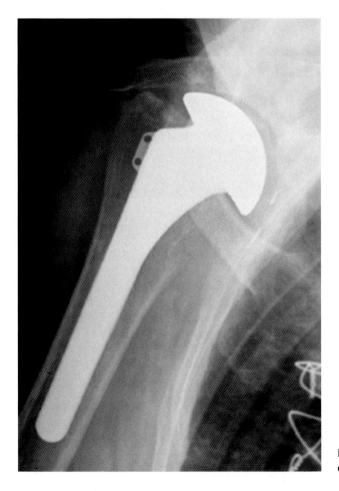

Figure 36-8   Osteolysis around both the glenoid and humeral components is strongly suggestive of infection.

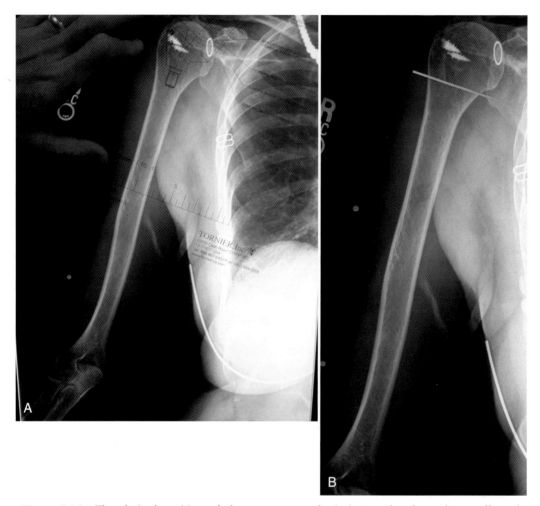

Figure 36-9 The desired position of the reverse prosthesis is templated on the unaffected humeral radiograph (**A**), and the level of the metaphyseal-diaphyseal junction of the humeral component is marked (**B**).

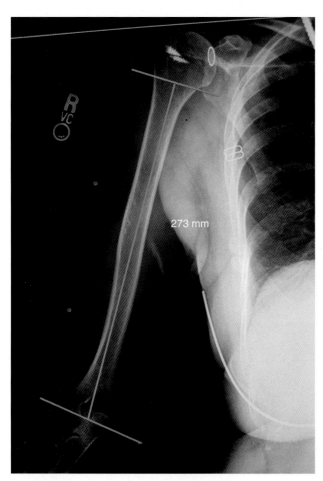

Figure 36-10 The distance from the transepicondylar axis at the elbow to the desired level of the metaphyseal-diaphyseal junction of the humeral component is measured.

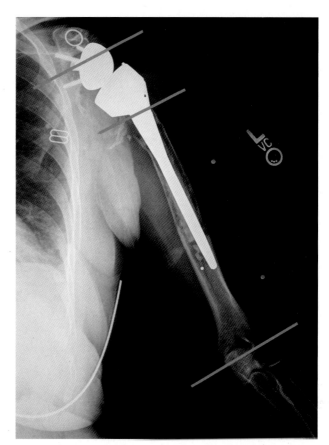

Figure 36-11 A mark is made at the same distance from the transepicondylar axis on the affected radiograph. A second mark is made at the most proximal extent of the humeral shaft.

seal-diaphyseal junction and the proximal extent of the humeral shaft is measured (Fig. 36-12). A ruler is used during surgery to measure the distance and mark the level on the humeral stem for the desired prosthetic position (Fig. 36-13). This technique of preoperative planning provides only a guideline and may be superseded by intraoperative observations.

Rarely, proximal humeral bone loss during revision surgery is sufficiently severe to necessitate use of a custom implant or proximal humeral composite bone graft. Templates are useful to determine whether existing prefabricated implants are sufficient or whether a custom-manufactured implant is required.

SECONDARY IMAGING

A computed tomographic arthrogram is obtained in all patients for evaluation of the rotator cuff tendons and musculature before revision shoulder arthroplasty (Fig. 36-14). This study further assists in evaluation of possible component loosening. Many patients exhibit radiolucent lines around the glenoid component after unconstrained total shoulder arthroplasty. Use of computed tomographic arthrography assists in determining whether these components are indeed loose by demonstrating radiographic contrast material around the base of the component (Fig. 36-15). Computed tomography also provides the greatest osseous detail of the glenoid and can show the presence and extent of bony glenoid deficiency. Bony deficiencies can occur after erosion from hemiarthroplasty (Fig. 36-16). In these cases the computed tomogram helps determine whether the existing glenoid bone is sufficient

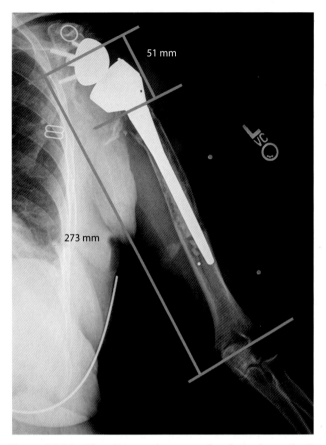

Figure 36-12   The distance between the desired prosthetic level at the metaphyseal-diaphyseal junction and the proximal extent of the humeral shaft is measured.

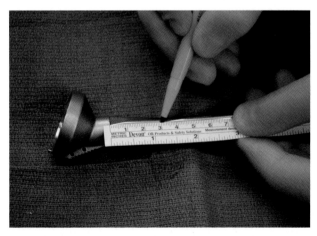

Figure 36-13   A ruler is used during surgery to measure the distance and mark the level on the humeral stem for the desired prosthetic position.

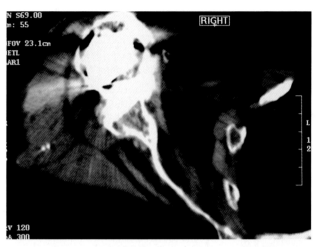

Figure 36-14   Evaluation of the rotator cuff tendons and musculature with computed tomographic arthrography.

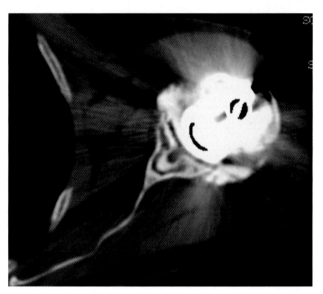

Figure 36-15   Glenoid component loosening identified on computed tomographic arthrography. Note the contrast material located around the keel of the glenoid component.

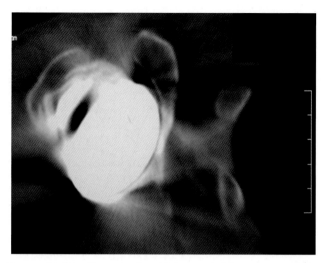

Figure 36-16 Central glenoid bony deficiency caused by glenoid erosion after hemiarthroplasty.

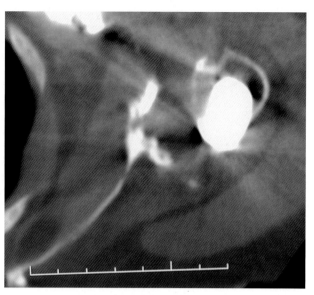

Figure 36-17 Bony glenoid deficiency caused by loosening of the glenoid component.

to allow implantation of a glenoid component. Bony deficiencies more commonly occur concomitantly with loosening of the glenoid component (Fig. 36-17). In these cases the computed tomogram allows the bony deficiency to be classified as contained or uncontained (Fig. 36-18).[1]

The rotator cuff is evaluated, including assessment of tendinous integrity and muscle quality (fatty infiltration). The condition of the long head of the biceps tendon is noted, particularly its position (centered, subluxated, dislocated, ruptured), to assist in identifying it at the time of surgery.

SPECIAL TESTS

In all candidates for revision shoulder arthroplasty, regardless of whether signs of infection are present, a preoperative infection workup is indicated, including hematologic evaluation consisting of a complete blood cell count with differential, a sedimentation rate, and C-reactive protein. Additionally, fluoroscopically guided shoulder aspiration performed at the time of computed tomographic arthrography is obtained and the specimen submitted for aerobic, anaerobic, fungal, and mycobacterial culture. If the findings are suggestive of infection (increased sedimentation rate,

increased C-reactive protein, leukocytosis, moderate to many leukocytes observed in aspirated joint fluid), intraoperative frozen histologic sections are planned at the time of shoulder arthroplasty. The patient is educated that the revision surgery may be staged if infection is further suspected by the results of intraoperative histologic tissue analysis. If the preoperative infection workup yields a positive culture from the aspirate, infection is considered present and the treatment plan proceeds accordingly. In all patients with an infected shoulder arthroplasty, consultation with an infectious disease specialist is obtained preoperatively.

Electromyography and nerve conduction studies are performed in any patient with a suggestion of neurologic deficiencies on physical examination. Specifically, all patients unable to reliably contract the deltoid should undergo neurologic testing before revision shoulder arthroplasty. If the deltoid is compromised, neurologic consultation is obtained. Revision shoulder arthroplasty is reserved until the time of deltoid/axillary nerve recovery. In patients with permanent deltoid insufficiency, revision arthroplasty is contraindicated and resection arthroplasty is considered.

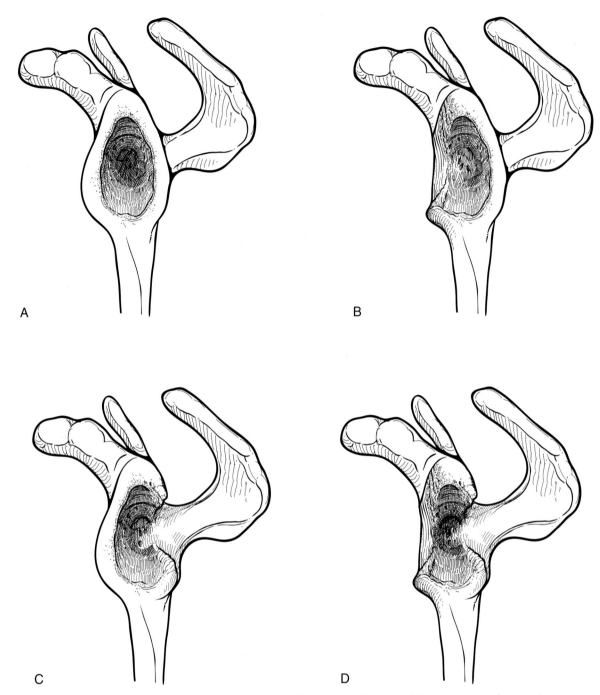

Figure 36-18   Classification of bony glenoid deficiency. **A,** Contained. **B,** Uncontained—anterior. **C,** Uncontained—posterior. **D,** Uncontained—combined.

REFERENCE

1. Antuna SA, Sperling JW, Cofield RH, Rowland CM: Glenoid revision surgery after total shoulder arthroplasty. J Shoulder Elbow Surg 2001;10:217-224.

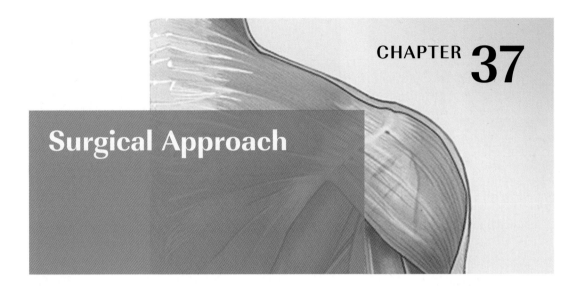

Surgical Approach

All revision shoulder arthroplasty in our practice is performed through a deltopectoral approach. The utilitarian nature of this approach makes it ideal for use in revision shoulder arthroplasty. The deltopectoral approach is easily extended into an anterolateral approach to the humeral diaphysis should it be necessary for extraction of a humeral component or for fixation of a periprosthetic fracture.

The most difficult portion of the deltopectoral approach performed in the revision scenario is dealing with scar tissue from previous surgery because it obscures the normal tissue planes easily identified during primary arthroplasty. The extent of scaring present and the amount of difficulty encountered in identifying soft tissue planes vary greatly among patients, and we have yet to identify any reliable preoperative factors to assist in determining which dissections will be especially difficult. Scarring may be present throughout the surgical approach and commonly obscures the deltopectoral interval, the plane between the pectoralis major and conjoined tendon of the short head of the biceps and coracobrachialis, and the plane between the conjoined tendon and the subscapularis. Additionally, subdeltoid adhesions are commonly present at the time of revision surgery.

When performing revision shoulder arthroplasty, the surgeon must be able to approach the humeral shaft, which is done by extending the deltopectoral approach into an anterolateral approach to the humeral diaphysis. Use of the extensile portion of this approach is necessary when performing a humeral osteotomy for removal of the humeral stem or in the operative treatment of a periprosthetic fracture. In these scenarios it is often necessary to perform some type of cerclage fixation of the humeral diaphysis.

Before performing cerclage fixation of the humeral diaphysis, it is mandatory that the radial nerve be identified so that it can be protected throughout this portion of the procedure. The surgeon must be able to perform radial nerve dissection to safely perform revision shoulder arthroplasty.

TECHNIQUE FOR THE DELTOPECTORAL APPROACH

The deltopectoral approach used for revision shoulder arthroplasty follows the same technical principles described for primary shoulder arthroplasty (see Chapter 8). Patient positioning is the same as for primary shoulder arthroplasty. Draping differs in revision arthroplasty in that the stockinet is placed only up to the elbow to allow distal extension of the surgical approach if necessary (Fig. 37-1). Any previous skin incisions are delineated with a sterile surgical marking pen (Fig. 37-2). This makes these incisional scars more visible after skin preparation and placement of the occlusive drape. The previous skin incision is used if possible. If the previous incision is topographically positioned within 5 cm of our standard deltopectoral skin incision as described in Chapter 8, we will use the previous incision site (Fig. 37-3). If the previous incision deviates substantially from our standard deltopectoral incision, we will make a new incision altogether. If the previous incision has resulted in a hypertrophic scar, the scar is elliptically excised with a no. 10 scalpel blade (Fig. 37-4). The incision extends for 10 to 15 cm, depending on the size of the patient. Occasionally, the original incision is longer than what we consider necessary. In that situation we use only a portion of the

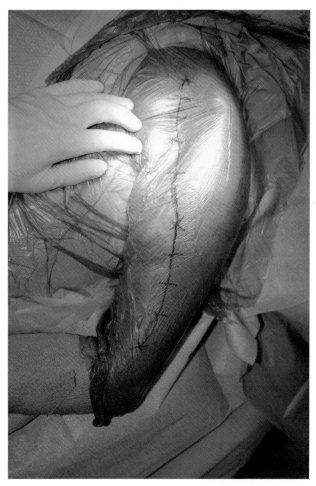

Figure 37-1   Draping for revision shoulder arthroplasty while leaving the distal part of the arm accessible to allow an extensile exposure.

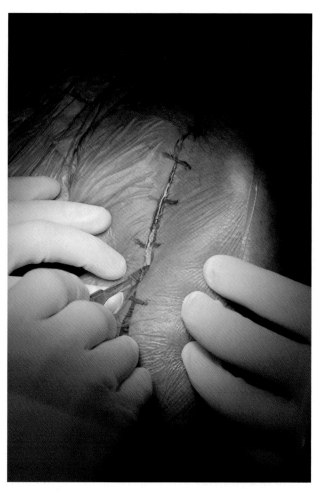

Figure 37-3   Use of the previous incision for the deltopectoral approach during revision shoulder arthroplasty.

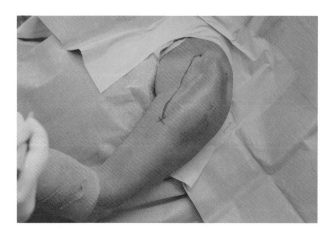

Figure 37-2   Previous incisions are marked before placing the occlusive drape.

original incision. To minimize hemorrhage, we use a needle tip electrocautery for subcutaneous dissection and for most of the deep dissection throughout the procedure. Medium-size skin rakes are used for retraction during this portion of the approach.

The cephalic vein, when present, is located to identify the interval between the deltoid and pectoralis major. In many cases the cephalic vein is not identified during revision shoulder arthroplasty. If such is the case, the deltopectoral interval can be readily located proximally by identifying a small triangular area devoid of muscle tissue between the proximal portions of the deltoid and pectoralis major muscles (Fig. 37-5). If located, the cephalic vein is dissected free of the pectoralis major muscle with Metzenbaum scissors. We prefer to retract the cephalic vein laterally with the deltoid because most of the branches of the cephalic vein are deltoid based. Medial retraction of the cephalic vein with the pectoralis major disrupts

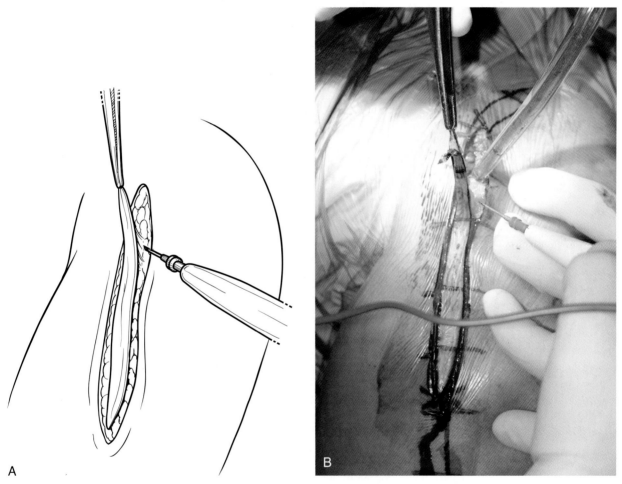

A

B

Figure 37-4 **A** and **B,** Excision of a previous hypertrophic skin scar.

Deltopectoral interval

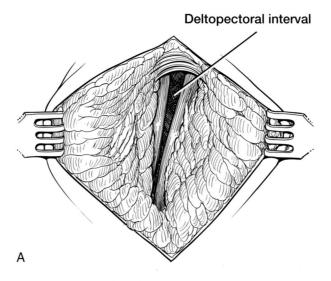

A

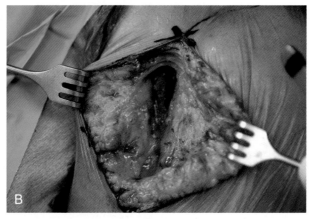

B

Figure 37-5 A and **B,** Identification of the deltopectoral interval proximally in a patient without an identifiable cephalic vein by locating the area proximally devoid of muscle.

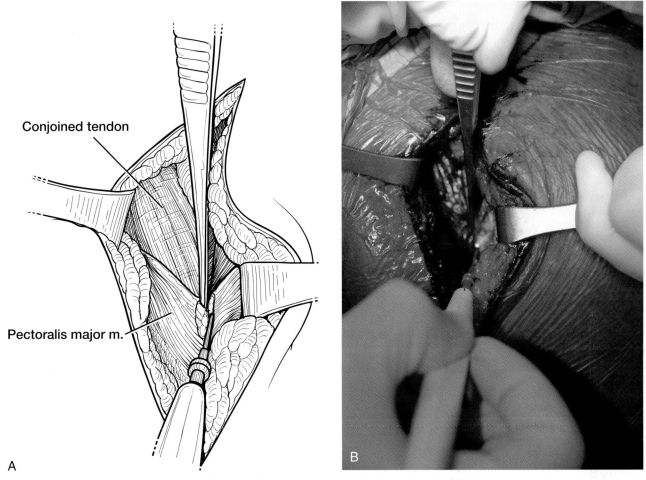

Conjoined tendon

Pectoralis major m.

A

B

Figure 37-6   **A** and **B,** Release of the superior aspect of the pectoralis major tendon to enhance exposure of the inferior subscapularis.

these deltoid branches and introduces unwanted hemorrhage.

The deltopectoral interval is developed through somewhat tedious dissection, depending on the severity of scarring, with a combination of Metzenbaum scissors and needle tip electrocautery. After the deltopectoral interval has been developed, Army-Navy retractors are used to maintain the interval. The humeral insertion of the pectoralis major tendon is identified. Dividing the superior centimeter of the pectoralis major tendon enhances exposure of the inferior aspect of the subscapularis and axillary nerve (Fig. 37-6). The deltoid is frequently adherent to the subdeltoid bursa and lateral aspect of the proximal humerus. If so, the deltoid is progressively released from the subdeltoid bursa with the electrocautery as the arm is progressively internally rotated (Fig. 37-7). A self-retaining cerebellar-type deltopectoral retractor is

inserted to maintain the deltopectoral interval. Next, the conjoined tendon is identified and traced proximally to its insertion on the coracoid process. Large curved Mayo scissors are used to create a space superior to the coracoid process by placing the scissors just over the top of the coracoid and spreading the blades open. The tip of a Hohmann retractor is placed in the space behind the base of the coracoid process to allow proximal retraction (Fig. 37-8). The pectoralis major muscle is frequently adherent to the conjoined tendon during revision shoulder arthroplasty. If this is the case, the pectoralis major muscle is released from the conjoined tendon with Metzenbaum scissors or a Cobb elevator (Fig. 37-9).

The arm is placed in an abducted and externally rotated position, and the apex that is formed by the insertions of the coracoacromial ligament and the conjoined tendon on the coracoid process is identified.

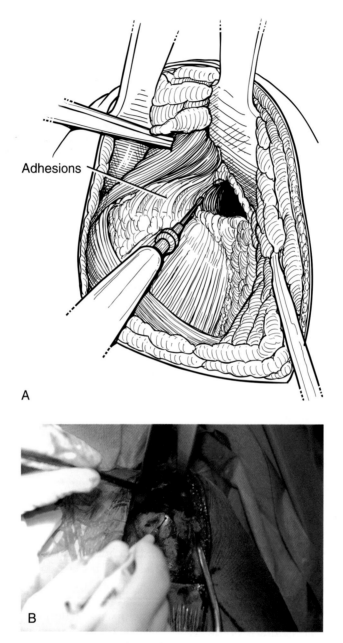

Figure 37-7 **A** and **B,** Release of subdeltoid adhesions.

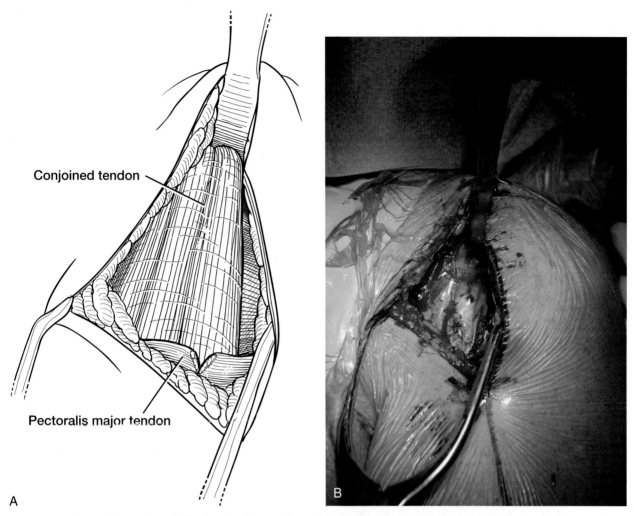

Conjoined tendon

Pectoralis major tendon

A

B

Figure 37-8 **A** and **B,** Proximal retraction with a Hohmann retractor behind the coracoid process.

This apex is developed with the needle tip electrocautery. If an unconstrained implant is planned, the coracoacromial ligament is retained. If a reverse prosthesis is the implant to be used in the revision, the coracoacromial ligament is released with the electrocautery to further enhance visualization, particularly if superior migration of the humerus is noted. The lateral aspect of the conjoined tendon is released with the electrocautery to expose the subscapularis tendon, if present. Scar tissue is nearly always present between the deep surface of the conjoined tendon and the anterior surface of the subscapularis tendon, and surgical release of the scar tissue is necessary. The release is performed carefully with Metzenbaum scissors or a Cobb elevator along the surface of the subscapularis tendon (Fig. 37-10). Extreme caution is exercised to avoid injury to the

musculocutaneous nerve, which may enter the coracobrachialis within 4 cm distal to the tip of the coracoid process. After this release, the conjoined tendon is retracted medially with a narrow Richardson retractor to expose the subscapularis tendon, when present. The anterior humeral circumflex vessels (the "three sisters") are usually absent at the time of revision shoulder arthroplasty. With the arm externally rotated, the anterior humeral circumflex vessels, when present, are suture-ligated together at the inferior border of the subscapularis with no. 0 dyed absorbable braided suture, as in cases of primary shoulder arthroplasty.

The axillary nerve is next identified through direct visualization. The narrow Richardson retractor is moved slightly inferiorly along the conjoined tendon

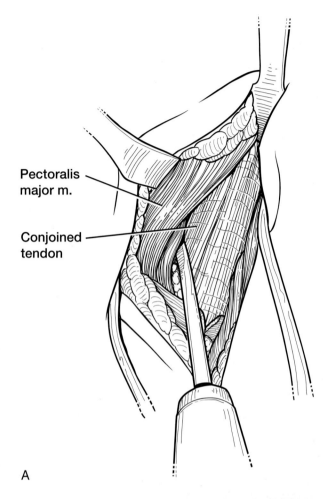

Pectoralis
major m.

Conjoined
tendon

A

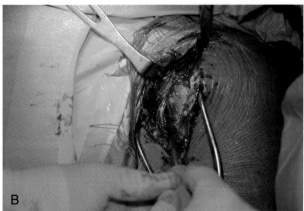

B

Figure 37-9 **A** and **B,** Release of the undersurface of the pectoralis major muscle from the underlying conjoined tendon.

to a point just below the inferior aspect of the subscapularis. The arm is flexed forward in neutral rotation, and blunt dissection is undertaken by spreading the tips of Metzenbaum scissors in the axillary fat inferior and deep to the subscapularis. Identification

of the axillary nerve helps protect it throughout the procedure.

In cases in which the subscapularis is intact, it is handled identically to cases of primary shoulder arthroplasty. Two stay sutures of no. 2 polyester are placed in the subscapularis tendon near the musculotendinous junction. The neck of the humeral prosthesis is identified and a scalpel is used to transect the subscapularis tendon and joint capsule along the prosthetic humeral neck. If permanent sutures from earlier subscapularis repair at the time of the previous arthroplasty are present and appear to be in the appropriate location along the prosthetic neck, they are used as a guide for subscapularis tenotomy (Fig. 37-11). The electrocautery replaces the scalpel at the inferior portion of the subscapularis to cauterize the previously ligated anterior humeral circumflex vessels, when present. A humeral head retractor is placed in the glenohumeral joint and used to retract the prosthetic humeral head posteriorly. Circumferential release of the subscapularis tendon is performed, along with release of the superior, middle, and inferior glenohumeral ligaments, as in unconstrained shoulder arthroplasty. The subscapularis is then tucked into the subscapularis fossa with forceps and held with a glenoid rim retractor. If a reverse prosthesis is to be used as the revision implant, no sponge is placed in the subscapularis fossa because insertion of the screws for fixation of the glenoid base plate risks entrapment of the sponge with screws as they penetrate the anterior scapular cortex. If the subscapularis tendon is not present, the remaining subscapularis bursa is excised to expose the glenohumeral joint, and the humeral head retractor and glenoid rim retractor are inserted. If present, the intra-articular portion of the long head of the biceps tendon is handled as described in Chapter 5 (tenotomy or tenodesis).

TECHNIQUE FOR EXTENSION OF THE DELTOPECTORAL APPROACH INTO AN ANTEROLATERAL APPROACH TO THE HUMERAL DIAPHYSIS

During revision shoulder arthroplasty it is frequently necessary to extend the deltopectoral approach distally to obtain access to the midhumeral diaphysis. The main indications for using an extensile approach in revision shoulder arthroplasty are extraction of a well-fixated humeral stem and management of periprosthetic fractures. The surgeon should be prepared to perform this extended approach for any revision shoulder arthroplasty.

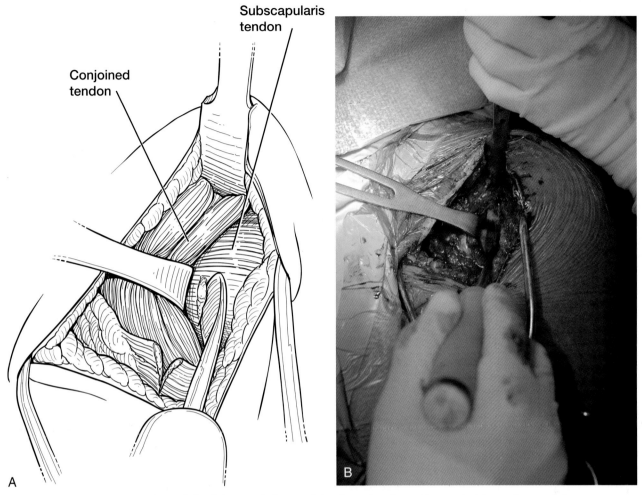

Conjoined tendon

Subscapularis tendon

A

B

Figure 37-10 **A** and **B,** Release of the conjoined tendon from the underlying subscapularis tendon.

After marking the primary incision site and the planned deltopectoral portion of the revision incision (these are often the same), the marking pen is used to delineate the proposed skin incision for extending the skin incision distally along the lateral border of the biceps brachii for an anterolateral approach to the humeral diaphysis (Fig. 37-12). Once it is determined that an extensile approach is necessary, the skin incision is extended with a no. 10 scalpel blade (Fig. 37-13). The needle tip electrocautery is used to dissect through subcutaneous tissue and around the lateral border of the biceps brachii (Fig. 37-14). The brachialis muscle is next encountered along the anterolateral humeral shaft. The brachialis is split longitudinally to expose the humeral shaft (Fig. 37-15). Subperiosteal dissection can be carried out around the humeral shaft if necessary to complete the exposure (Fig. 37-16). More proximally, the humeral insertion of the deltoid should be identified and protected (Fig. 37-17).

In some cases, particularly those involving a periprosthetic fracture, it may be necessary to place cerclage cables around the humeral shaft in the middle

Text continued on p. 398

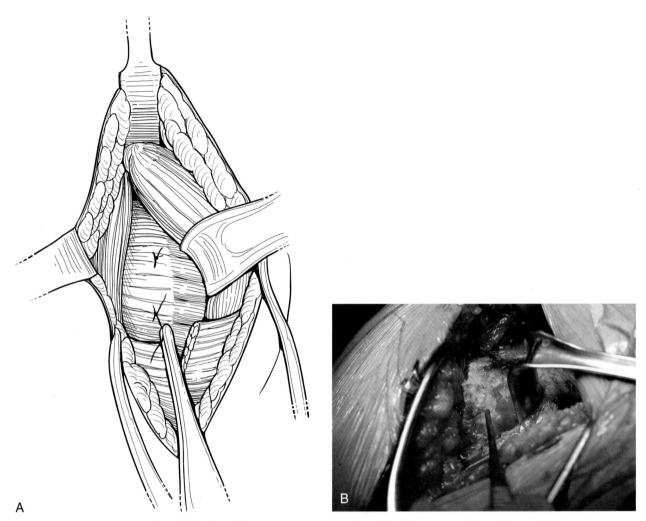

A

B

Figure 37-11   **A** and **B,** Line of permanent sutures placed during repair of the subscapularis at the time of primary arthroplasty.

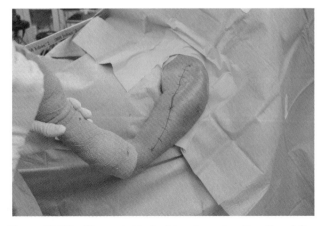

Figure 37-12   Planned skin incision for extending the delto-pectoral approach into an anterolateral approach to the humeral shaft.

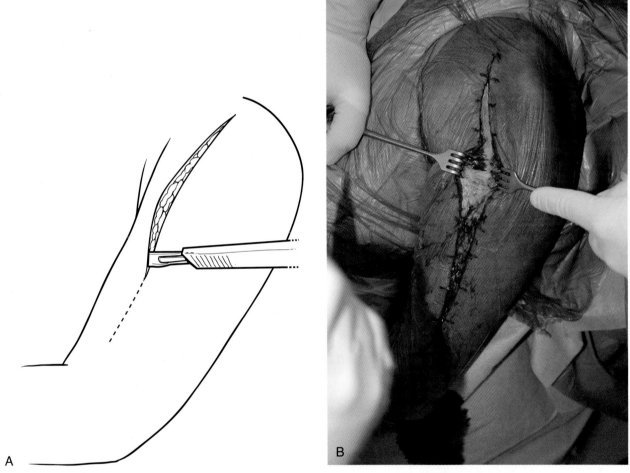

A

B

Figure 37-13 A and **B,** Extension of the skin incision for the anterolateral approach to the humeral shaft.

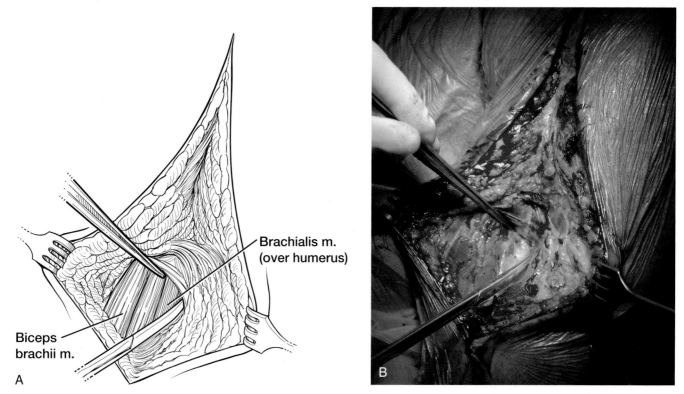

Brachialis m.
(over humerus)

Biceps
brachii m.

A

B

Figure 37-14   A and **B,** Dissection lateral to the biceps brachii.

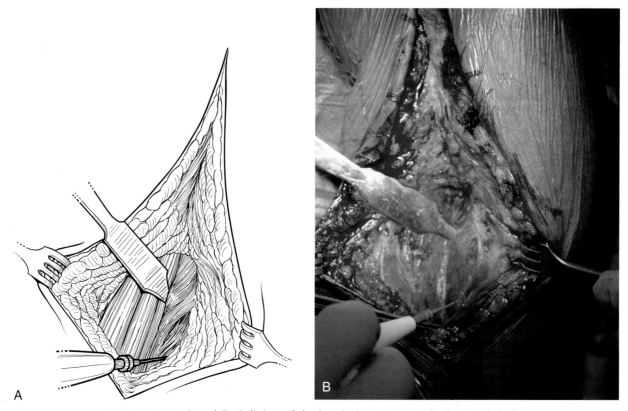

A

B

Figure 37-15   A and **B,** Splitting of the brachialis to expose the humeral shaft.

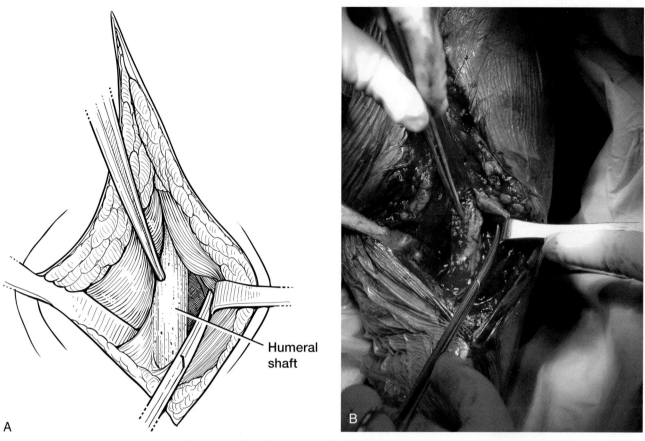

Figure 37-16 **A** and **B,** Completed exposure of the humeral shaft during revision shoulder arthroplasty.

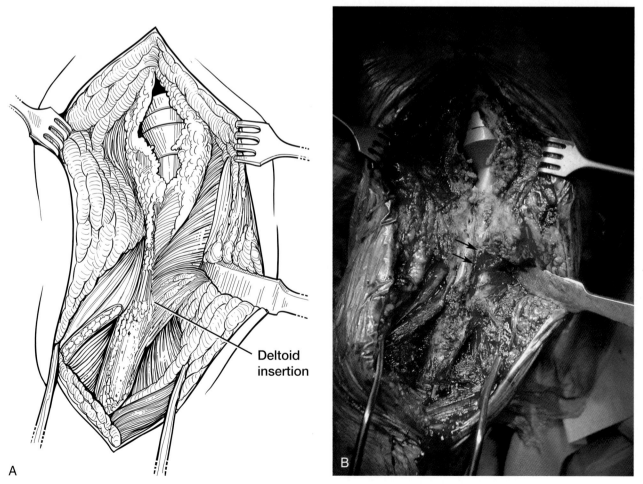

Figure 37-17 **A** and **B,** The humeral insertion of the deltoid (*arrows*) is protected during the extensile approach used for revision shoulder arthroplasty.

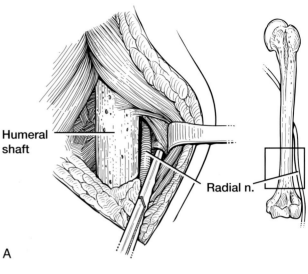

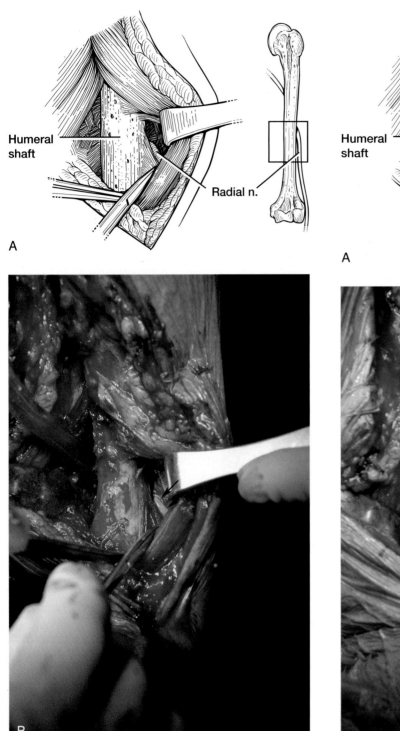

Figure 37-18   **A** and **B,** The radial nerve (*arrows*) is identified between the brachialis and brachioradialis distally in the incision.

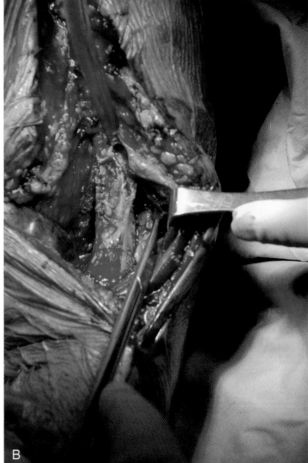

Figure 37-19   **A** and **B,** The radial nerve is traced proximally and protected throughout the procedure.

diaphysis. In such cases the radial nerve should be visualized and protected to avoid transection or incarceration by a cable. In these cases it is easiest to identify the radial nerve distally and trace its course proximally and posteriorly. The nerve is identified just proximal to the elbow as it courses between the brachialis and brachioradialis muscles (Fig. 37-18). From this point it is traced proximally and protected from any cerclage devices placed around the humeral diaphysis (Fig. 37-19).

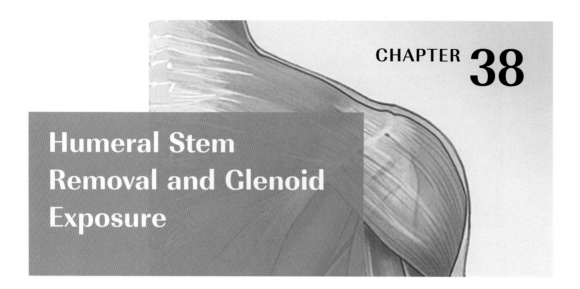

CHAPTER 38

Humeral Stem Removal and Glenoid Exposure

Humeral stem removal can be simple or one of the most difficult and time-consuming aspects of revision shoulder arthroplasty. Preoperative planning becomes very important in facilitating removal of the humeral stem during revision shoulder arthroplasty. Whereas relatively smooth press-fit humeral stems may be easy to remove, extensively porous-coated stems can be especially difficult to extract, particularly when they have been inserted with bone cement. Identification of the brand and type of implant used in the primary shoulder arthroplasty by radiographs or the primary arthroplasty operative report (or both) allows the surgeon to have an instrument set available to assist in extraction of the humeral implant (Fig. 38-1). Controlled extraction of the humeral implant, even if a humeral osteotomy is required, is certainly preferable to an intraoperative fracture of the proximal humerus caused by ill-fated attempts at extracting a well-fixated humeral stem without performing an osteotomy.

Once the humeral stem is removed, glenoid exposure proceeds in much the same manner as for primary shoulder arthroplasty (see Chapter 10). This chapter details our techniques for humeral stem removal and glenoid exposure during revision shoulder arthroplasty.

TECHNIQUE FOR HUMERAL STEM REMOVAL

Tenotomy of the subscapularis with subsequent release of the superior, middle, and inferior glenohumeral ligaments (see Chapters 9 and 37) is performed if the subscapularis is intact. If the subscapularis is absent, any subscapularis bursa is excised to expose the anterior aspect of the humeral head component (Fig. 38-2).

A humeral head retractor is placed for retraction of the proximal humerus posteriorly (Fig. 38-3). If this provides sufficient visualization of the anterior glenoid and inferior capsule, inferior capsular release is performed, as described in the following section on glenoid exposure. Frequently, because of its size, however, the humeral implant sufficiently hinders glenoid visualization to prevent inferior capsular release. In these cases it is necessary to remove the humeral stem before proceeding with glenoid exposure.

The proximal humerus must be dislocated before attempts at removal of the humeral stem. The dislocation must be done with great care to avoid humeral injury. Frequently, capsular stiffness prevents dislocation by simple external rotation and extension of the arm. If this maneuver is not initially successful, a humeral-based inferior capsular release is performed (Fig. 38-4). Progressive release of the inferior medial capsule from the humerus with the needle tip electrocautery allows dislocation of the proximal humerus. Care must be taken to keep the electrocautery in contact with the humerus to avoid injury to the axillary nerve. Dislocation maneuvers must be done slowly and with great care in revision cases to prevent humeral fracture because the humerus is often osteopenic and compromised (Fig. 38-5).

Once the humerus has been dislocated, the humeral head portion of the arthroplasty is circumferentially exposed by removing any fibrous tissue at its margins with the needle tip electrocautery (Fig. 38-6). Nearly all implants currently encountered during revision surgery have a modular head fixed onto a stem via a Morse taper mechanism. It is important, however, for a surgeon unfamiliar with the type of implant being

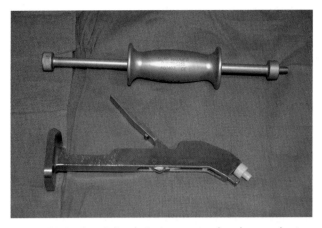

Figure 38-1 Specialized instruments for humeral stem extraction specific for a single brand and model of humeral implant.

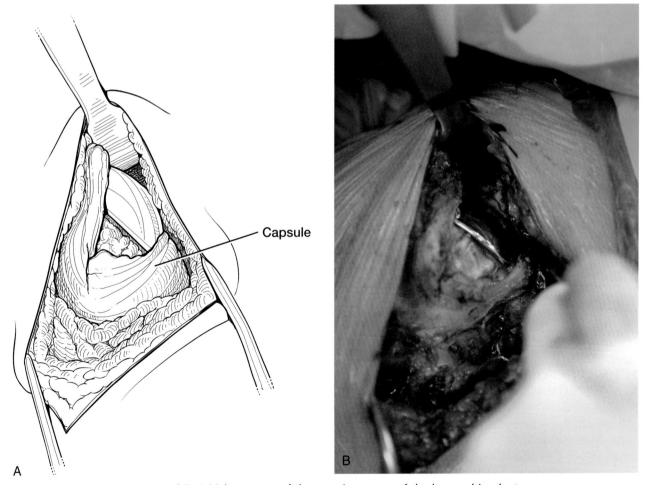

Figure 38-2 **A** and **B,** Initial exposure of the anterior aspect of the humeral implant.

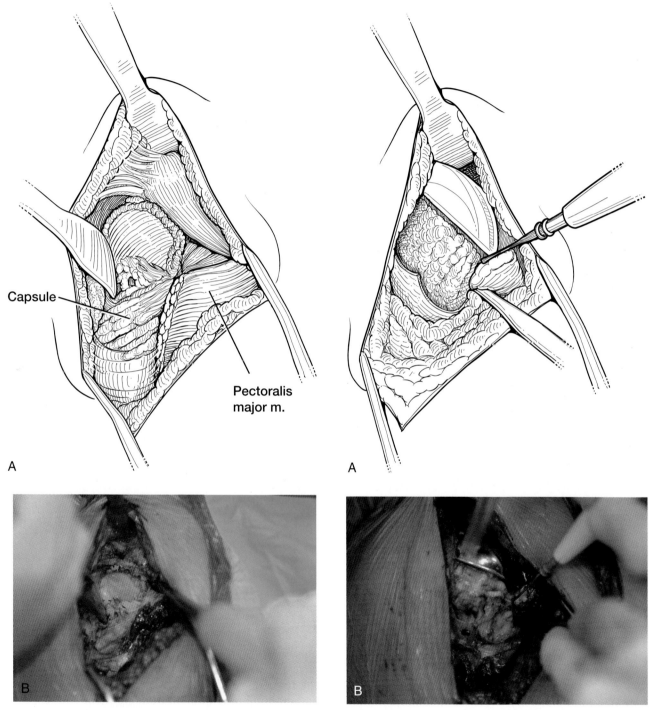

Figure 38-3 **A** and **B,** Retraction of the proximal humerus posteriorly with a humeral head retractor before extraction of the primary humeral prosthesis.

Figure 38-4 **A** and **B,** Performance of a humeral-based inferior capsular release with the needle tip electrocautery to allow dislocation of the proximal humerus.

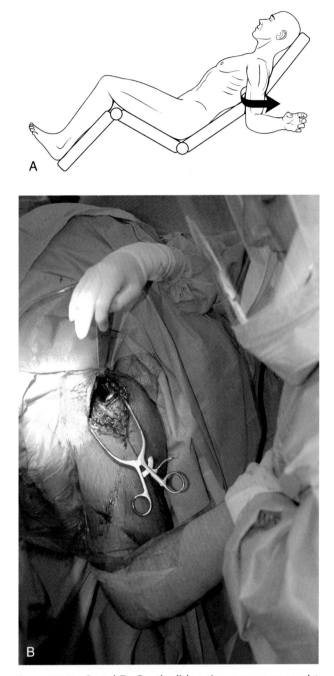

Figure 38-5 **A** and **B,** Gentle dislocation maneuver consisting of external rotation and extension of the arm.

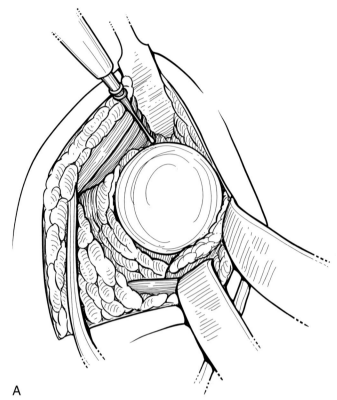

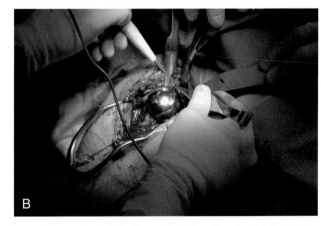

Figure 38-6 **A** and **B,** Once the glenohumeral joint is dislocated, any fibrous tissue at the margins of the humeral implant proximally is removed with the electrocautery.

removed to obtain any information available about the implant from the manufacturer. The surgeon must discover whether the implant is modular or monoblock and whether any accessory mechanisms have been used to fix the humeral head to the stem portion of the component (i.e., a threaded screw was used to further secure the Morse taper in some early modular designs; Fig. 38-7). If the humeral component is

modular with only Morse taper fixation of the humeral head portion to the stem portion of the component, the humeral head is usually easily removed by disimpacting the humeral head from the stem with a Cobb elevator at the inferior aspect of the humeral head component (Fig. 38-8). Often, fibrous tissue covers the proximal aspect of the stem portion of the component (Fig. 38-9). This fibrous tissue is completely removed with the needle tip electrocautery to delineate the peripheral proximal portion of the stem circumferen-

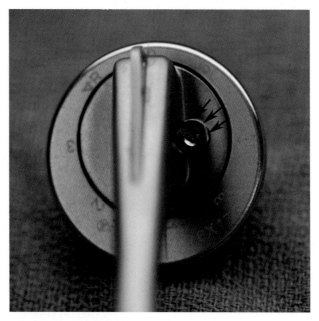

Figure 38-7 The Aequalis cemented stem (Tornier, Inc., Minneapolis, MN) has an accessory screw (*arrows*) available to further secure the Morse taper fixation of the humeral head portion of the implant to the stem portion of the implant.

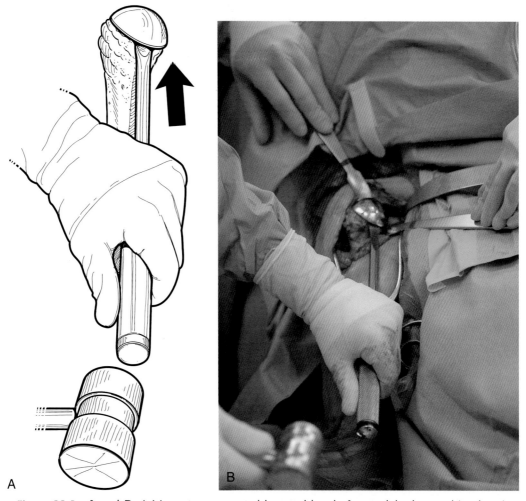

Figure 38-8 **A** and **B**, A Morse taper–secured humeral head of a modular humeral implant is usually easily removed with a Cobb elevator as an impactor.

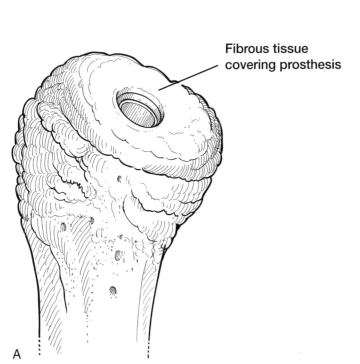

Fibrous tissue
covering prosthesis

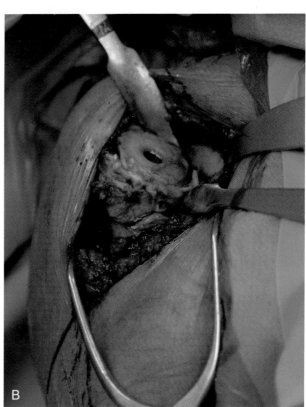

Figure 38-9 **A** and **B,** Fibrous tissue covering the proximal aspect of the stem portion of the humeral prosthesis after removal of a modular humeral head.

tially (Fig. 38-10). The condition of the superior and posterior rotator cuff tendons can be evaluated at this point (Fig. 38-11).

After all soft tissue has been released peripherally from the proximal aspect of the stem portion of the implant, the extraction device specific for the implant, if available, is attached (Fig. 38-12). Attempts are made with the extraction device (generally with an attached slap hammer). If attempts to extract the implant are initially unsuccessful, the extraction device is removed and small, thin osteotomes are used to delicately separate the proximal humerus from the proximal aspect of the humeral implant (Fig. 38-13). The extraction device is reattached and additional attempts are made to remove the humeral component. If these attempts

are unsuccessful, a humeral osteotomy is performed for removal of the humeral implant (see later).

If no extraction device for the type of implant being removed exists, small, thin osteotomes are used to delicately separate the proximal humerus from the proximal aspect of the humeral implant after all soft tissue has been released peripherally from the proximal portion of the stem portion of the implant. A large Cobb elevator is used to disimpact the humeral implant from the proximal humerus by striking it at its medial portion (Fig. 38-14). The Cobb elevator is directed as parallel as possible to the humeral implant stem. If attempts at implant extraction are unsuccessful with this technique, humeral osteotomy should be performed.

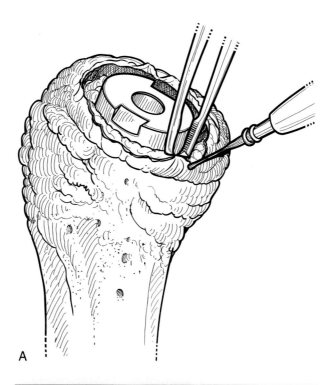

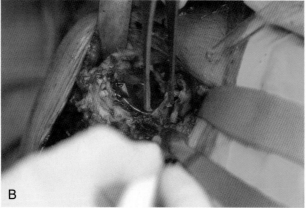

Figure 38-10   **A** and **B,** Removal of the fibrous tissue covering the proximal aspect of the stem portion of the humeral prosthesis with a needle tip electrocautery.

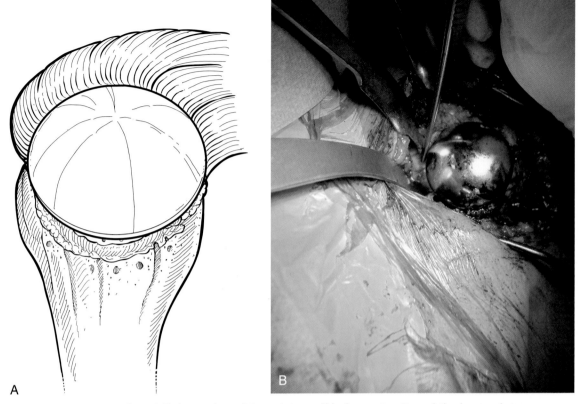

Figure 38-11 **A** and **B,** Inspection of the rotator cuff before extraction of the humeral stem.

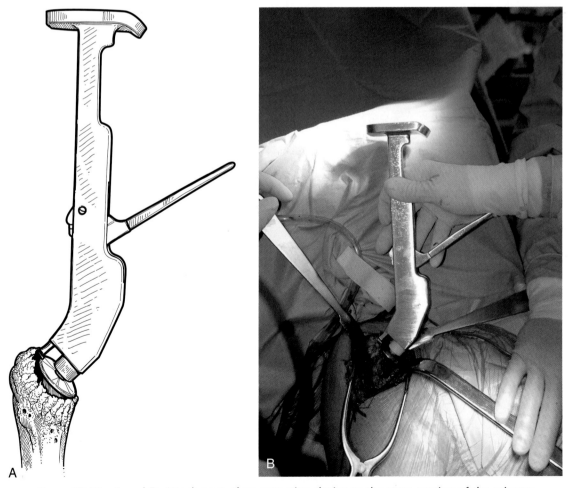

Figure 38-12 **A** and **B,** Attachment of an extraction device to the stem portion of the primary humeral stem.

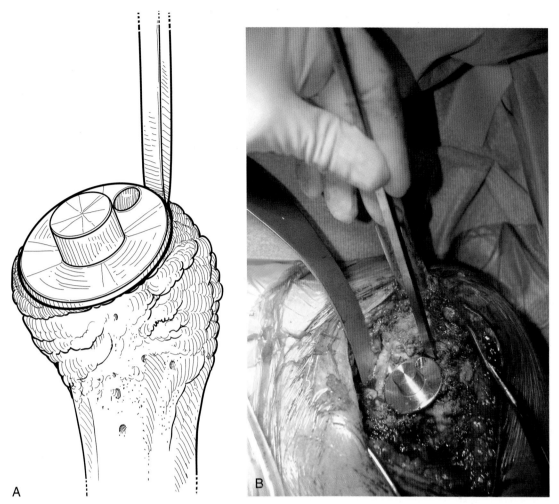

Figure 38-13 **A** and **B,** Small, thin osteotomes are used to delicately separate the proximal humerus from the proximal aspect of the humeral implant.

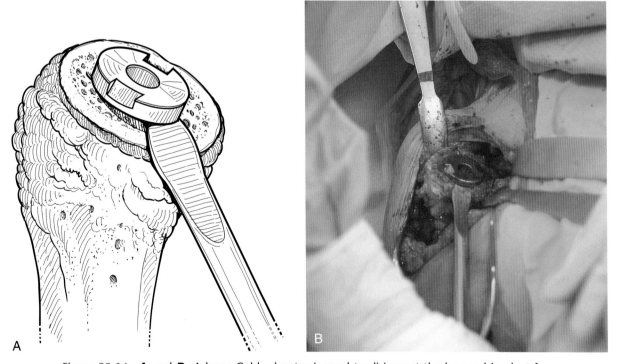

Figure 38-14 **A** and **B,** A large Cobb elevator is used to disimpact the humeral implant from the proximal humerus by striking it at its medial portion.

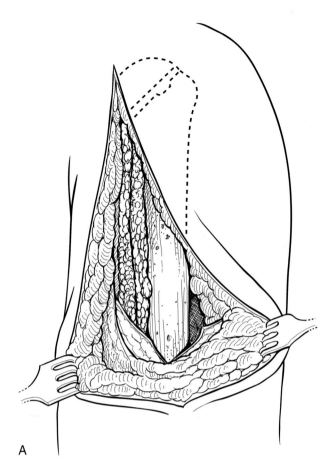

A

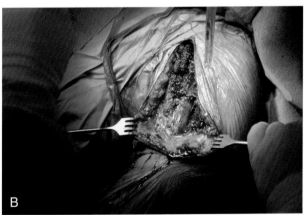

B

Figure 38-15 **A** and **B,** Exposure of the humerus in preparation for humeral osteotomy.

Humeral Osteotomy

Once the necessity for humeral osteotomy is established, the surgical approach is extended distally, as detailed in Chapter 37. The humerus is exposed from its proximal aspect to the area distal to the pectoralis major insertion (Fig. 38-15). The planned osteotomy site is demarcated with the needle tip electrocautery

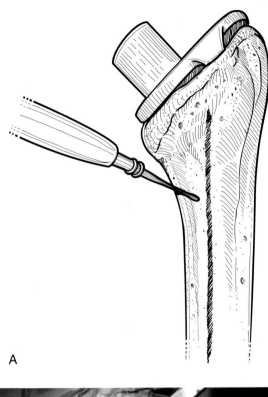

A

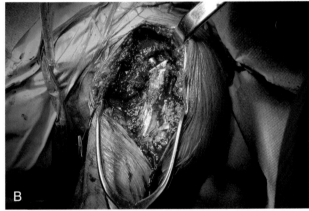

B

Figure 38-16 **A** and **B,** The planned osteotomy site is demarcated with a needle tip electrocautery.

and extended along the anterior humerus by starting just medial to the bicipital groove and continuing distally between the pectoralis major insertion and the deltoid insertion (Fig. 38-16). The distal extent of the osteotomy is determined by the length of the humeral stem to be removed.

Before performing the osteotomy, cerclage cables are placed for subsequent osteotomy fixation. Depending on the length of the osteotomy, we place two or three cables composed of a nylon monofilament core wrapped in braided ultrahigh-molecular-weight polyethylene (Kinamed Inc., Camarillo, CA). The cables are placed subperiosteally with the cable-passing instrumentation provided (Fig. 38-17). In cases in which the

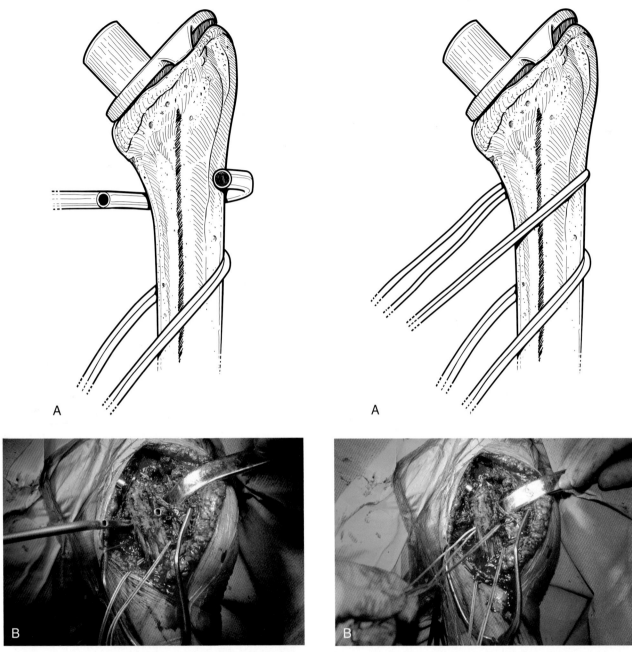

A

A

B

B

Figure 38-17 **A** and **B,** Placement of cables for later fixation of the humeral osteotomy.

Figure 38-18 **A** and **B,** Final placement of the cables, which are held temporarily with Kocher clamps.

osteotomy extends beyond the junction of the proximal third and middle third of the humeral shaft, the radial nerve must be identified and protected before passing cables posterior to the humerus (see Chapter 37). Once the cables are passed, the free ends of each cable are clamped together with Kocher clamps (Fig. 38-18).

A unicortical humeral osteotomy is performed by penetration of the anterior cortex with a sagittal saw along the humerus at the demarcated osteotomy site down to the humeral implant (Fig. 38-19). A $1^1/_2$-inch straight osteotome is impacted into the osteotomy site proximally (Fig. 38-20). The osteotome is turned to open the osteotomy by plastically deforming the proximal humerus (Fig. 38-21). The humeral stem can then be removed with the extraction instrumentation provided or by disimpaction with a Cobb elevator, as described earlier (Fig. 38-22).

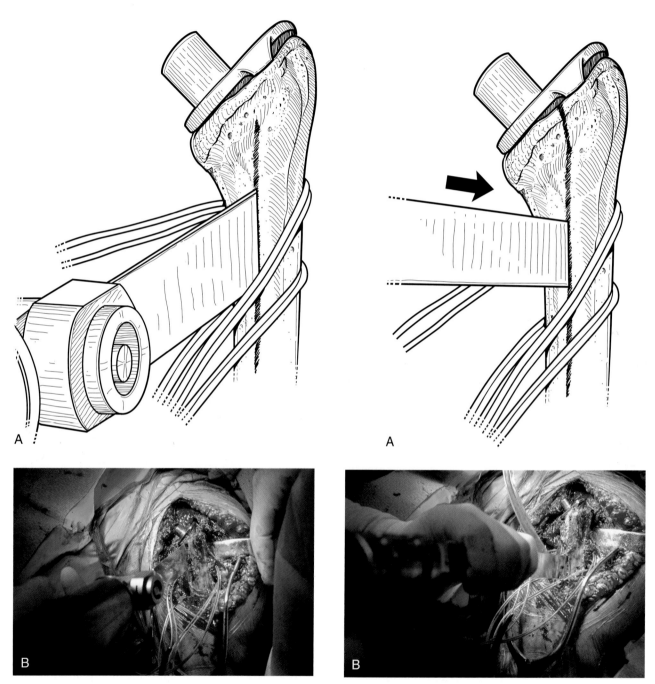

Figure 38-19 **A** and **B,** The osteotomy is performed with a saw along the anterior humerus.

Figure 38-20 **A** and **B,** An osteotome is impacted into the osteotomy site proximally.

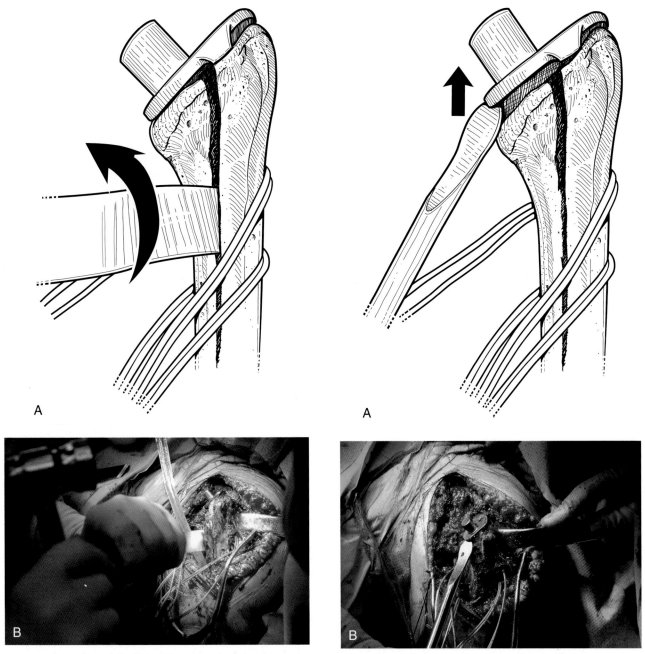

Figure 38-21 **A** and **B,** The osteotome is turned to open the osteotomy site by plastic deformation.

Figure 38-22 **A** and **B,** The humeral stem is removed.

After the humeral stem and any necessary cement (see later) are removed, the osteotomy must be fixated. This is performed by first preparing the proximal humerus for insertion of the revision humeral component with the instrumentation provided. The trial

humeral stem is inserted and the cables are tightened with the tensioning device provided (Fig. 38-23). The cables are tightened in a distal-to-proximal direction. In cases in which the native humeral cortex is excessively thin, fresh frozen allograft cortical struts

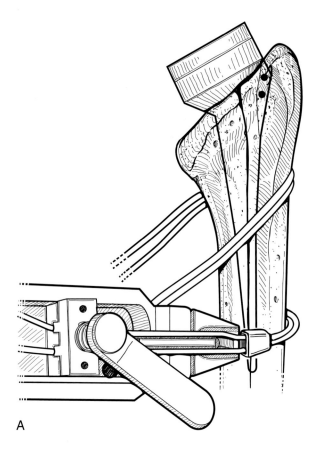

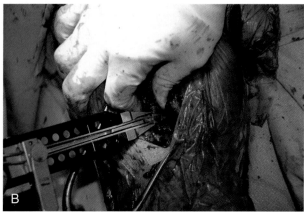

Figure 38-23 **A** and **B,** The cables are tightened over the trial stem.

are placed around the native humerus beneath the cables before tightening to provide additional support to the proximal humerus (Fig. 38-24).

Cement Removal

When removing a cemented humeral stem, residual cement is removed for two reasons—if it is loose within the humerus and if it prevents insertion of the revision humeral stem. Any residual cement that is well fixed

within the humeral canal and does not interfere with insertion of the revision humeral stem is left in place. The revision humeral stem can be successfully fixated into a stable residual cement mantle.[1]

Loose cement within the humeral canal is easily removed with pituitary-type forceps (Fig. 38-25). Removing cement that is well fixed within the humeral canal to make room for the revision humeral component is more challenging. We use a set of specialized cement-removing osteotomes (Moreland osteotomes) that come in a variety of shapes and sizes (Fig. 38-26). A combination of curved and straight Moreland osteotomes is used to remove the proximal cement mantle (Fig. 38-27). Any cement fragments that fall into the humeral canal are removed with pituitary forceps. Only enough cement is removed to permit insertion of the revision humeral stem. The trial stem is inserted intermittently during the cement removal process to evaluate the sufficiency of cement removal.

Occasionally, it is necessary to remove a distal cement plug to permit insertion of the revision humeral stem. If this is the case, it will often be necessary to perform a humeral osteotomy to permit removal of the cement plug without perforating and damaging the humeral diaphysis. Once the humeral osteotomy is performed and extended distal to the cement plug, the osteotomy is plastically opened distally with an osteotome and the cement plug is removed from the humeral canal with pituitary forceps. If a cement restrictor is present, it is removed with the pituitary forceps.

TECHNIQUE FOR GLENOID EXPOSURE

After the humeral component is removed, attention is turned to glenoid exposure. In cases in which no glenoid component has previously been implanted, any remaining labrum is excised from the base of the coracoid process extending inferiorly to the 5 o'clock position in a right shoulder (7 o'clock in a left shoulder) with the needle tip electrocautery. This allows identification of the osseous anterior margin of the glenoid. In nearly all cases, proper exposure of the glenoid requires release of the inferior capsule. The tip of the electrocautery is used to release the inferior capsule directly off the rim of the glenoid bone, just as in primary total shoulder arthroplasty. To help prevent injury to the axillary nerve, the tip of the electrocautery should be kept in contact with glenoid bone. This release is extended sufficiently medially to completely transect the capsule and expose the muscular fibers of the triceps inserting on the inferior osseous glenoid. The amount of posterior subluxation present on preoperative secondary imaging studies

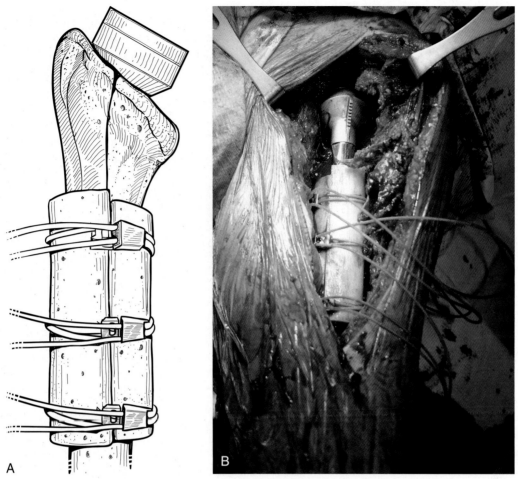

Figure 38-24 **A** and **B,** Cortical allograft struts can be used to reinforce the proximal humerus in patients with severe osteopenia.

(computed tomography, magnetic resonance imaging) determines the posterior extent of release. In shoulders without posterior subluxation, the release continues posteriorly to the 8 o'clock position for right shoulders (4 o'clock position for left shoulders). In shoulders that have preexisting posterior subluxation, either with or without posterior glenoid erosion, the release continues initially to only the 6 o'clock position. These patients often have a distended posterior capsule, so no more release is performed than is absolutely necessary to avoid compromising these posterior structures further. If release to only the 6 o'clock position proves inadequate later in the procedure during glenoid reaming, the release can be extended at that time. A

Cobb elevator can be used to check the release for completeness.

If a glenoid component has previously been placed, removal is usually simple because most of these components are loose in the revision scenario. After the humeral component has been removed, the proximal humerus is retracted posteriorly with a humeral head retractor. Soft tissue is removed circumferentially from around the glenoid component with the needle tip electrocautery (Fig. 38-28). The inferior capsule is released just as in cases in which no glenoid component has previously been placed. Once the periphery of the glenoid component has been cleared of soft tissue, a half-inch curved osteotome is used to lever

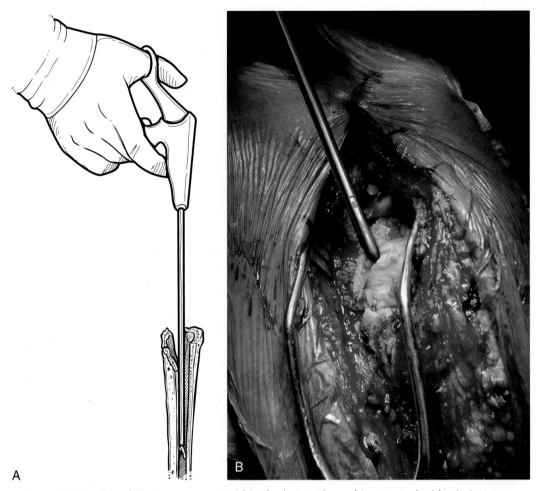

Figure 38-25   **A** and **B,** Loose cement within the humeral canal is removed with pituitary-type forceps.

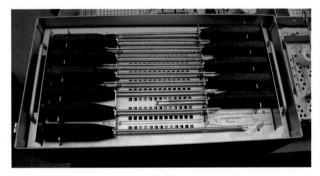

Figure 38-26   Cement removal osteotomes.

the glenoid component gently out of the native glenoid (Fig. 38-29). The majority of cemented glenoid components come out with the cement still bonded to the implant (Fig. 38-30). Loose cement fragments and fibrous tissue are removed with forceps and a rongeur.

Any residual cement fixed to the native glenoid is removed with a quarter-inch straight osteotome. Only when all residual cement and fibrous tissue have been removed can the osseous defect in the remaining native glenoid be properly evaluated and classified as contained or uncontained (Fig. 38-31).

SPECIAL SITUATIONS

Periprosthetic Fracture

If a periprosthetic fracture is encountered either preoperatively or intraoperatively, the fracture site may be used for removal of the humeral stem. The radial nerve must be identified and protected. Working through the fracture site, the humeral stem may be removed by striking the distal tip of the humeral com-

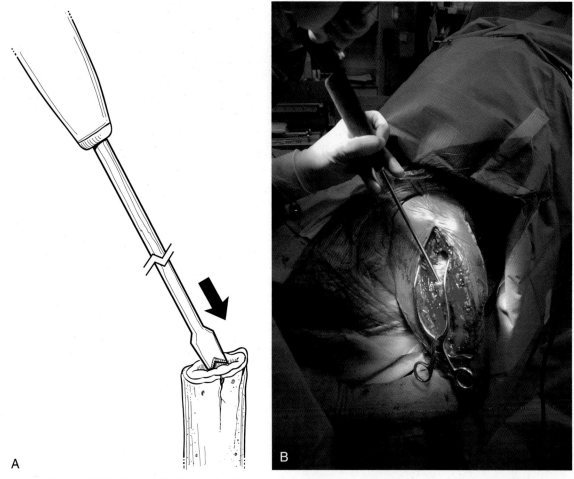

Figure 38-27 **A** and **B,** Removal of the proximal cement mantle with specialized osteotomes.

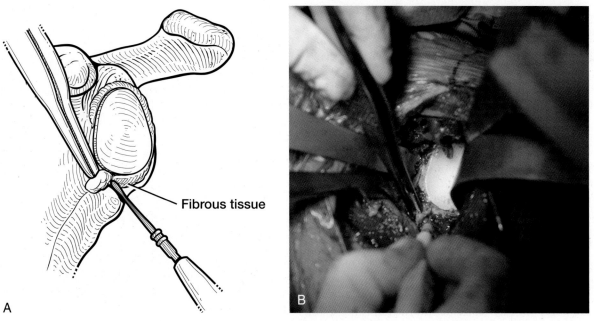

Fibrous tissue

Figure 38-28 **A** and **B,** Soft tissue is removed circumferentially from around the glenoid component.

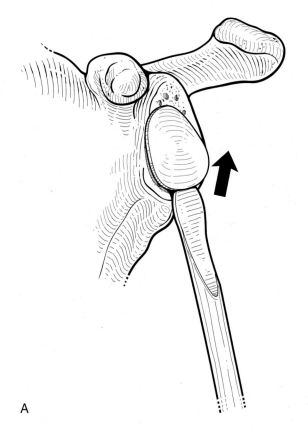

A

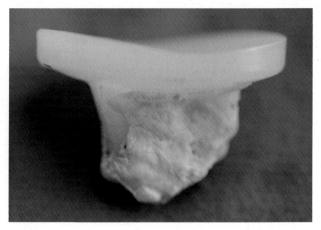

Figure 38-30 The majority of cement usually remains bonded to the implant.

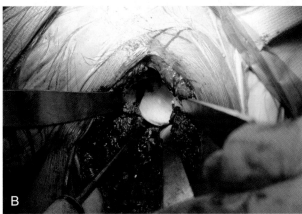

B

Figure 38-29 **A** and **B,** A curved osteotome is used to gently lever the glenoid implant from the native glenoid bone.

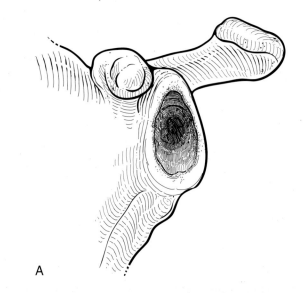

A

ponent with a mallet and bone tamp (Fig. 38-32). This should be performed only after proper exposure plus release of the proximal humerus has been achieved. This technique may eliminate the need for a humeral osteotomy.

Infection

In cases of confirmed or suspected infection (based on the preoperative infection workup; see Chapter 36), no preoperative antibiotics are administered. Once the

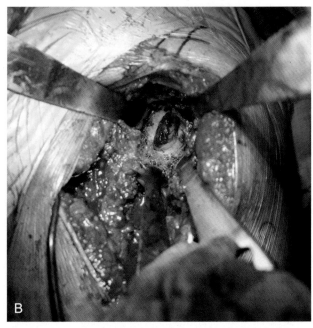

B

Figure 38-31 **A** and **B,** Osseous defect remaining in the glenoid after removal of the glenoid component and cement.

416

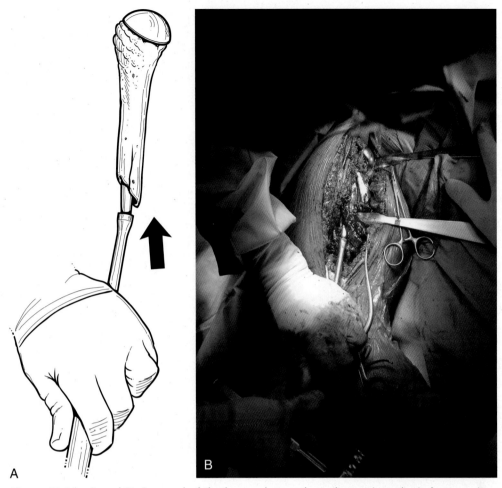

Figure 38-32 **A** and **B,** Removal of the humeral stem through a periprosthetic fracture site.

glenohumeral joint is opened, samples are taken for multiple cultures, including aerobic, anaerobic, fungal, and mycobacterial. We routinely use both swabs and fragments of soft tissue for analysis. Once these samples are taken for culture, standard perioperative antibiotics are administered.

In cases of possible or suspected infection (preoperative aspiration negative, but other indicators of infection present), multiple synovial biopsy samples are submitted for intraoperative frozen section evaluation. While the pathologist is evaluating the tissue, the procedure continues with removal of the primary components. If findings on frozen section are indicative of infection (more than five polymorphonuclear leukocytes per high-power field in five consecutive fields) or in the case of confirmed infection (positive culture on preoperative aspirates), the components are removed and an antibiotic-impregnated polymethylmethacrylate cement spacer shaped like a humeral hemiarthroplasty is inserted as the first stage of a two-stage revision (Fig. 38-33).[2] We are more aggressive in cement removal from the proximal humerus in cases of infection and remove as much cement from the primary arthroplasty as possible without severely damaging the proximal humerus. Additionally, in all cases of suspected infection, thorough irrigation is performed with at least 9 L of antibiotic-impregnated sterile saline (50,000 units bacitracin per liter sterile normal saline) introduced with a pulse lavage irrigator. Any necrotic-appearing tissue is sharply débrided.

The cement spacer is created with fast-setting bone cement (DePuy 2, DePuy, Inc., Warsaw, IN). Two grams of vancomycin powder is mixed into each bag of cement. Two bags of cement are usually required for an average-size patient. In patients allergic to vancomycin, 2.4 g of tobramycin powder is mixed into each bag of cement. As the cement becomes doughy, it is introduced into the proximal humerus and shaped into a humeral head.

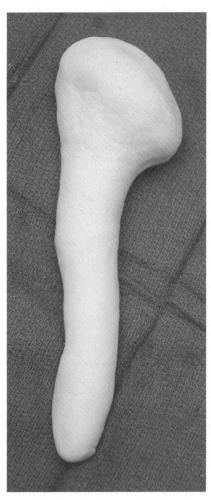

Figure 38-33   Antibiotic cement spacer used in staged revision arthroplasty after infection.

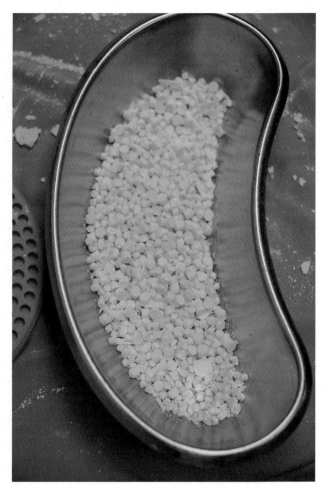

Figure 38-34   Absorbable antibiotic-impregnated pellets used for the treatment of an infected arthroplasty in a patient who is not a candidate for a staged revision arthroplasty.

Occasionally, we treat a patient with a chronically infected shoulder arthroplasty who is not a candidate for staged revision arthroplasty. In this case we treat the patient by removing the prosthetic implants, performing irrigation and débridement, and implanting antibiotic-impregnated absorbable calcium sulfate pellets (Stimulan, Biocomposites, Ltd., Wilmington, NC). A 10-cc package of pellets is mixed with 1 g of vancomycin or with 1.2 g of tobramycin for a vancomycin-allergic patient. Two 10-cc packages are usually sufficient to fill to the defect left by removal of the implant (Fig. 38-34).

REFERENCES

1. Walch G, Edwards TB, Boulahia A: Revision of the humeral stem: Technical problems and complications. In Walch G, Boileau P, Molé D (eds): 2000 Prostheses d'Epaule . . . Recul de 2 à 10 Ans. Paris, Sauramps Medical, 2001, pp 443-454.
2. Feldman DS, Lonner JH, Desai P, Zuckerman JD: The role of intraoperative frozen sections in revision total joint arthroplasty. J Bone Joint Surg Am 1995;77: 1807-1813.

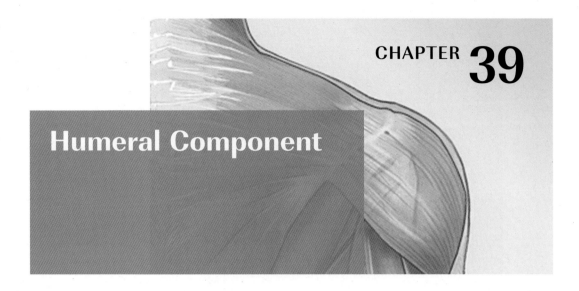

CHAPTER 39

Humeral Component

Reconstruction of the proximal humerus can be a very difficult aspect of revision shoulder arthroplasty. During extraction of the previous humeral stem, every effort should be made to preserve as much native proximal humeral bone as possible (see Chapter 38). The overall condition of the proximal humerus and rotator cuff plays a significant role in determining the type of implant to be used in revision surgery (unconstrained versus semiconstrained). In cases in which the rotator cuff is largely functional, preservation of the greater and lesser tuberosities helps dictate which type of revision implant to use during revision surgery. Once the type of revision implant to be used is selected, preparation of the proximal humerus and implantation of the humeral component proceed just as for primary arthroplasty. This chapter details our techniques for reconstruction and preparation of the proximal humerus and implantation of the humeral component in revision shoulder arthroplasty.

TECHNIQUE FOR PREPARATION OF THE PROXIMAL HUMERUS

Preparation of the proximal humerus is largely dependent on the residual osseous anatomy of the proximal humerus after the previously placed humeral stem has been extracted. In cases in which extraction of the previous humeral stem was relatively uncomplicated, with minimal compromise of the proximal humeral metaphysis and tuberosities, preparation of the proximal humerus can be straightforward and similar to proximal humeral preparation for primary shoulder arthroplasty. In cases in which the proximal humeral osseous anatomy has been compromised either before or during extraction of the humeral stem, preparation of the proximal humerus becomes substantially more complicated.

When proximal humeral osseous anatomy is well preserved, proximal humeral preparation for either an unconstrained stem or a reverse stem is performed similar to cases of primary arthroplasty.

Unconstrained Humeral Stem

In cases in which we are going to implant an unconstrained proximal humeral stem, we prefer to implant a stem with geometry designed originally for use in proximal humeral fractures. This cemented stem design allows a good fit into the humeral metaphysis and comes in a variety of lengths. This allows the surgeon to treat periprosthetic fractures or bypass the distal aspect of a humeral diaphyseal osteotomy used for extraction of the humeral stem (Fig. 39-1).

For this revision stem, no metaphyseal broaching is necessary. The diaphysis is progressively reamed with the hand reamers provided (Fig. 39-2). Frequently, after removing an uncemented humeral stem, a small pedestal of bone exists in the intramedullary canal at the level just distal to the tip of the original humeral stem (Fig. 39-3). It is easy to tap the smallest diaphyseal reamer through this osseous pedestal. Subsequent reamers pass through this area without difficulty.

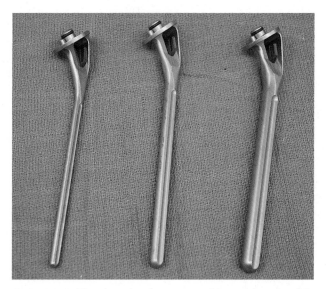

Figure 39-1 Unconstrained stems used in revision shoulder arthroplasty.

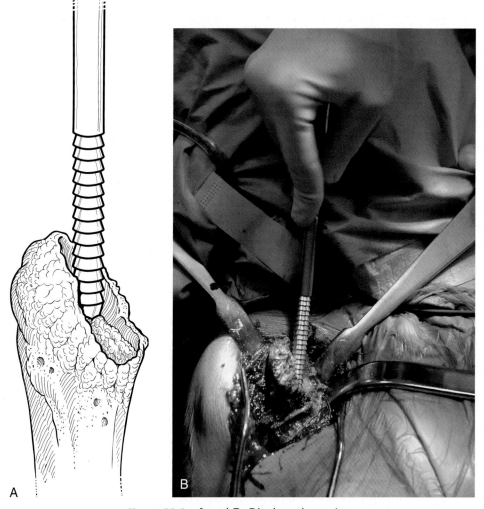

Figure 39-2 **A** and **B,** Diaphyseal reaming.

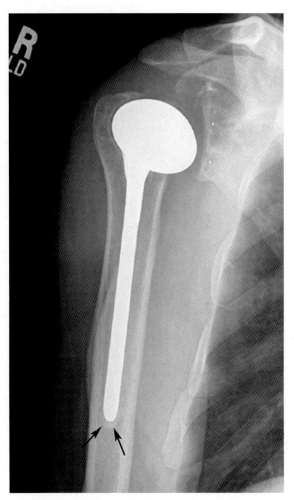

Figure 39-3   Pedestal of intramedullary cortical bone (*arrows*) distal to the tip of an uncemented humeral stem.

Once a humeral stem diameter of appropriate size is selected, the trial humeral stem is inserted by impacting the stem into the proximal humerus (Fig. 39-4). Effort is made to impact the stem laterally into the tuberosities (Fig. 39-5). It is not necessary to broach the humeral metaphysis because the bone in this area is relatively soft and compresses sufficiently to allow full seating of the implant. On occasion, the metaphyseal bone will be moderately to severely osteopenic, and the trial humeral stem will fall into the medial portion of the metaphysis (Fig. 39-6). This "loose fit" hinders testing of the trial implant. The trial may be stabilized within the proximal humerus in this scenario by wrapping a sterile sponge (or portion of a sterile sponge) around the metaphyseal portion of the trial implant before placing it in the humeral canal (Fig. 39-7).

Once the trial humeral stem is securely placed in the proximal humerus, a humeral head implant of appropriate size is selected. The prosthetic head should provide adequate coverage of the proximal humeral metaphysis but not overhang the humerus at any portion. The system that we use allows variable medial-to-lateral and anterior-to-posterior offset. The prosthetic humeral head is placed on the trial humeral stem at the various offset positions to allow selection of the best offset index (Fig. 39-8). Once the proper index has been selected, the glenohumeral joint is reduced and humeral version is judged. With the arm in neutral rotation, the center of the prosthetic humeral head should align with the center of the glenoid, provided that osseous glenoid morphology is intact and does not demonstrate a nonconcentric wear pattern (Fig. 39-9). In cases with nonconcentric glenoid mor-

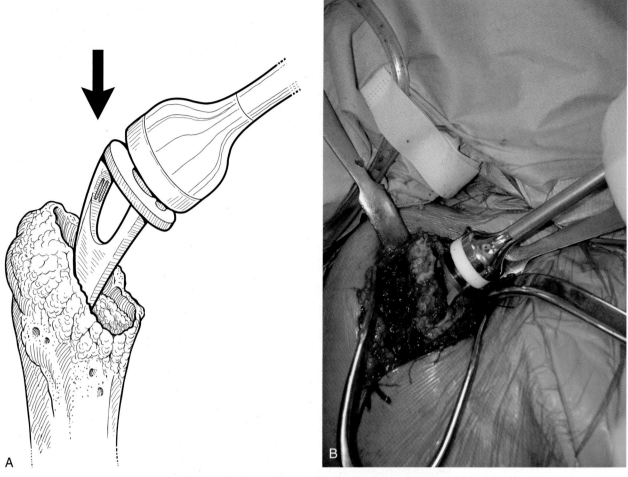

Figure 39-4 **A** and **B,** Impaction of the trial humeral stem into the proximal humerus.

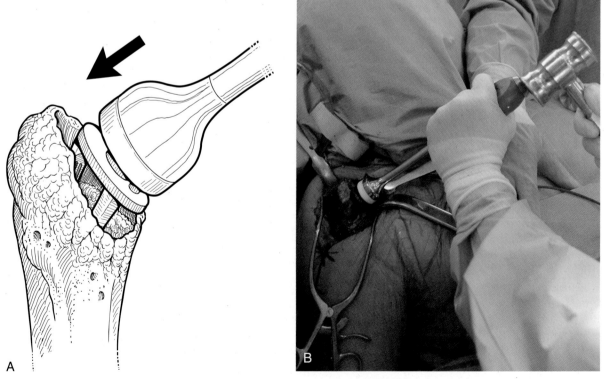

Figure 39-5 **A** and **B,** The trial humeral stem is impacted laterally into the greater tuberosity.

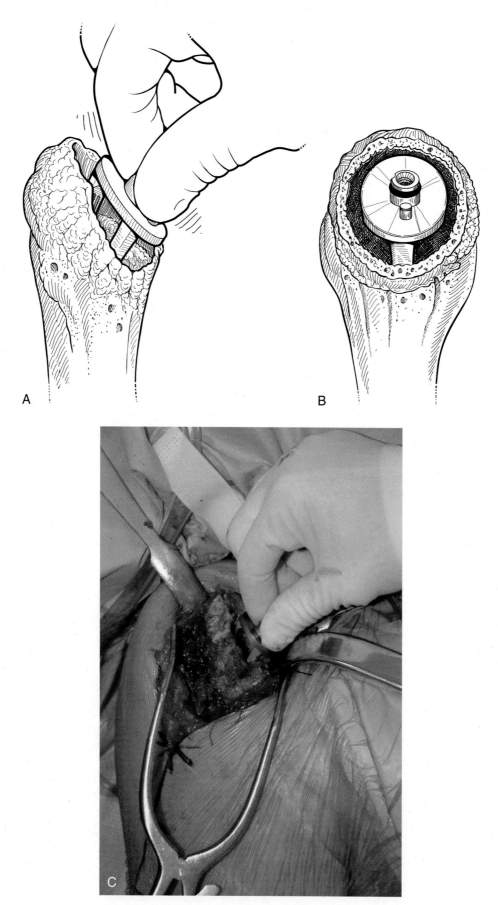

Figure 39-6 **A** to **C,** Humeral stem poorly filling the proximal humerus.

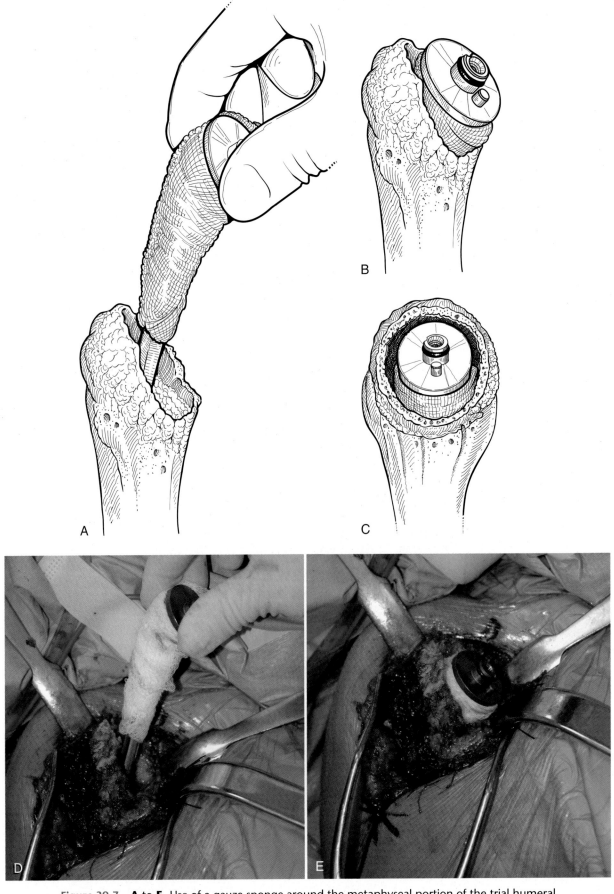

Figure 39-7 **A** to **E,** Use of a gauze sponge around the metaphyseal portion of the trial humeral stem to allow easier trial insertion of the revision implants.

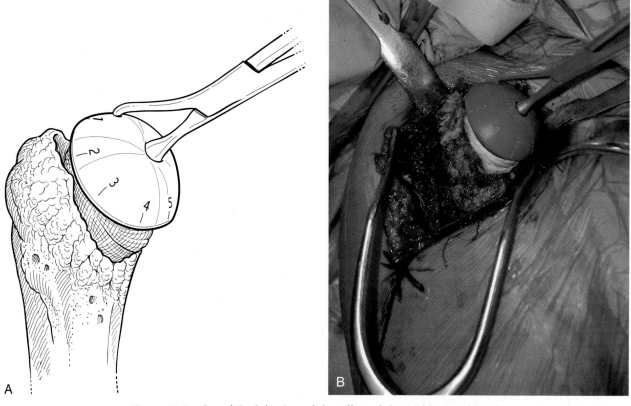

Figure 39-8 **A** and **B,** Selection of the offset of the trial humeral head.

phology or cases in which the osseous glenoid is compromised, we judge humeral version by placing the prosthesis in approximately 30 degrees of retroversion relative to the long axis of the forearm (Fig. 39-10). If the version of the trial humeral stem is unacceptable, the humeral trial is removed and humeral version changed by revising the original plane of humeral head resection by way of a revision humeral cut to introduce more retroversion or anteversion, as deemed appropriate by the trial glenohumeral reduction. The trial humeral implant is reinserted and the trial reduction repeated to ensure that humeral version has been corrected acceptably.

Reverse-Design Humeral Stem

In cases in which a reverse-design humeral implant is to be used as the revision humeral stem and the osseous

proximal humerus is relatively preserved, the epiphysis, metaphysis, and diaphysis are prepared in much the same way as for insertion of a reverse prosthesis as a primary implant. The epiphyseal reamer is first used to create a place for the proximal portion of the humeral implant (Fig. 39-11), after which the metaphyseal hand reamer is used (Fig. 39-12). Progressive diaphyseal reaming is then performed, with penetration of any osseous pedestal present in the humeral canal (Fig. 39-13). The trial humeral stem is assembled by using an implant diameter corresponding to the largest-diameter diaphyseal reamer that was used. The trial humeral implant is placed in approximately 10 degrees of humeral retroversion by using the forearm referencing insertion instrument and is fully impacted (Fig. 39-14). The position of the fin is marked on the proximal humerus with the electrocautery (Fig. 39-15).

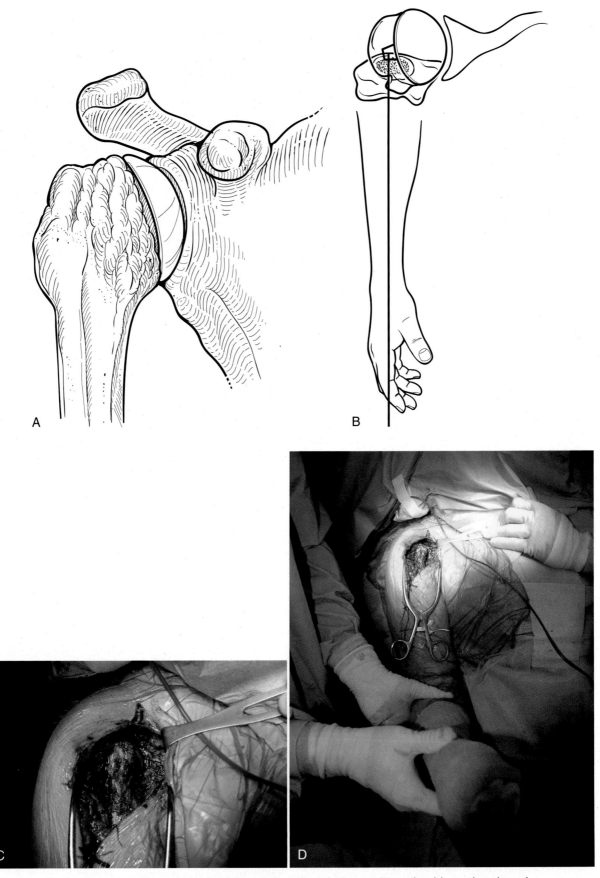

Figure 39-9 **A** to **D,** Judgment of humeral version during revision shoulder arthroplasty by ensuring that the prosthetic head is centered in the glenoid with the arm in neutral rotation.

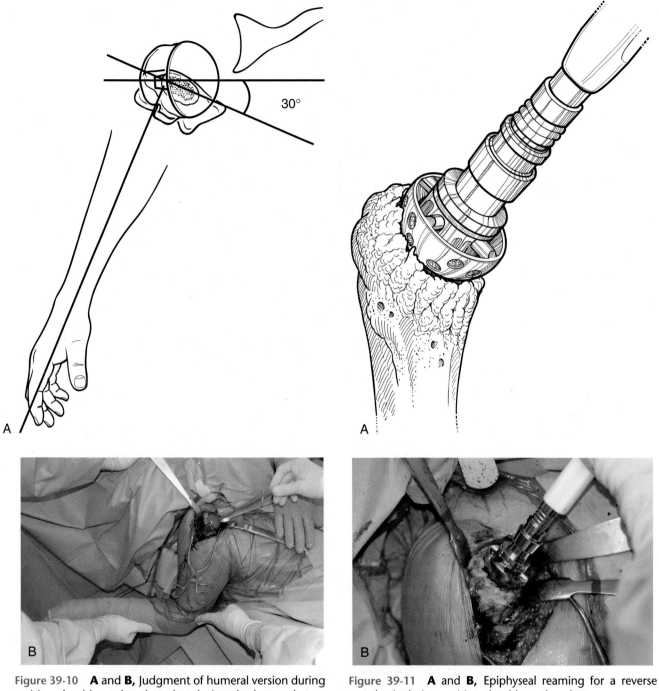

Figure 39-10 **A** and **B,** Judgment of humeral version during revision shoulder arthroplasty by placing the humeral stem in 30 degrees of retroversion relative to the long axis of the forearm. This technique is used in patients with nonconcentric glenoid wear or in those with glenoid osseous deficiency.

Figure 39-11 **A** and **B,** Epiphyseal reaming for a reverse prosthesis during revision shoulder arthroplasty.

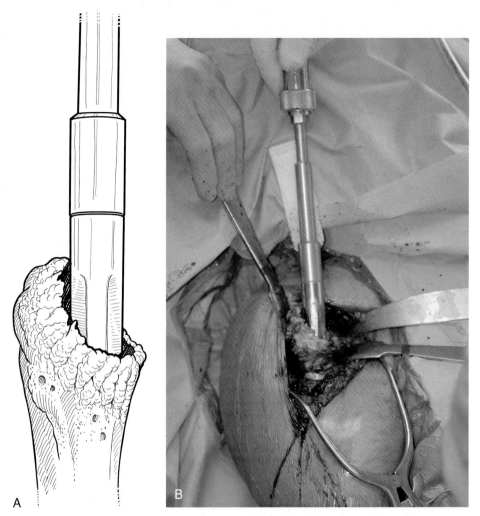

Figure 39-12 **A** and **B,** Metaphyseal reaming for a reverse prosthesis during revision shoulder arthroplasty.

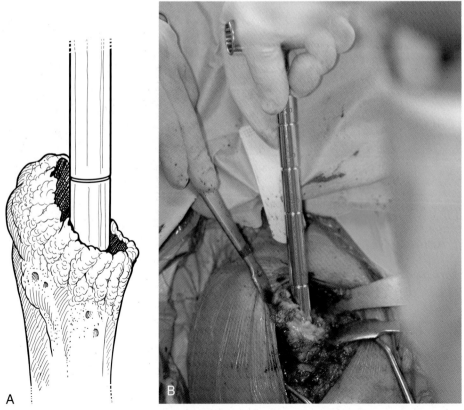

Figure 39-13 **A** and **B,** Diaphyseal reaming for a reverse prosthesis during revision shoulder arthroplasty.

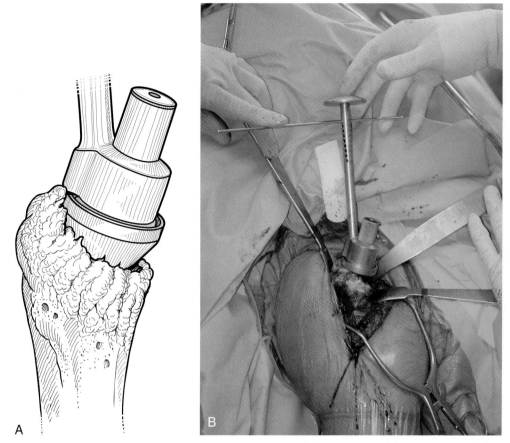

Figure 39-14 **A** and **B,** Insertion of the trial humeral component during revision shoulder arthroplasty with a reverse prosthesis.

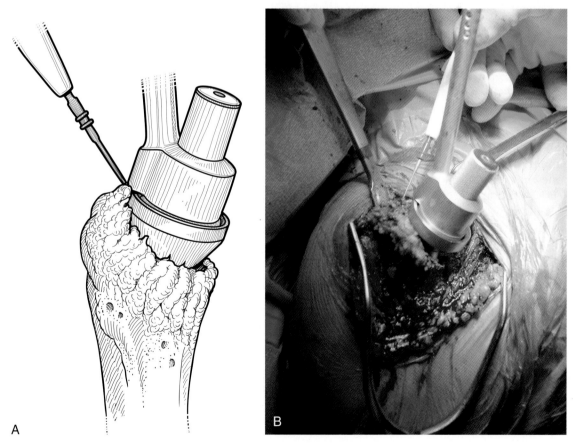

Figure 39-15 **A** and **B,** Marking retroversion of the humeral component during revision shoulder arthroplasty with a reverse prosthesis.

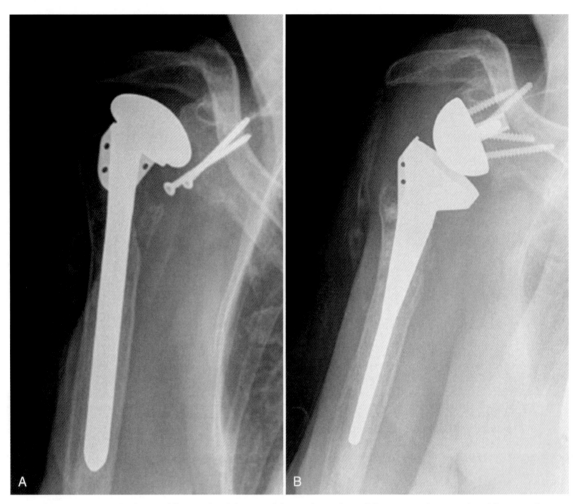

Figure 39-16 Patient with proximal humeral bone loss that did not require proximal humeral bone graft reconstruction before (**A**) and after (**B**) revision arthroplasty with a reverse prosthesis.

Revision cases with proximal humeral insufficiency may require proximal humeral osseous reconstruction with a bone graft. In general, in any case in which the rotator cuff insertion is compromised and glenoid bone stock allows, we will use a reverse prosthesis for revision arthroplasty. In cases of proximal humeral insufficiency limited to the proximal humeral metaphysis, no bone graft is indicated because the reverse prosthesis can be implanted into the intact humeral diaphysis (Fig. 39-16). In cases in which proximal humeral bone loss extends distally and compromises the proximal humeral diaphysis, bone graft reconstruction of the proximal humeral diaphysis is indicated (Fig. 39-17). In many cases, only a portion of the proximal humeral diaphysis is deficient (anterior or posterior). For this reason we prefer to reconstruct only the portion that is deficient and leave any native bone intact. Fresh frozen cortical strips of

allograft tibia are used for the reconstruction (Fig. 39-18). The residual diaphysis is reamed with the hand reamers.

Depending on the length of the humeral defect, we place two or three cables composed of a nylon mono-filament core wrapped in a braided ultrahigh-molecu-lar-weight polyethylene (Kinamed, Inc., Camarillo, CA) subperiosteally around the residual native humerus with the cable-passing instrumentation provided (Fig. 39-19). One or two allograft strips are trimmed to fit the diaphyseal defect and placed in the defect. The trial humeral stem is placed in the humeral diaphysis, and the allograft is placed in the diaphyseal defect (Fig. 39-20). The cables are tightened in a distal-to-proximal direction with the tensioning device (Fig. 39-21). The humeral stem is removed while leaving the recon-structed proximal humerus, and attention is turned to the glenoid, if indicated (Fig. 39-22).

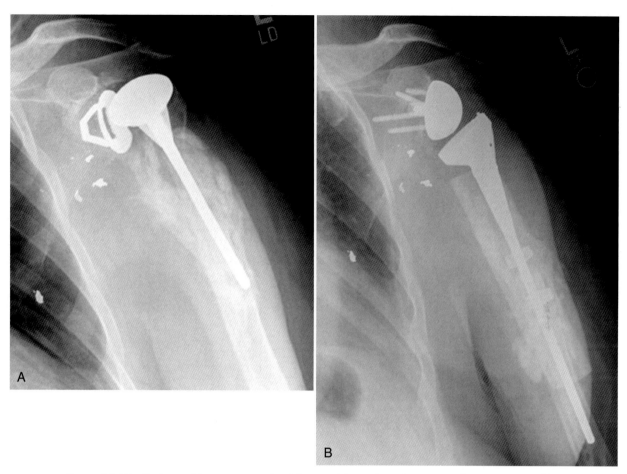

Figure 39-17   Patient with severe proximal humeral bone loss that required proximal humeral bone graft reconstruction before (**A**) and after (**B**) revision arthroplasty with a reverse prosthesis.

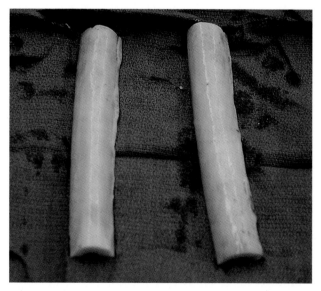

Figure 39-18   Fresh frozen allograft tibial strips used in proximal humeral reconstruction.

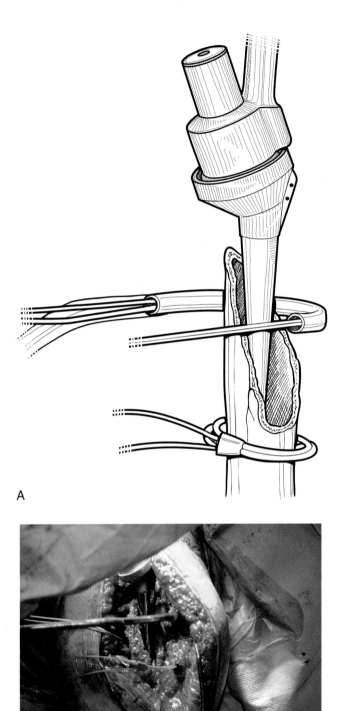

Figure 39-19   A and **B,** Passage of fixation cables to secure the allograft during proximal humeral reconstruction.

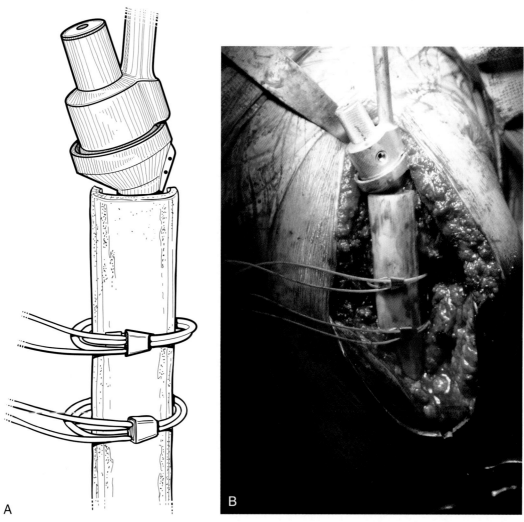

Figure 39-20   **A** and **B,** Placement of the allograft strip over the diaphyseal defect during proximal humeral reconstruction.

In cases in which a proximal humeral osteotomy has been performed for removal of the humeral stem, the cerclage cables are secured before removal of the trial humeral stem (see Chapter 38). In cases in which the native humeral cortex is excessively thin, fresh frozen allograft cortical struts are placed around the native humerus beneath the cables before tightening them to provide additional support for the proximal humerus, as shown in Chapter 38. The trial humeral stem is removed and attention is turned to the glenoid, if indicated.

TECHNIQUE FOR INSERTION OF A REVISION HUMERAL STEM

Once any glenoid pathology has been addressed, the humeral stem may be implanted. We cement the humeral stem in nearly all revision cases. In cases in which an unconstrained shoulder arthroplasty is to be implanted, the trial stem is replaced after any glenoid procedure is completed and glenohumeral stability is evaluated. With the arm externally rotated approximately 30 degrees, force is applied in a posterior direction to the proximal humerus, as with primary unconstrained shoulder arthroplasty. The prosthetic humeral head should subluxate posteriorly approximately 30% to 50% of its diameter and spontaneously reduce on release of the posteriorly directed force. If spontaneous reduction does not occur, posterior capsulorrhaphy may be necessary, as described in Chapter 13. Conversely, if posterior translation of at least 30% of the diameter of the humeral head is not possible, posterior capsular release may be necessary.

Once the shoulder is properly balanced, the humeral implant is cemented into place. Before insertion of the humeral stem, a cement restrictor is placed 1 cm distal

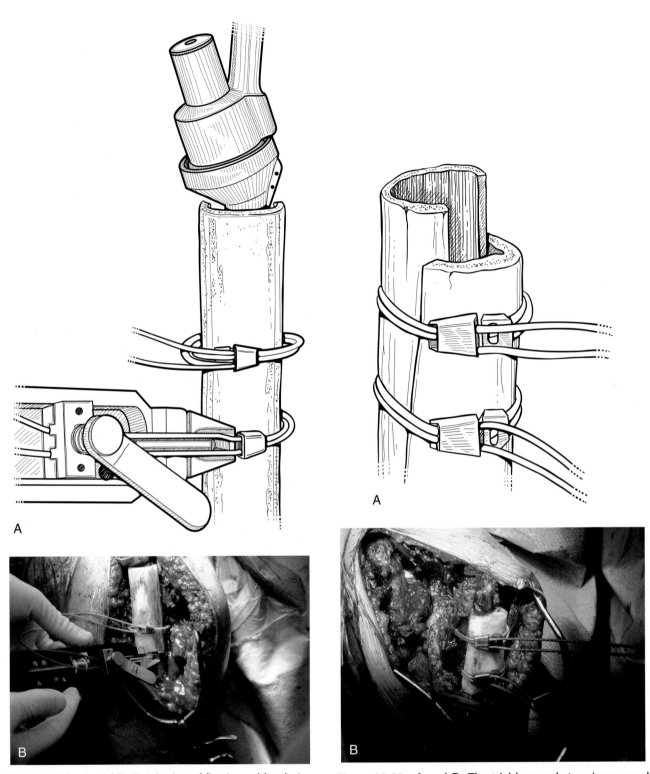

Figure 39-21 A and B, Tensioning of fixation cables during proximal humeral reconstruction.

Figure 39-22 A and B, The trial humeral stem is removed while leaving the reconstructed proximal humerus.

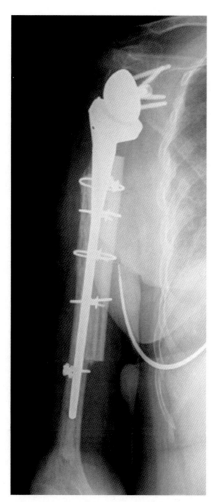

Figure 39-23 Case not requiring the use of a cement restrictor.

to the distal-most extent of the stem with an insertion device, except in cases in which a long-stem humeral implant that extends distally to the humeral isthmus is used, in which case no cement restrictor is placed (Fig. 39-23). Three no. 2 nonabsorbable braided sutures are placed first through the humeral stump of the subscapularis tendon, into the lesser tuberosity, and out through the intramedullary canal of the humerus for later use in reattachment of the subscapularis, as in cases of primary unconstrained shoulder arthroplasty (Fig. 39-24). These sutures are tagged with three different types of hemostats to identify the sutures as superior, middle, and inferior (we use a curved Kelly hemostat superiorly, a mosquito hemostat on the middle suture, and a regular hemostat inferiorly). The humeral canal is irrigated with sterile saline and dried with suction and gauze sponges. Two packages of bone cement (we prefer to use DePuy 2 bone cement [DePuy, Inc., Warsaw, IN] because of its accelerated curing time of less than 8 minutes) impregnated with 4 g of vancomycin powder (or 4.8 g of tobramycin powder in

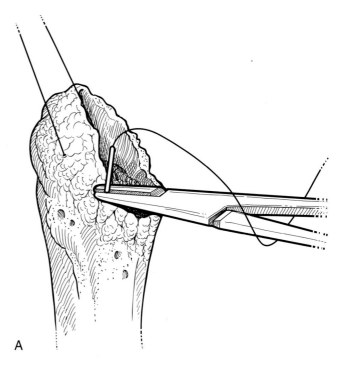

A

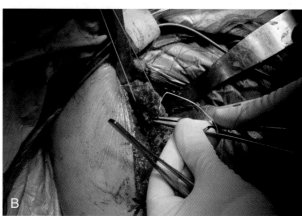

B

Figure 39-24 **A** and **B,** Transosseous sutures placed before insertion of the humeral stem for later use in reattachment of the subscapularis.

patients with vancomycin allergy) are introduced with a modified catheter tip syringe (Fig. 39-25). The canal is filled with cement and the assembled humeral stem is seated with an impactor while making sure to lateralize the humeral stem (Fig. 39-26). It is not necessary to pressurize the cement. Excess cement is removed with a Freer elevator. The cement is allowed to cure before reducing the glenohumeral joint. The subscapularis is repaired with the previously placed transosseous sutures, as in cases of primary shoulder arthroplasty.

When implanting a reverse prosthesis during revision shoulder arthroplasty, we reinsert the trial humeral stem with the 6-mm polyethylene insert after complet-

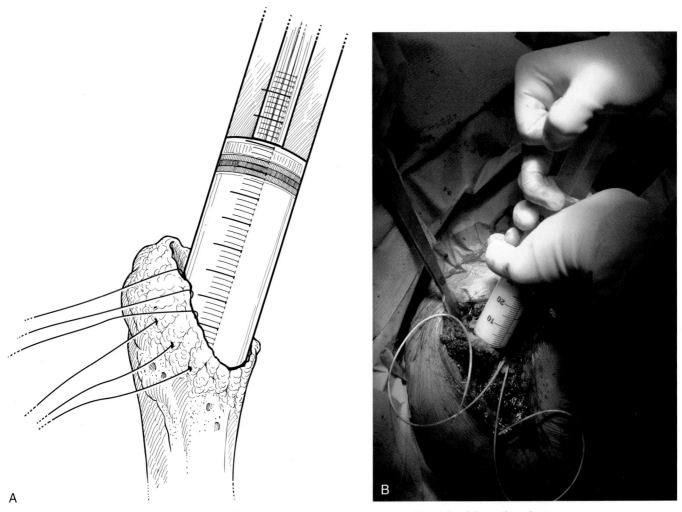

A

B

Figure 39-25   A and **B,** Insertion of cement during revision shoulder arthroplasty.

ing implantation of the glenoid component and reduce the prosthetic glenohumeral joint. With longitudinal traction placed on the arm, the humeral component is manually telescoped maximally out of the humerus to the glenoid component (Fig. 39-27), and the level of the trial humeral implant with respect to the proximal humerus is marked (Fig. 39-28). The distance between the metaphyseal-diaphyseal prosthetic junction and the mark made with respect to the proximal humerus is compared with the distance templated preoperatively (see Chapter 36) to evaluate restoration of appropriate humeral length. This enables an estimation of the appropriate level at which to cement the humeral component. If the humeral component is cemented too distally within the humerus, adequate tension may not be obtainable. Conversely, if the humeral component is cemented too proximally

within the humerus, the prosthetic joint may be irreducible.

Once the desired level at which to cement the humeral implant has been selected, preparation is made to insert the humeral prosthesis. Before insertion of the humeral stem, a cement restrictor is placed 1 cm distal to the distal-most extent of the stem with an insertion device, except in cases in which a long-stem humeral implant that extends distally to the humeral isthmus is used, in which case no cement restrictor is placed. If the subscapularis tendon is present and reparable, three no. 2 nonabsorbable braided sutures are placed first through the humeral stump of the subscapularis tendon, into the lesser tuberosity, and out through the intramedullary canal of the humerus for later use in reattachment of the subscapularis, as in cases of primary and revision unconstrained shoulder

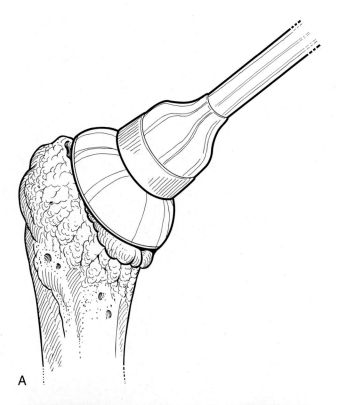

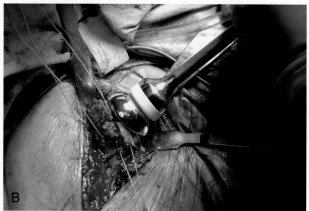

Figure 39-26   A and **B,** The humeral stem is held laterally as the cement cures.

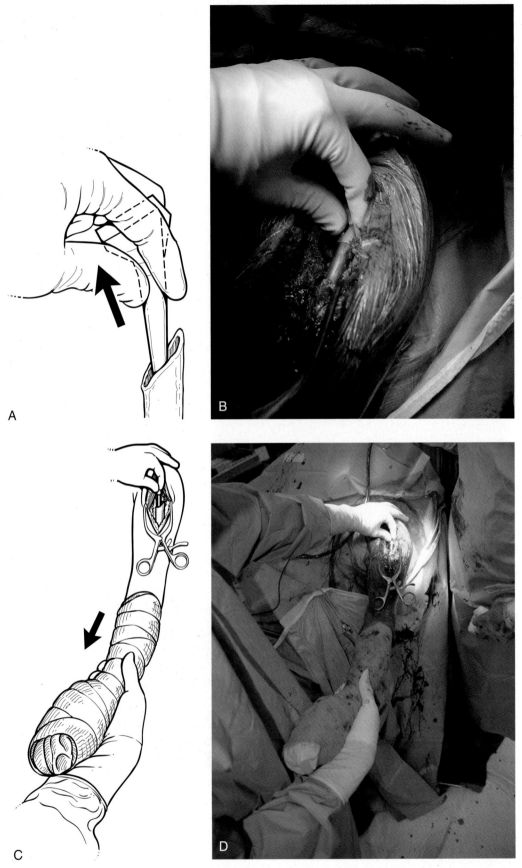

Figure 39-27 **A** and **B,** Judgment of the appropriate level at which to insert a reverse-prosthesis humeral component during revision shoulder arthroplasty. **C** and **D,** With longitudinal traction placed on the arm, the humeral component is manually telescoped maximally out of the humerus to the glenoid component.

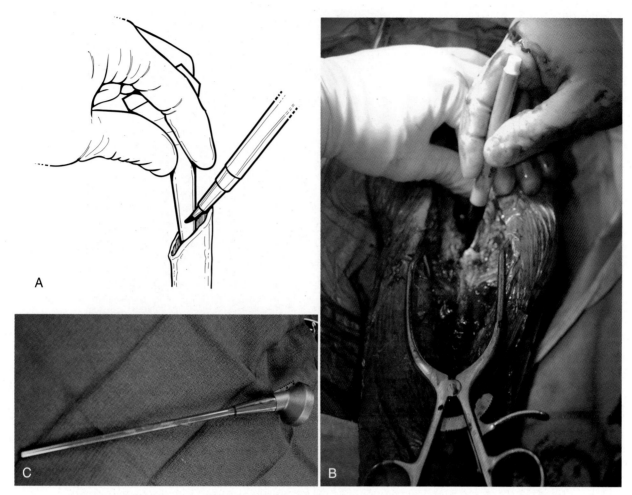

Figure 39-28 **A** to **C,** Judgment of the appropriate level at which to insert a reverse-prosthesis humeral component during revision shoulder arthroplasty. The level of the trial humeral implant is marked with respect to the proximal humerus.

arthroplasty, as previously described. The humeral canal is irrigated with sterile saline and dried with suction and gauze sponges.

The final humeral implant is cemented into place with antibiotic-impregnated cement via the technique previously described in this chapter. The cement is allowed to cure before reducing the glenohumeral joint. Once the humeral component has been cemented into place within the humerus (see Chapter 28), trial insertion of the various implants commences, as described in Chapter 30. In revision cases, no pistoning is accepted between the humeral and glenoid components. Additionally, we often use a "shoe horn" instrument to aid in reduction by levering the humerus distally to engage the glenoid (Fig. 39-29). Once appropriate tension has been obtained, the final polyethylene insert is placed, as described in Chapter 30.

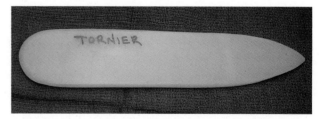

Figure 39-29 "Shoe horn" instrument used to reduce the reverse prosthesis during revision shoulder arthroplasty.

SPECIAL SITUATIONS

Periprosthetic Fracture

In cases of periprosthetic fracture, the fracture must be reduced before placement of the revision humeral stem. The fracture and associated structures (i.e., the

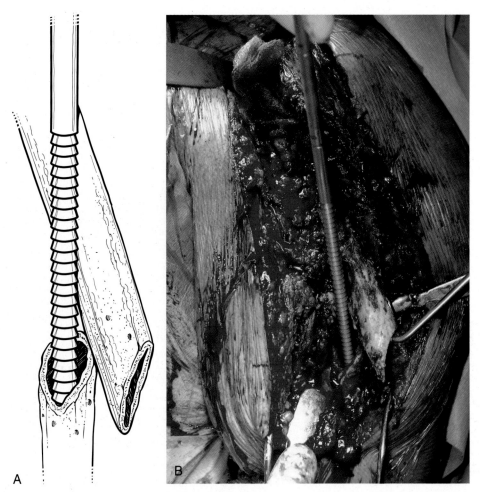

Figure 39-30   A and **B,** The humerus distal to the fracture site is reamed with diaphyseal reamers introduced at the fracture site.

radial nerve) are exposed as detailed in Chapter 37. The humerus distal to the fracture site is reamed with the diaphyseal reamers introduced at the fracture site (Fig. 39-30). The humerus proximal to the fracture site is prepared with the instrumentation provided for the selected humeral stem. It is often helpful to stabilize the proximal humeral fragment with a bone clamp during preparation of the proximal humerus (Fig. 39-31).

Once the proximal humerus has been prepared, the fracture is reduced and the trial humeral stem is placed. A humeral stem that bypasses the distal extent of the fracture by a minimum of two cortical diameters is selected (Fig. 39-32).[1] The position of the humeral stem within the humerus is noted after trial reduction and stability testing, as previously described. Fresh frozen cortical strips of allograft tibia are used on each side of the humerus and centered at the fracture site. We place two or four cables composed of a nylon monofilament core wrapped in a braided ultrahigh-molecular-weight polyethylene (Kinamed Inc., Camarillo, CA) subperiosteally around the residual native humerus with the cable-passing instrumentation provided while taking care to avoid the radial nerve posteriorly (Fig. 39-33). The cables are tightened with the tensioning device, the humeral stem is removed, and the periprosthetic fracture is left reduced (Fig. 39-34). The humeral canal is irrigated with sterile saline and dried with suction and gauze sponges. The final humeral implant is cemented into place with antibiotic-impregnated cement via the technique previously described in this chapter (Fig. 39-35). The cement is allowed to cure before reducing the glenohumeral joint.

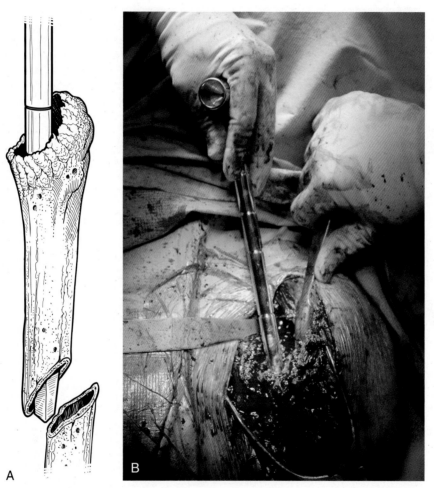

Figure 39-31 A and **B,** The humerus proximal to the fracture site is prepared with the instrumentation provided for the selected humeral stem.

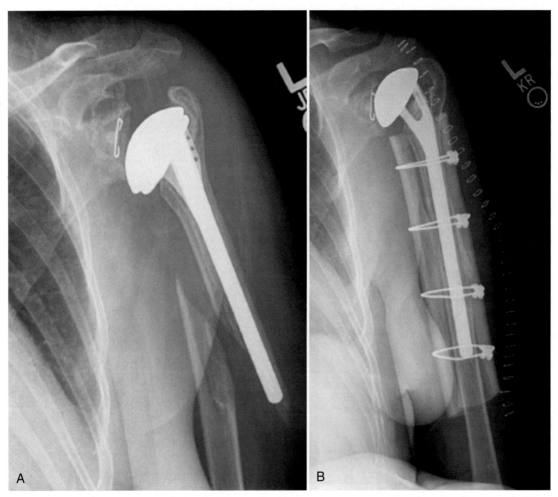

Figure 39-32   A, Preoperative radiograph. **B,** The humeral stem selected should bypass the distal extent of the fracture by a minimum of two cortical diameters.

Figure 39-33 **A** and **B,** Cables placed for fixation of a cortical strip allograft during treatment of a periprosthetic humeral fracture by revision arthroplasty.

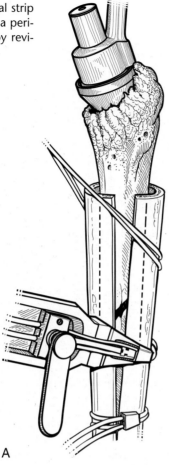

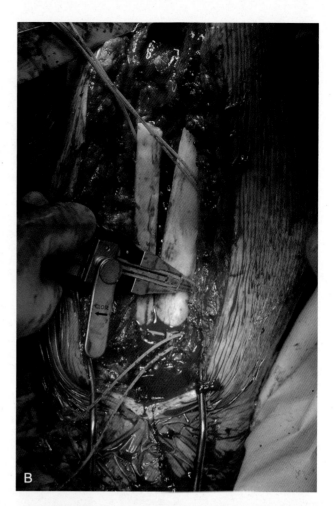

Figure 39-34 **A** and **B,** The humeral stem is removed, leaving the periprosthetic fracture reduced.

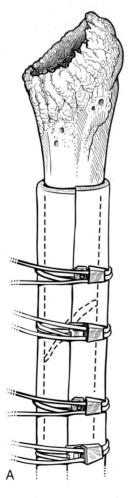

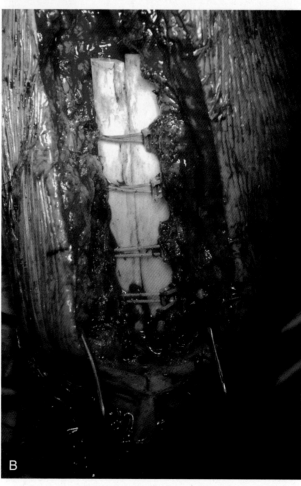

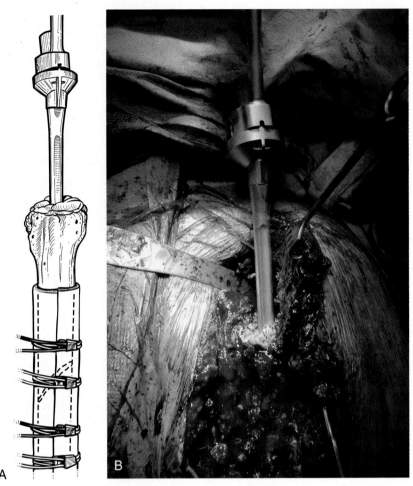

Figure 39-35 **A** and **B,** The final humeral implant is cemented into place with antibiotic-impregnated cement.

REFERENCE

1. Johansson JE, McBroom R, Barrington TW, Hunter GA: Fractures of the ipsilateral femur in patients with total hip replacement. J Bone Joint Surg Am 1981;61:1435-1442.

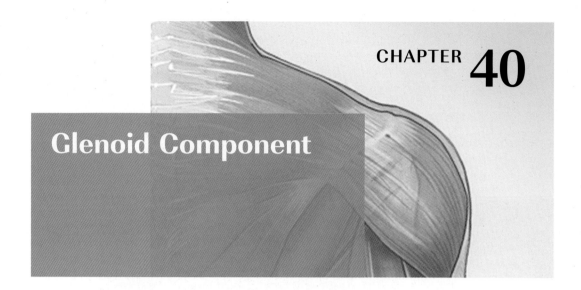

CHAPTER **40**

Glenoid Component

Problems with the glenoid are a common indication for revision arthroplasty. Such problems include failure of previously implanted glenoid components from total shoulder arthroplasty and osseous glenoid erosion after hemiarthroplasty. Frequently, glenoid problems involve substantial osseous compromise and require complex reconstruction. The ability to deal with these glenoid problems is necessary to successfully treat many cases of failed shoulder arthroplasty. Treatment of the various types of glenoid problems are addressed in detail in this chapter.

GLENOID REVISION NOT REQUIRING A BONE GRAFT

Glenoid erosion after hemiarthroplasty is a common indication for revision arthroplasty and occurs in two situations: (1) in patients with rotator cuff deficiency and superior glenoid erosion coupled with static superior (or anterior superior) humeral migration (Fig. 40-1) and (2) in patients with an intact rotator cuff and painful symptomatic humeral erosion that is central, anterior, or posterior (Fig. 40-2). Usually, the erosion is not severe enough to require a bone graft, but the surgeon should first determine the severity of the osseous glenoid defect with a preoperative computed tomogram (Fig. 40-3).

Unconstrained Shoulder Arthroplasty Cases Not Requiring a Glenoid Bone Graft

In patients with glenoid erosion after hemiarthroplasty and a functional rotator cuff, revision surgery from hemiarthroplasty to total shoulder arthroplasty is per-

formed similar to cases of primary unconstrained shoulder arthroplasty. In such cases, if the humeral component is properly sized and positioned, the surgeon may be able to retain the humeral stem while performing revision surgery. This almost always necessitates changing the humeral head of the modular implant. It is important to know preoperatively the type of implant that the patient had and the radius of curvature of the various head sizes of this implant. A different brand of glenoid component can be coupled with the previous humeral head component if prosthetic mismatch can be calculated and respected during revision arthroplasty (see Chapter 12 for discussion of prosthetic mismatch and its implications in unconstrained shoulder arthroplasty). In general, radial mismatch of greater than 5.5 mm and less than 10 mm should be respected and the glenoid component size selected accordingly. If the humeral component is not properly sized or positioned or if adequate glenoid exposure cannot be obtained because of the humeral stem, the humeral component should be removed as described in Chapter 38.

Once glenoid exposure is achieved, implantation of a glenoid component proceeds as in cases of primary unconstrained arthroplasty with either a keeled or pegged glenoid component (Fig. 40-4). The technique for insertion of an unconstrained glenoid component is detailed in Chapter 12.

Reverse Shoulder Arthroplasty Cases Not Requiring a Glenoid Bone Graft

In patients with glenoid erosion after hemiarthroplasty and a nonfunctional rotator cuff, revision surgery from hemiarthroplasty to reverse shoulder arthroplasty is

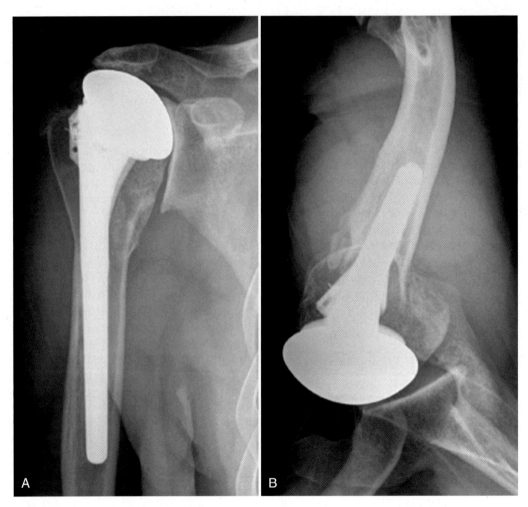

Figure 40-1   A and **B,** Anterior superior escape of a hemiarthroplasty without significant glenoid bone loss.

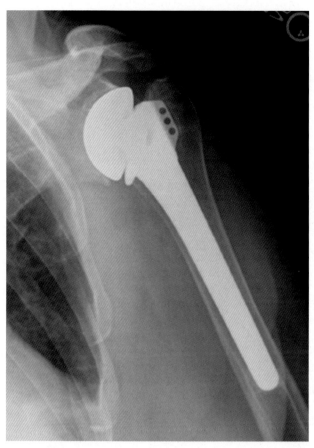

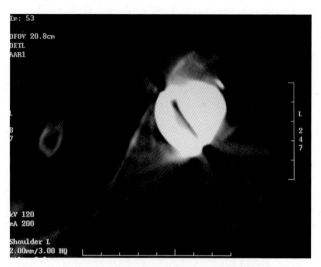

Figure 40-3 Preoperative tomogram of a patient after hemiarthroplasty demonstrating central erosion of the glenoid but with sufficient glenoid bone stock remaining to allow placement of a glenoid component without bone grafting of the glenoid.

Figure 40-2 Painful central glenoid erosion after hemiarthroplasty.

performed similar to cases of primary reverse shoulder arthroplasty. In such cases the hemiarthroplasty component is removed and the glenoid exposed as described in Chapter 38. Implantation of a reverse glenoid component proceeds as in cases of primary reverse arthroplasty, as described later in this chapter and in detail in Chapter 29.

GLENOID REVISION REQUIRING A BONE GRAFT

In cases of hemiarthroplasty with moderate to severe glenoid osseous erosion and in cases of failure of a primary glenoid component, reconstruction of the glenoid with an autogenous iliac crest structural bone graft is indicated.[1] Our previous experience with cancellous bone grafts, allografts, and bone graft substitutes resulted in a high rate of graft resorption and led us to the technique that we now use.

Unconstrained Shoulder Arthroplasty Cases Requiring a Glenoid Bone Graft

Rarely, moderate to severe osseous insufficiency of the glenoid occurs after hemiarthroplasty of the shoulder, and poor glenoid bone stock prohibits insertion of an unconstrained glenoid component (Fig. 40-5). In these cases two options exist: (1) conversion to resection arthroplasty by simple removal of the humeral component and (2) glenoid reconstruction with an iliac crest bone graft. Similarly, in patients with a failed glenoid component (loosening, component fracture), options include resection arthroplasty, removal of the glenoid component with retention of the humeral component, and glenoid reconstruction with an iliac crest bone graft (Fig. 40-6). We tell patients selected for glenoid reconstruction that we anticipate a second-stage operation for insertion of a polyethylene glenoid component once it is confirmed with computed tomography that the bone graft has been incorporated (Fig. 40-7), which occurs approximately 6 months after bone graft reconstruction. In patients who desire conversion to resection arthroplasty or removal of the glenoid component (usually elderly patients seeking only pain relief), this is easily accomplished by removing the humeral stem or glenoid component, or both, as described in Chapter 38 (Fig. 40-8).

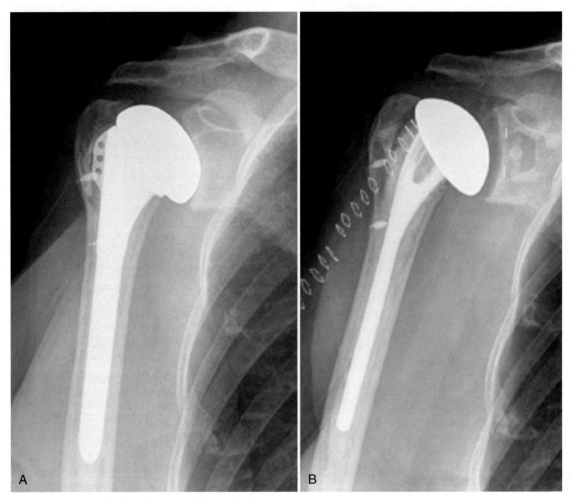

Figure 40-4   Pre-revision (**A**) and post-revision (**B**) radiographs of a patient with conversion of a hemiarthroplasty to a total shoulder arthroplasty.

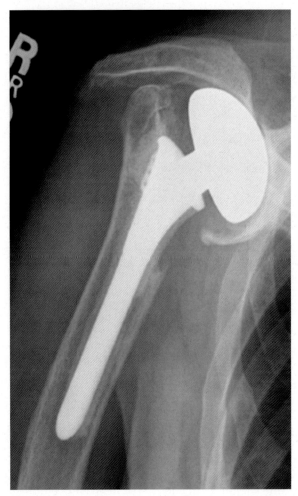

Figure 40-5 Patient with severe glenoid erosion after hemi-arthroplasty prohibiting simple insertion of a glenoid component.

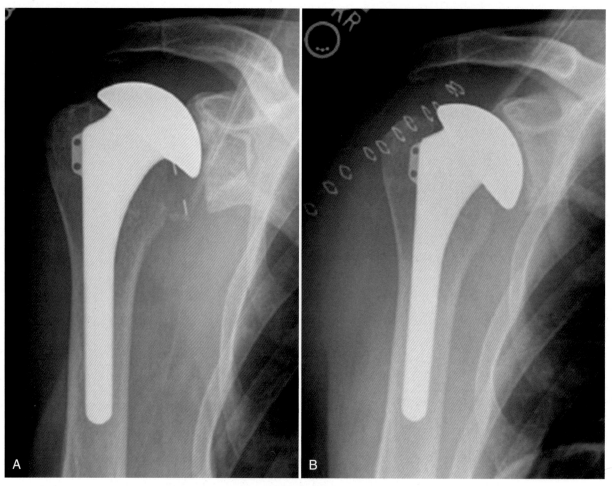

Figure 40-6   In patients with a failed glenoid component (loosening, component fracture) (**A**), options include resection arthroplasty, removal of the glenoid component with retention of the humeral component, and glenoid reconstruction with an iliac crest bone graft (**B**).

For glenoid reconstruction, an autogenous iliac crest bone graft is first harvested, as described later in this chapter. The glenoid is exposed, as previously described. Any soft tissue covering the remaining osseous glenoid is removed to define the limits of the glenoid osseous margins (Fig. 40-9). The area of deficiency is identified. If the deficiency is central, it may be possible to fashion the bone graft to fit the defect via an interference fit and eliminate the need for internal fixation (Fig. 40-10). For peripheral deficits, it is necessary to secure the bone graft with internal fixation to avoid migration. In anterior or posterior osseous insufficiency, we usually opt for cannulated, partially threaded 4.0-mm-diameter screws with washers placed through the bone graft and into the intact osseous glenoid. In central glenoid osseous insufficiency (not amenable to interference fit of the bone graft) and superior glenoid osseous insufficiency, we opt for graft

fixation with 1.5 × 60-mm bioabsorbable fixation pins (SmartPin, Linvtec, Inc., Largo, FL).

Contained Osseous Deficit
For interference-fit fixation of a central osseous deficit, the defect is prepared by lightly abrading the glenoid surface with a 5-mm round burr (Fig. 40-11). The tricortical iliac crest bone graft is trimmed with a cutting rongeur to a shape similar to the defect and slightly larger (Fig. 40-12). Cancellous bone is placed in the central defect, and the tricortical segment of the bone graft is placed in the defect and impacted into place with a large bone tamp until it is flush with the intact glenoid surface (Fig. 40-13). Care is taken to orient the tricortical graft so that a cortical surface faces laterally (Fig. 40-14). If the bone graft is not secured by interference fit, bioabsorbable fixation pins are used to prevent migration of the bone graft. This is done by first fixing

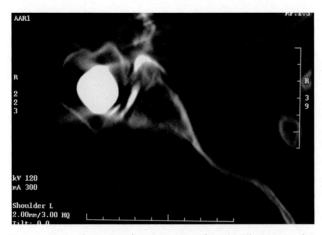

Figure 40-7 Computed tomogram showing incorporation of an iliac crest bone graft used for reconstruction of the glenoid.

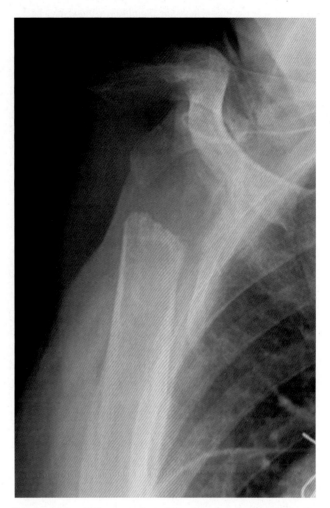

Figure 40-8 Patient undergoing resection arthroplasty for pain relief after failed shoulder arthroplasty.

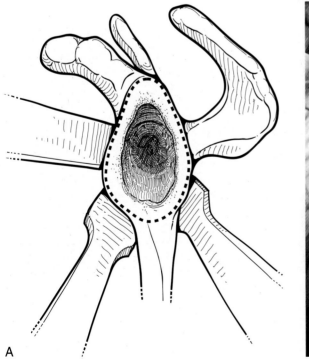

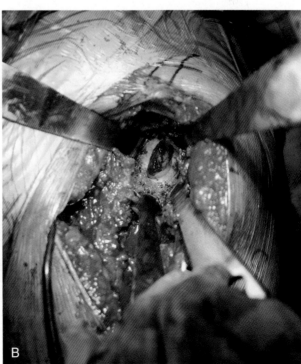

Figure 40-9 **A** and **B,** The margins of the osseous glenoid are defined before reconstruction of the glenoid.

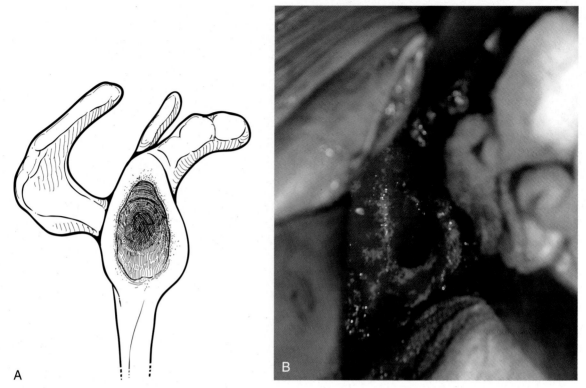

Figure 40-10   A and **B,** Central glenoid deficiency that can be treated by bone graft reconstruction with interference-fit fixation.

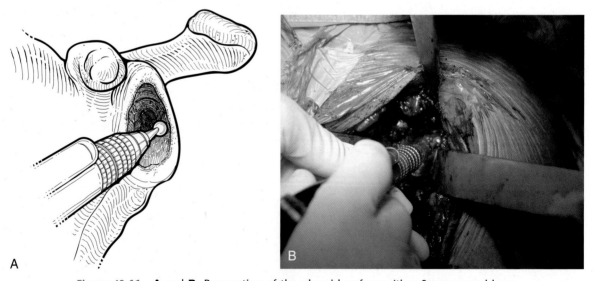

Figure 40-11   A and **B,** Preparation of the glenoid surface with a 5-mm round burr.

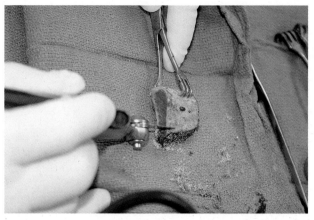

Figure 40-12   Contouring of the iliac crest bone graft before insertion into the glenoid cavity.

the graft with two 0.062-inch Kirschner wires placed through the bone graft and into the native glenoid medially. These wires are intentionally placed so that they are not parallel to one another (Fig. 40-15). One of the wires is removed, and a bioabsorbable pin is advanced into the hole left by the Kirschner wire with the insertion device (Fig. 40-16). Another wire is used to create another hole in a direction and orientation different from that of the previous two holes, and another bioabsorbable pin is placed (Fig. 40-17). This process is repeated until a minimum of four pins have been placed. To enhance fixation, we avoid placing any of the pins parallel to one another. The residual pin tips are clipped flush with the bone graft with a

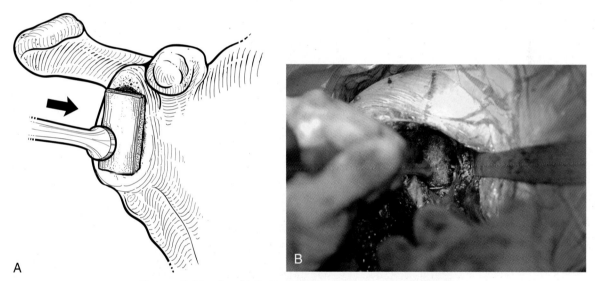

A

B

Figure 40-13   **A** and **B,** Impaction of the glenoid bone graft.

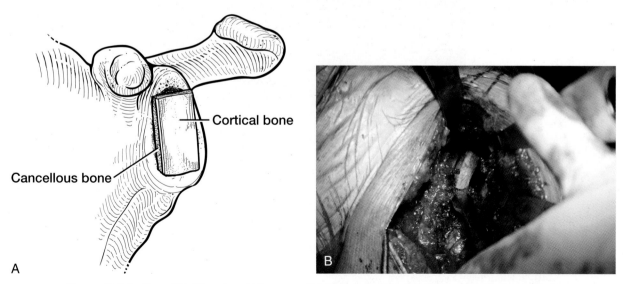

Cortical bone

Cancellous bone

A

B

Figure 40-14   **A** and **B,** The glenoid bone graft is inserted with a cortical surface facing laterally to resist medialization of the humeral head.

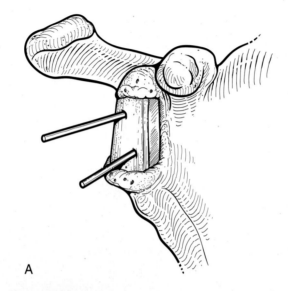

A

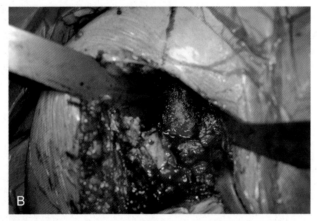

B

Figure 40-15   **A** and **B,** Kirschner wires placed before insertion of bioabsorbable pins for bone graft fixation.

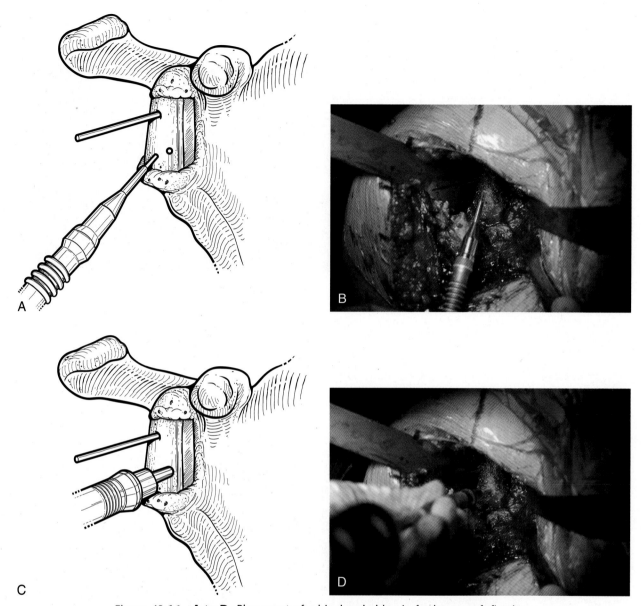

Figure 40-16   **A** to **D,** Placement of a bioabsorbable pin for bone graft fixation.

large rongeur to complete fixation of the bone graft (Fig. 40-18). This same technique is used for superior defects. After contouring the bone graft to fit the defect and preparation of the base of the defect, the graft is fixated with multiple bioabsorbable pins (Fig. 40-19).

Uncontained (Anterior or Posterior) Osseous Deficit

In cases of anterior or posterior glenoid insufficiency requiring bone graft reconstruction, the tricortical iliac crest bone graft is contoured to fit the defect with a cutting rongeur so that a cortical surface faces laterally (Fig. 40-20). Two guide wires for 4.0-mm screws are placed across the graft and the glenoid vault and into

the opposite cortex of the native glenoid (Fig. 40-21). Care is taken to direct the guide wires so that they do not violate the central portion of the glenoid vault and thereby prohibit later placement of a glenoid component (Fig. 40-22). For anterior glenoid insufficiency, these guide wires can be placed through the deltopectoral approach. For posterior glenoid insufficiency, the guide wires are placed percutaneously from the posterior aspect of the shoulder (Fig. 40-23). Screw lengths are measured from the guide wire (Fig. 40-24). The drill provided is used over the guide wire (Fig. 40-25). The proper size screw with washer is placed over the guide wire and advanced until fully seated (Fig. 40-26).

Text continued on p. 460

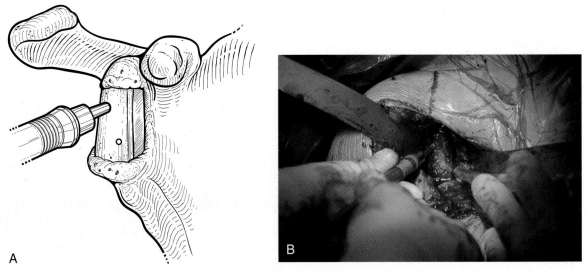

A

B

Figure 40-17 **A** and **B,** Placement of a second bioabsorbable pin for bone graft fixation. The pin is not placed parallel to the initial pin.

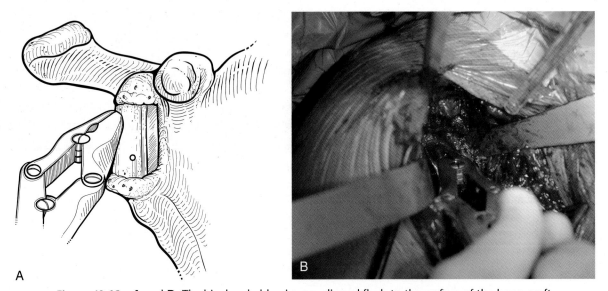

A

B

Figure 40-18 **A** and **B,** The bioabsorbable pins are clipped flush to the surface of the bone graft with a rongeur.

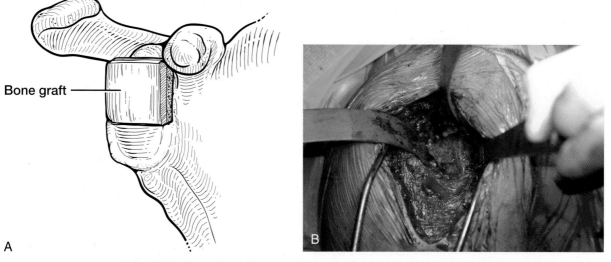

Figure 40-19 **A** and **B,** Final glenoid bone graft construct after fixation with bioabsorbable pins to fill a superior glenoid defect.

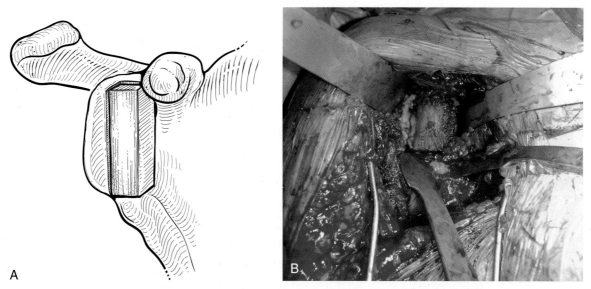

Figure 40-20 **A** and **B,** Placement of a glenoid bone graft to fill an anterior glenoid defect.

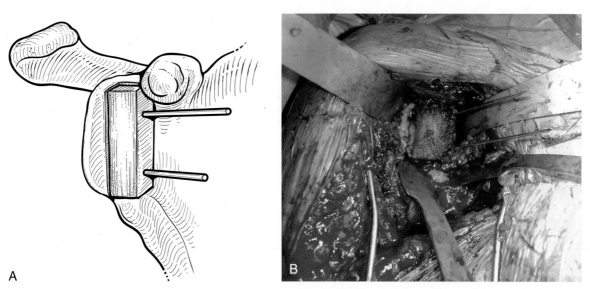

Figure 40-21 **A** and **B,** Placement of guide wires for the 4.0-mm cannulated screws used for bone graft reconstruction of an anterior glenoid defect.

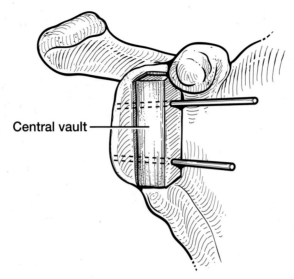

Central vault

Figure 40-22 Guide wires are placed so that the central portion of the glenoid vault is not violated and later placement of the glenoid component prohibited.

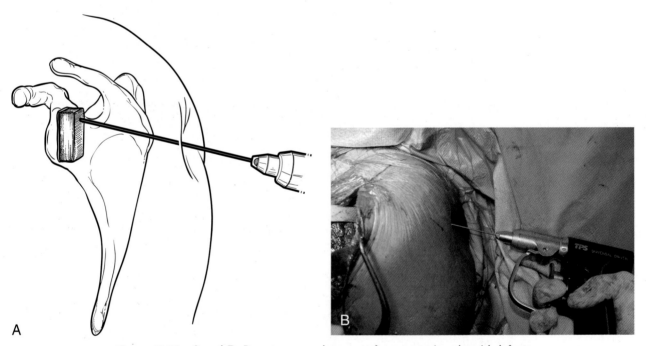

A

B

Figure 40-23 **A** and **B,** Percutaneous placement for a posterior glenoid defect.

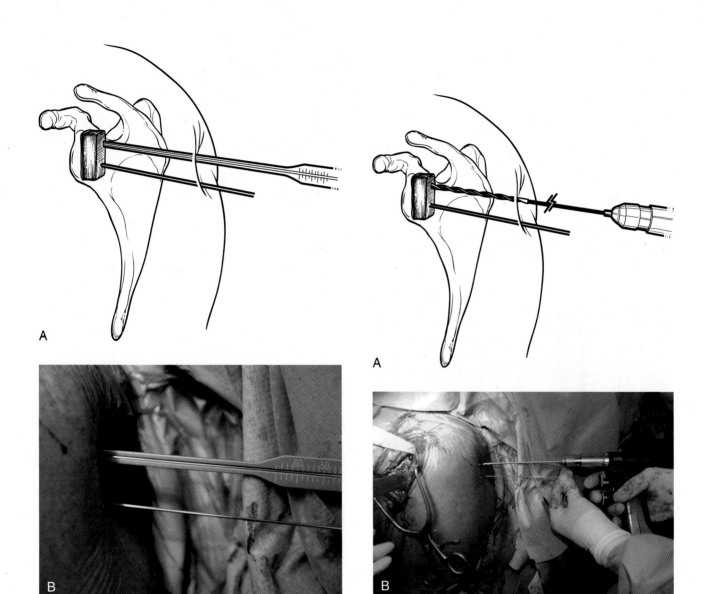

Figure 40-24   **A** and **B,** Measurement of screw length from the guide wires.

Figure 40-25   **A** and **B,** Drilling the holes for the cannulated screws over the guide wires.

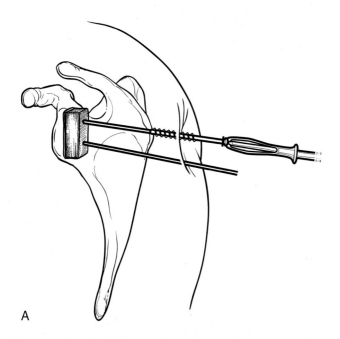

A

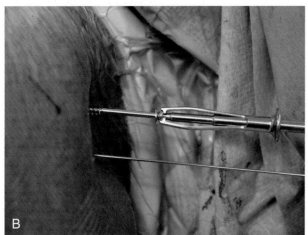

B

Figure 40-26 A and **B,** Fixation of the bone graft with screws and washers.

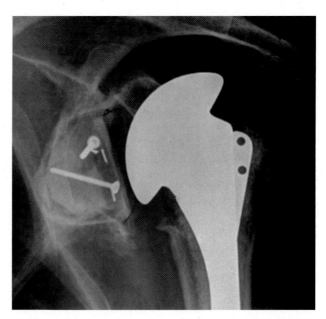

Figure 40-27 Failure of the glenoid component after attempted single-stage reconstruction of the glenoid with an iliac crest bone graft and placement of an unconstrained shoulder arthroplasty.

When performing bone graft reconstruction of the glenoid, we avoid simultaneous implantation of an unconstrained glenoid component. Single-stage implantation of a glenoid component after reconstruction of the glenoid with a bone graft has resulted in an unacceptably high rate of failure of the glenoid component (Fig. 40-27). In this scenario we will offer the patient implantation of a glenoid component 6 months after glenoid reconstruction if a computed tomogram confirms incorporation of the bone graft and sufficient glenoid bone stock to allow insertion of a glenoid component (Fig. 40-28). In this situation, placement of the revision glenoid component is performed as in cases of primary glenoid resurfacing (see Chapter 12). Occasionally in young patients, we

will perform fascia lata glenoid resurfacing at the time of glenoid reconstruction (Fig. 40-29; see Chapter 34).

Reverse Shoulder Arthroplasty Cases Requiring a Glenoid Bone Graft

Cases in which a primary hemiarthroplasty is to be revised to a reverse prosthesis occasionally require bone grafting of the glenoid. The defect is usually superior in cases of rotator cuff deficiency but may be anterior or posterior in cases of prosthetic instability after hemiarthroplasty (Fig. 40-30). Similarly, cases with a failed glenoid component and rotator cuff insufficiency are an indication for glenoid reconstruction and placement of a reverse prosthesis (Fig. 40-31). The same techniques used for glenoid reconstruction with an autogenous iliac crest bone graft for unconstrained shoulder arthroplasty are performed. The main difference between revision with a reverse prosthesis and revision with an unconstrained prosthesis in this scenario is the potential ability to perform a single-stage procedure when using the reverse prosthesis. If the majority of the central post of the reverse prosthesis base plate can be implanted into native glenoid bone, the reverse prosthesis can be implanted as a single-stage procedure (Fig. 40-32). An alternative base plate designed for revision surgery is available. This base plate has a central post that is 1 cm longer than the standard base plate. This extra length allows

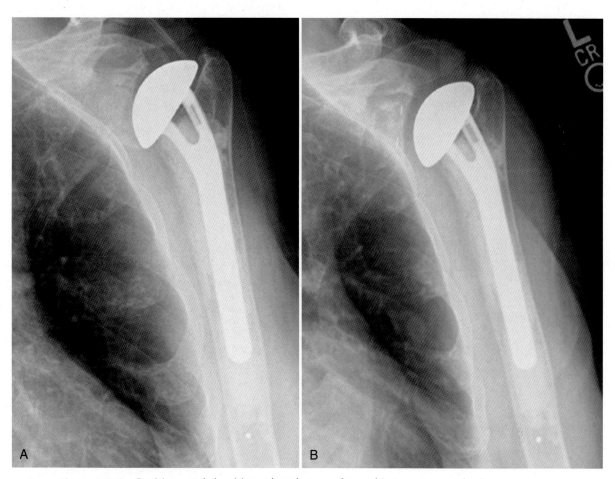

Figure 40-28 Revision total shoulder arthroplasty performed in two stages. The first stage consisted of glenoid reconstruction with a bone graft (**A**). The second stage involved implantation of a glenoid component 6 months after reconstruction of the osseous glenoid (**B**).

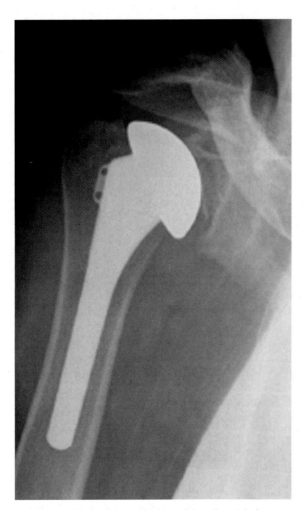

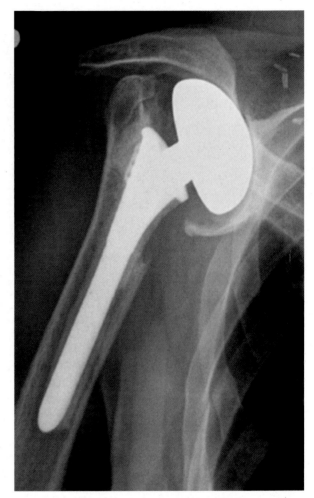

Figure 40-29   Biologic resurfacing of the glenoid after reconstruction of the osseous glenoid with a bone graft. It was performed as a single-stage procedure.

Figure 40-30   Failed hemiarthroplasty evaluated for conversion to a reverse prosthesis. The glenoid bone erosion necessitates osseous glenoid reconstruction with an iliac crest bone graft.

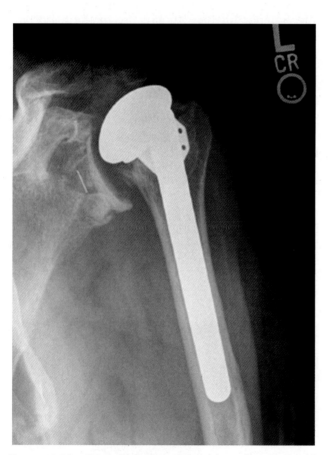

Figure 40-31 Case of failed total shoulder arthroplasty with rotator cuff insufficiency.

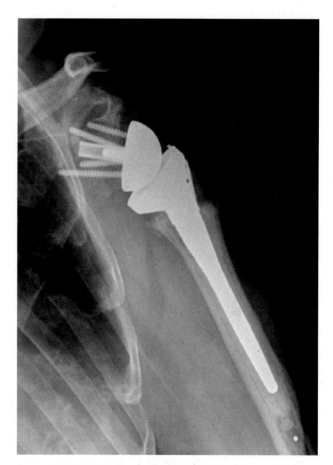

Figure 40-32 Case in which the majority of the central post of the reverse prosthesis base plate can be seated into native glenoid bone and allow single-stage revision.

seating of the central post of the base plate into native glenoid bone with the use of a reconstructive bone graft (Fig. 40-33).

After glenoid reconstruction with an autogenous iliac crest bone graft as described previously, preparation of the glenoid and insertion of the glenoid component are performed. As with primary reverse shoulder arthroplasty, we avoid using a Fukuda glenohumeral retractor during implantation of the reverse prosthesis because the base plate fixation screws may incarcerate

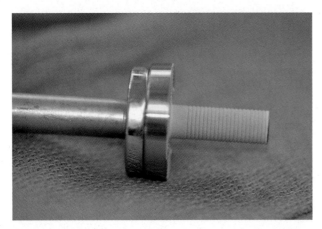

Figure 40-33 Revision base plate component with a longer central post to allow placement of the central post into native glenoid bone in the revision scenario.

the retractor. A hole is drilled with the inferior referencing guide provided (Fig. 40-34). In cases in which there is good fixation of the bone graft, reaming is performed by placing slight inferior pressure on the reamer to introduce approximately 10 degrees of inferior tilt to the surface of the glenoid, as in cases of primary reverse shoulder arthroplasty. To help avoid fracture, the reamer is always started before contacting the bone and then gradually and gently advanced to engage the bone and ream it to a flat surface. If the bone graft fixation is thought to be tenuous, a hand burr is used to flatten the glenoid surface and introduce inferior tilt (Fig. 40-35). Use of the hand burr avoids the chance that the glenoid reamer will catch the edge of the glenoid bone graft and disrupt it. Once reaming is complete, the cortical aperture of the glenoid hole is open to a slightly larger diameter (7.6 mm) to accommodate the central peg of the glenoid base plate (Fig. 40-36).

Insertion of the glenoid component of a reverse prosthesis proceeds as in cases of primary reverse shoulder arthroplasty. The glenoid base plate is oriented and introduced with the insertion handle (Fig. 40-37). A mallet is used to impact the base plate until it is flush with the glenoid bone circumferentially. The insertion handle is disengaged from the base plate and the base plate is checked to ensure that it has been completely seated with the tips of vascular forceps in each hole (Fig. 40-38). If any concern exists over

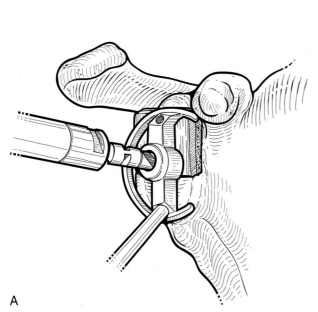

A

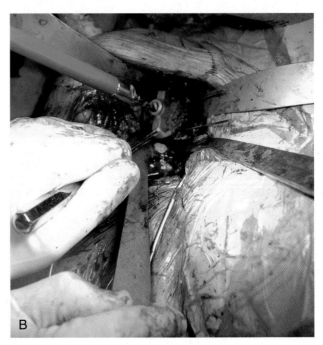

B

Figure 40-34 **A** and **B,** Creation of a central glenoid drill hole with the inferior referencing guide after glenoid reconstruction.

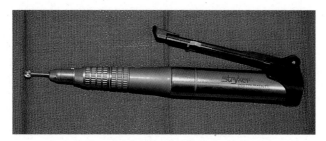

Figure 40-35 Hand burr used to prepare the glenoid surface if the bone graft fixation is thought to be tenuous.

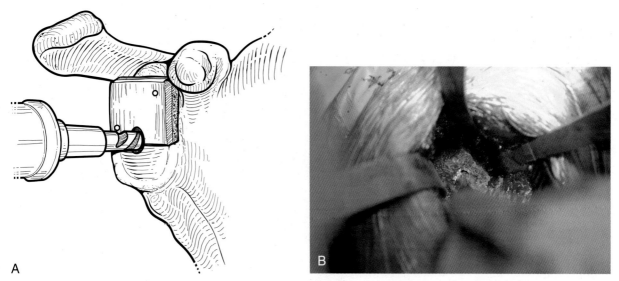

Figure 40-36 A and **B,** Opening of the central hole to accommodate the central post of the base plate.

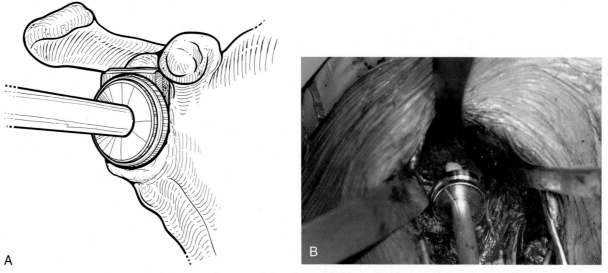

Figure 40-37 A and **B,** Introduction of the glenoid base plate into the reconstructed and prepared glenoid.

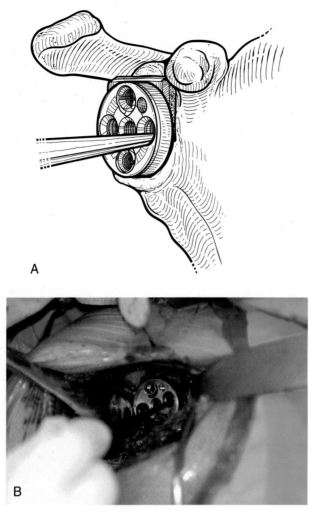

Figure 40-38   A and **B,** Checking to ensure complete seating of the base plate.

incomplete seating of the base plate, a smooth large tamp may be used to further impact the base plate. Additionally, the peripheral inferior rim of the base plate should be confirmed to be in contact with underlying glenoid. In some cases of glenoid reconstruction, small voids may remain in the surface of the glenoid beneath the base plate (Fig. 40-39). Such voids can be accepted if they are small, with no further treatment required.

The next step involves screw insertion to complete fixation of the base plate via the same technique used during primary reverse shoulder arthroplasty (see Chapter 29). The inferior screw is placed first to ensure maintenance of inferior tilt of the glenoid component. A drill guide is placed in the inferior hole of the base plate. A drill (3.0-mm bit) is used through the guide to create a bicortical hole (Fig. 40-40). The direction of the drill should be chosen to maximize screw length so that the strongest fixation possible is provided. This is usually done by directing the drill halfway between the perpendicular and the maximal inferior direction allowed by the mechanical constraints of the base plate. After the second cortex is penetrated with the drill, a depth gauge is used to determine screw length.

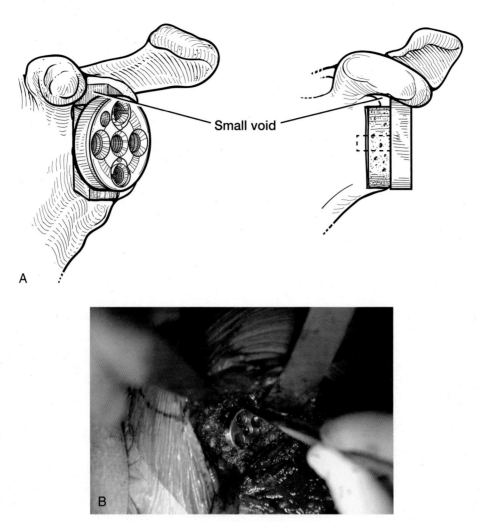

Figure 40-39 **A** and **B,** Small void under the base plate. It is not necessary to treat this small void.

A 4.5-mm screw is introduced and tightened until just before the threaded screw head engages the washer of the base plate. If the threaded head of the inferior screw engages the base plate washer, no further compression between the base plate and glenoid bone can be obtained. The drilling trajectory for the superior locking screw is directed toward the base of the coracoid process. The process of using the depth gauge is repeated for the superior locking screw. The superior screw is then inserted, once again making sure to not engage the base plate when the screw is advanced.

For the anterior and posterior screws, the drill is typically angled toward the central peg of the glenoid base plate and passes just superior or inferior to the central peg to perforate the opposite cortex (i.e., the anterior drill hole passes just superior to the central peg and perforates the posterior cortex deep within the glenoid vault, and the posterior drill hole passes just inferior to the central peg and perforates the anterior cortex deep within the glenoid vault). The depth gauge is used for selection of screw length, and the anterior and posterior screws are inserted and fully tightened to provide compression between the base plate and the glenoid bone. After the anterior and posterior screws are fully seated, the inferior and then superior screws are fully tightened so that they engage and complete fixation of the base plate (Fig. 40-41). Occasionally, the anterior or posterior screw will not obtain satisfactory osseous purchase because of underlying osteopenia. In

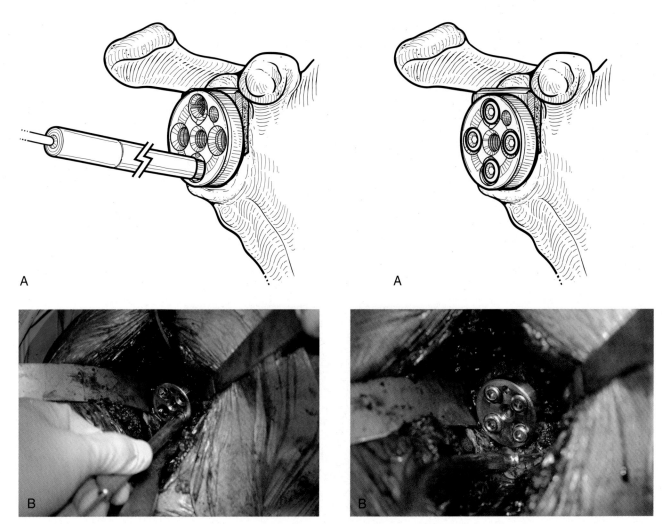

Figure 40-40   **A** and **B,** Drilling holes for the screws of the base plate.

Figure 40-41   **A** and **B,** Completed base plate fixation in the reconstructed glenoid.

this case the screw is left in place to provide interference-type resistance to loosening of the glenoid component.

The periphery and central hole of the base plate are cleared of soft tissue and blood, and the glenosphere component is positioned on the base plate with a screw driver used as an insertion device. The glenosphere attaches to the base plate via a peripheral rim Morse taper and is further secured with a central safety screw. The glenosphere is impacted into place with the impaction device, and the safety fixation screw is advanced to complete insertion of the glenoid component (Fig. 40-42).

After insertion of the glenoid component is complete, consideration can be given to performing a single-stage procedure. If the majority of the central post of the reverse prosthesis base plate (either standard- or long-post base plate) is implanted into native glenoid bone, the reverse prosthesis can be implanted as a single-stage procedure and attention directed toward insertion of the humeral component (Fig. 40-43). If the central post of the base plate is not well seated in native glenoid bone, a staged procedure should be performed. In this scenario, the humeral implant is not inserted. Six months after the first stage, the humeral component is implanted at the second stage (Fig. 40-44).

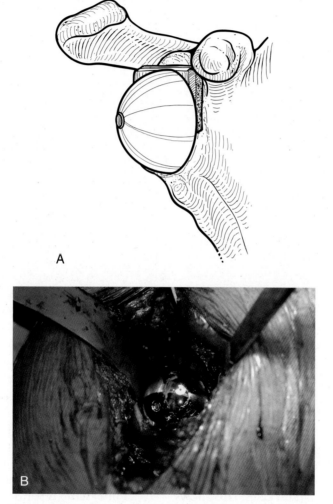

A

B

Figure 40-42 **A** and **B,** Completed glenoid component construct after insertion of the glenosphere.

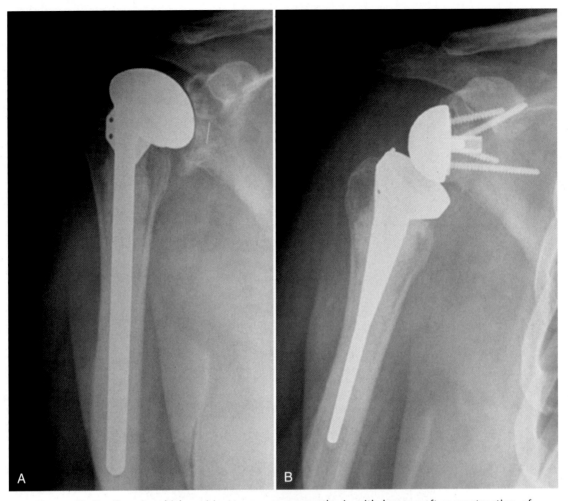

Figure 40-43 Case in which revision to a reverse prosthesis with bone graft reconstruction of the glenoid was performed as a single stage. **A,** Pre-revision. **B,** Post-revision.

TECHNIQUE FOR HARVEST OF AUTOGENOUS ILIAC CREST BONE GRAFT

In cases requiring reconstruction of the osseous glenoid, we use an autogenous anterior iliac crest tricortical bone graft. The iliac crest contralateral to the operative shoulder is selected in most cases. This allows easier surgical preparation and draping and, more importantly, permits more than one surgical team (if available) to work simultaneously. In our institution, one surgeon will frequently harvest the bone graft while the other surgeon performs the surgical approach on the operative shoulder. Exceptions occur when the patient has previously had an anterior bone graft harvested on the contralateral side (although this does not represent an absolute contraindication if harvesting took place longer than 1 year previously and radiographs show reconstitution of the anterior iliac crest bone stock) or when the patient specifically requests that we use bone from the iliac crest ipsilateral to the operative shoulder.

The operative shoulder is prepared as described in Chapter 4. The area of the entire contralateral iliac crest is prepared. The skin is initially cleaned with isopropyl alcohol, after which a povidone-iodine (Betadine) scrub is performed. The surgical area is then dried with towels and painted with a Betadine preparative solution (Fig. 40-45). In patients with allergy or hypersensitivity to Betadine, the scrub is performed with a 4% chlorhexidine gluconate solution (Betasept). The solution is removed with sterile water and an isopropyl alcohol preparation is applied. The area is draped with sterile towels secured to the skin with skin staples (Fig. 40-46). The contralateral shoulder is routinely draped as described in Chapter 4. The anterior iliac crest is palpated through the drapes and a hole is cut in the drapes with bandage scissors (Fig. 40-47). Any residual Betadine is dried at the surgical site. An

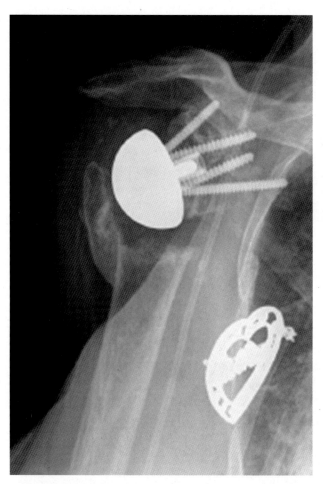

Figure 40-44 Intermediate stage of a two-stage revision to a reverse prosthesis.

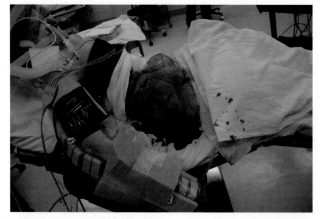

Figure 40-45 Skin preparation of the iliac crest bone graft harvest site.

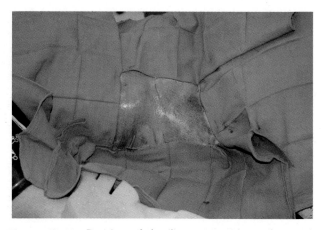

Figure 40-46 Draping of the iliac crest with sterile towels held with skin staples.

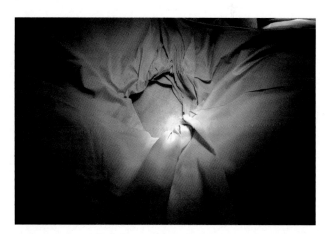

Figure 40-47 A hole is cut through the drapes over the iliac crest to allow exposure of the harvest site.

occlusive adhesive drape is applied to the surgical site. We prefer the occlusive drape to be impregnated with Betadine; however, in patients with Betadine allergy or hypersensitivity, we use a non–Betadine-impregnated version of the same drape. Completed draping of the iliac crest harvest site is shown in Figure 40-48.

An incision is made with a no. 10 scalpel blade centered over the iliac crest, starting 4 cm posterior to the palpated anterior superior iliac spine and extending 8 cm posteriorly along the iliac crest (Fig. 40-49). It is important not to extend the incision anteriorly to avoid injury to the lateral femoral cutaneous nerve. A needle tip electrocautery is used to dissect through the subcutaneous tissue down to the periosteum of the iliac crest (Fig. 40-50). Exposure is maintained with a self-retaining retractor. The periosteum of the iliac

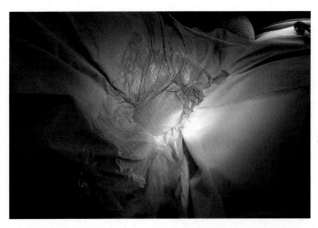

Figure 40-48 Completed skin preparation and draping of the iliac crest harvest site.

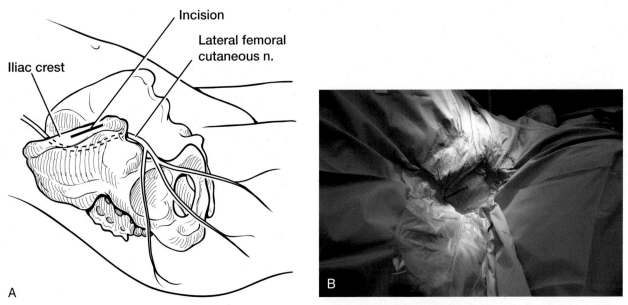

Incision

Lateral femoral cutaneous n.

Iliac crest

A

B

Figure 40-49 **A** and **B**, Skin incision for harvesting the anterior iliac crest.

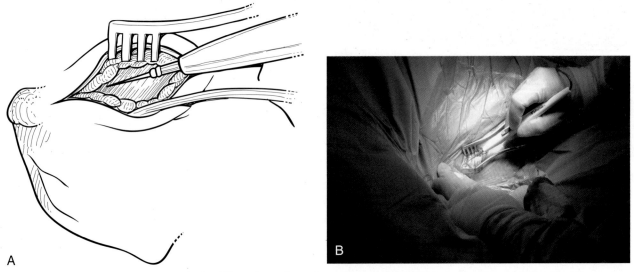

A

B

Figure 40-50 **A** and **B**, Dissection through subcutaneous tissue with the needle tip electrocautery.

Periosteum

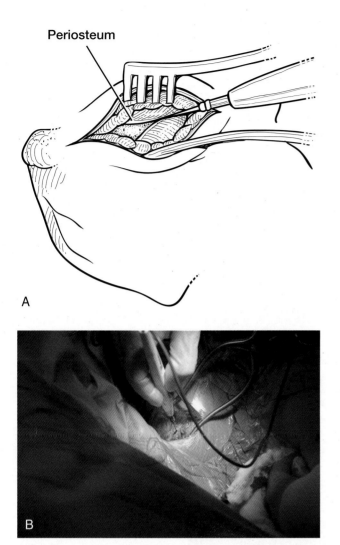

Figure 40-51 **A** and **B,** The periosteum of the iliac crest is divided with the electrocautery.

Outer table

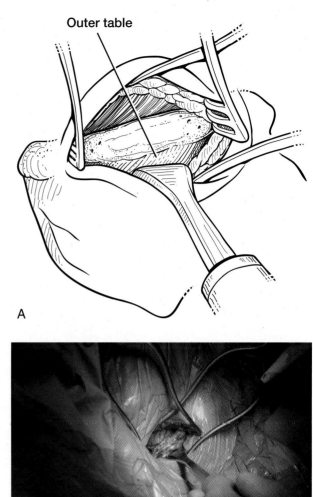

Figure 40-52 **A** and **B,** A Cobb elevator is used to expose the inner and outer tables of the iliac crest.

crest is divided along the longitudinal axis of the iliac crest with the electrocautery and progressively elevated (Fig. 40-51). A Cobb elevator is used to expose the inner and outer tables of the iliac crest (Fig. 40-52). Hohmann-type retractors are placed on each side of the iliac crest to maintain exposure (Fig. 40-53). A 1-inch straight osteotome is used to cut the iliac crest transversely in two places with a 3-cm-long intervening segment (Fig. 40-54). The osteotome is advanced to a depth of at least 2 cm in each location (Fig. 40-55). A 1-inch curved osteotome is used to connect the two vertical cuts in the iliac crest and free the tricortical bone graft (Fig. 40-56). The bone graft is held with a Lahey-type clamp before its final removal to avoid inadvertent contamination.

The tricortical bone graft is placed on the back table and the underlying cancellous bone graft removed

from the pelvis with curettes of various size and shape (Fig. 40-57). The bone graft site is irrigated with antibiotic-impregnated sterile saline (50,000 units bacitracin per liter sterile normal saline) via a bulb syringe. If the bone at the iliac crest harvest site continues to bleed, a medium closed suction drain is placed and maintained until the first postoperative day (Fig. 40-58). The periosteum is closed with no. 0 braided absorbable sutures in an interrupted technique. Subcutaneous tissue is closed with 2-0 braided absorbable sutures in an interrupted technique. The skin is closed with 3-0 monofilament absorbable sutures in a running subcuticular technique. Steri-Strips and a sterile dressing are applied (Fig. 40-59).

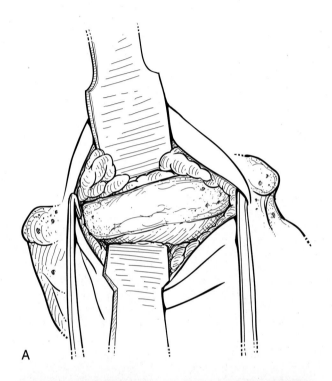

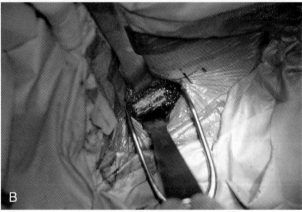

Figure 40-53 **A** and **B,** Hohmann-type retractors are used to maintain exposure of the iliac crest.

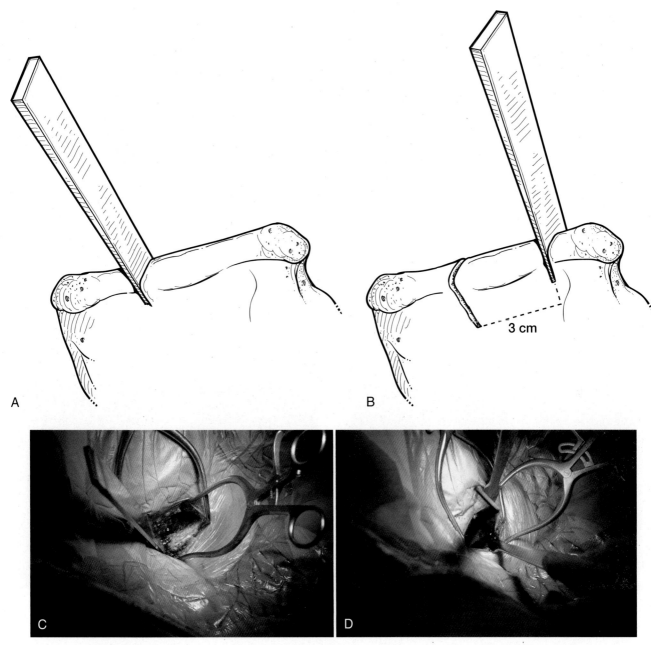

Figure 40-54 A to D, Vertical cuts are made in the iliac crest 3 cm apart with a 1-inch osteotome.

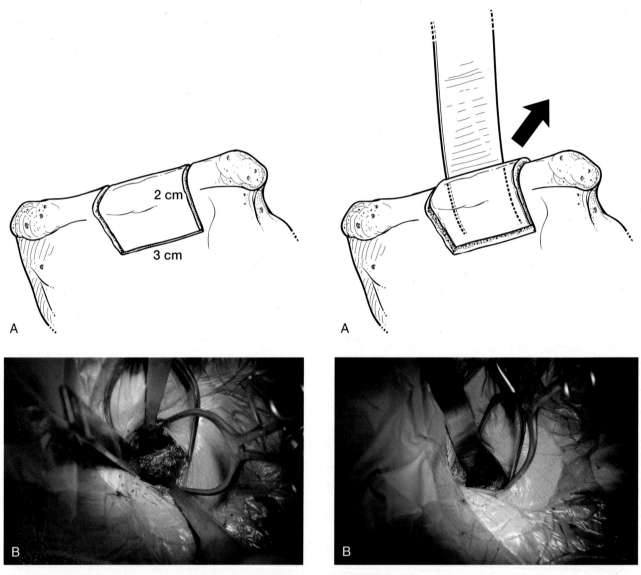

Figure 40-55 **A** and **B,** The vertical cuts continue until they are 2 cm in depth.

Figure 40-56 **A** and **B,** A 1-inch curved osteotome is used to connect the two vertical cuts in the iliac crest and free the tricortical bone graft.

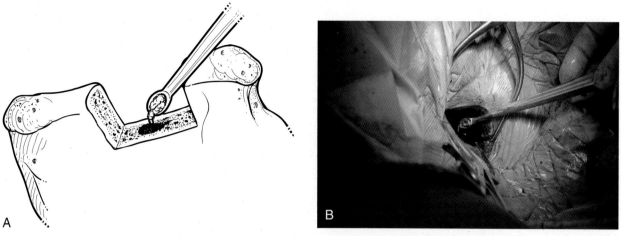

Figure 40-57 **A** and **B,** Removal of cancellous bone with a curette.

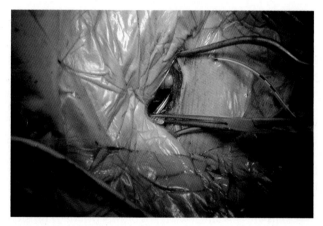

Figure 40-58 Placement of a medium closed suction drain in the iliac crest harvest site.

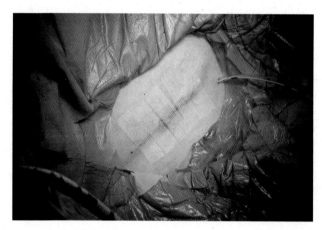

Figure 40-59 Final closure of the iliac crest harvest site.

REFERENCE

1. Neyton L, Walch G, Nové-Josserand L, Edwards TB: Glenoid corticocancellous bone grafting after glenoid component removal in the treatment of glenoid loosening. J Shoulder Elbow Surg 2006;15:173-179.

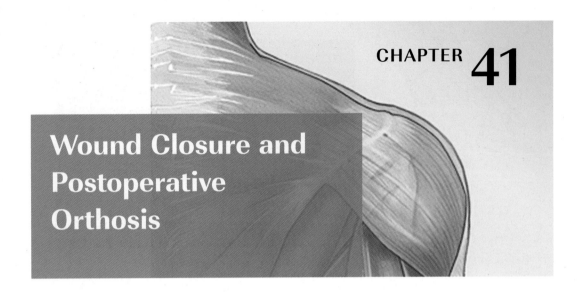

CHAPTER **41**

Wound Closure and Postoperative Orthosis

The final steps in revision arthroplasty are wound closure and placement of the postoperative orthosis. Wound closure after revision arthroplasty is performed similar to that for other arthroplasty cases. Revision shoulder arthroplasty often involves larger skin incisions, which can make wound closure an arduous task. The type of revision arthroplasty performed dictates the type of postoperative orthosis used and the duration of its use.

TECHNIQUE FOR WOUND CLOSURE

After reduction of the implant and closure of the subscapularis, if present, the wound is irrigated with 800 mL of antibiotic-impregnated sterile saline (50,000 units bacitracin per liter sterile normal saline) via a bulb syringe. The wound is checked to ensure that adequate hemostasis has been achieved. The electrocautery is used as necessary to minimize any residual hemorrhage. A medium-size closed suction drain is placed to help prevent postoperative hematoma formation in all cases in which a reverse prosthesis has been used, as described in Chapter 31.

Wound closure is initiated by reapproximation of the deep fascial layer with no. 0 braided absorbable suture in an interrupted figure-of-eight technique. As in cases of primary shoulder arthroplasty, we do not close the deltopectoral interval. The subcutaneous fascia is reapproximated with 2-0 braided absorbable suture in an interrupted figure-of-eight technique. The skin is reapproximated with skin staples (Fig. 41-1). We use skin staples in most revision cases because

closure with subcuticular suture can be difficult in the presence of dermal scarring from a previous incision. Additionally, the incision for revision shoulder arthroplasty can be large, especially if an extended approach is required. Use of skin staples facilitates closure of these large incisions (Fig. 41-2).

After skin closure is completed, the drain, if used, is checked to ensure that its position has been maintained. The occlusive draping is carefully removed from the site at which the drain tubing exits the skin. The skin in this area is cleaned and dried. Half-inch Steri-Strips are wrapped around the drain tubing to fix the drain to the skin and prevent inadvertent removal of the drain; we use two or three Steri-Strips (Fig. 41-3).

More of the occlusive draping is removed adjacent to the incision, and the skin is cleansed of blood with a saline-soaked sponge and then dried. Sterile gauze is placed over the incision, and a sterile absorbent pad is placed over the gauze. The dressing is secured with 3-inch foam tape. If applicable, the remainder of the surgical drain is connected to the drainage tube, and the suction function of the drain is activated. The remaining surgical drapes are then removed.

When used, the surgical drain is removed the day after surgery regardless of the amount of drainage recorded. The dressing is maintained in place until postoperative day 3, at which time it is removed. After removal of the dressing, the patient is allowed to shower, but submerging the incision in a bathtub is prohibited until 2 weeks postoperatively. The skin staples are removed 2 weeks postoperatively in the outpatient clinic (Fig. 41-4).

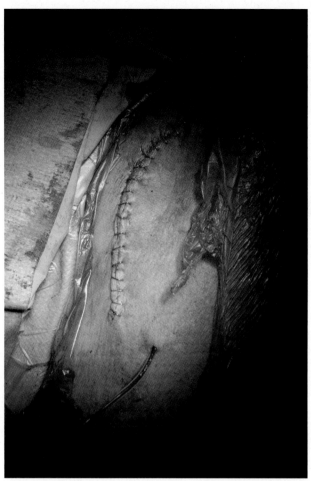

Figure 41-1   Skin closure with staples.

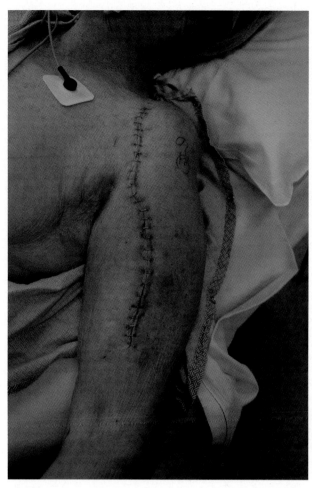

Figure 41-2   Extensile approach closed with skin staples.

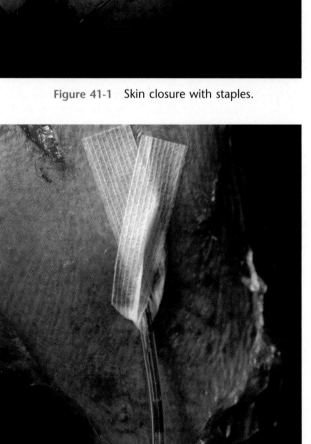

Figure 41-3   Steri-Strips hold the drain tube in place to prevent premature removal.

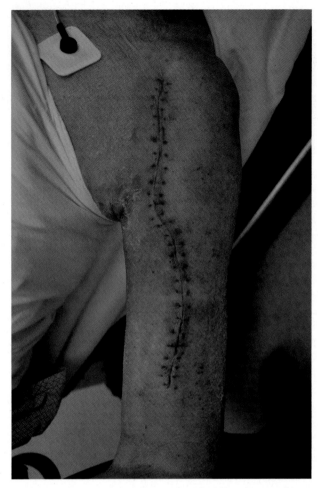

Figure 41-4   Incision after removal of the skin staples.

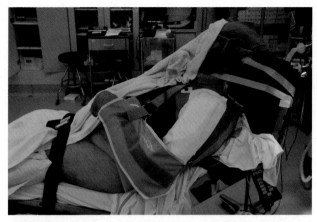

Figure 41-5   Neutral-rotation brace used after selected cases of revision shoulder arthroplasty.

POSTOPERATIVE ORTHOSIS

The postoperative orthosis is placed immediately after the dressing in the operating room. For unconstrained revision arthroplasty without a posterior capsulorrhaphy, we use a simple sling that the patient can discontinue as comfort allows within 2 to 4 weeks. For revision arthroplasty with a reverse prosthesis and unconstrained revision arthroplasty requiring an associated posterior capsulorrhaphy, we use a neutral-rotation sling (Ultrasling, Donjoy, Inc., Vista, CA; Fig. 41-5). The patient is allowed to remove the sling for performance of hand, wrist, and elbow mobility exercises and for hygiene.

For revision with a reverse prosthesis, the duration for which the orthosis is maintained is determined by the presence or absence of humeral metaphyseal bone loss. In uncomplicated cases with sufficient metaphyseal bone, the sling is discontinued and physical therapy initiated 3 weeks postoperatively. In cases of humeral metaphyseal bone loss, the sling is maintained for an additional week, and physical therapy is initiated 4 weeks postoperatively.

In unconstrained revision arthroplasty requiring an associated posterior capsulorrhaphy, the neutral-rotation sling is maintained for 4 weeks to protect the posterior capsulorrhaphy. Patients are allowed to remove the sling only for hygiene and rehabilitation exercises. Details of the postoperative rehabilitation regimen are provided in Chapter 43.

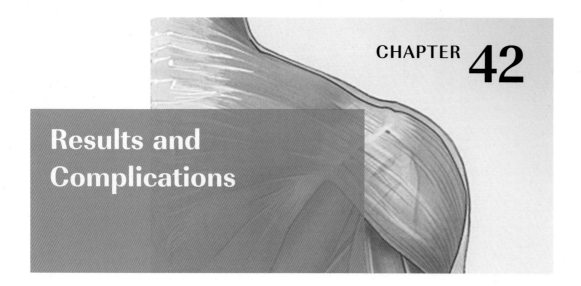

CHAPTER 42

Results and Complications

The results of revision shoulder arthroplasty are as variable as the indications for which it is performed. In general, outcomes after revision shoulder arthroplasty are less satisfactory than those after primary shoulder arthroplasty. Because of the paucity of results of revision shoulder arthroplasty reported in the literature, this chapter reports the results of revision shoulder arthroplasty by drawing from our own experience. Additionally, the most frequent complications and their treatment are outlined.

RESULTS

The results of revision shoulder arthroplasty are hard to examine because of the diversity of indications for which revision is performed. A simple indication such as converting a hemiarthroplasty to a total shoulder arthroplasty for symptomatic glenoid erosion would logically yield a better outcome than would implantation of a revision shoulder arthroplasty for a chronic infection after multiple irrigation and débridement sessions. Unfortunately, the relative rarity of revision shoulder arthroplasty prevents definitive conclusions regarding outcomes. Table 42-1 details the results of revision shoulder arthroplasty from our prospective database initiated in 2003. This table expresses the results in terms of active mobility; patient satisfaction; the Constant score, a shoulder-specific outcomes device incorporating pain, mobility, activity, and strength; and the age- and gender-adjusted Constant score.[1,2]

INTRAOPERATIVE COMPLICATIONS

Intraoperative complications are common during revision shoulder arthroplasty and may be divided into complications involving the humerus, glenoid, musculotendinous soft tissues (rotator cuff), and neurovascular structures.

Humerus

Intraoperative complications involving the humerus are common. The most frequent humeral complication is iatrogenic fracture, which usually occurs during an overly aggressive dislocation maneuver without previous adequate soft tissue release or during extraction of a well-fixed humeral stem. Patients with osteopenia and those with severe preoperative stiffness are most at risk for this complication. These fractures may occur at the humeral diaphysis or proximally and involve the tuberosities. Fractures involving the diaphysis should be reduced and a long-stem humeral implant placed. Allograft struts and cerclage cables may be added in patients with severe osteopenia (Fig. 42-1).

Intraoperative fractures involving the greater or lesser tuberosities (or both) usually occur during removal of the humeral stem. Many of these fractures can be successfully stabilized by suture fixation. If a tuberosity fracture is not satisfactorily stable despite suture fixation, use of a reverse prosthesis is considered as the revision implant.

Table 42-1 **RESULTS OF REVISION SHOULDER ARTHROPLASTY CLASSIFIED BY THE TYPE OF REVISION IMPLANT SELECTED IN THE AUTHORS' PROSPECTIVE DATABASE FROM 2003 TO 2006**

Type of Revision Prosthesis	Absolute Constant Score (Points)		Adjusted Constant Score (%)		Active Forward Flexion (Degrees)		Active External Rotation (Degrees)		Excellent/ Good Subjective Results (%)
	Preoperative	Postoperative	Preoperative	Postoperative	Preoperative	Postoperative	Preoperative	Postoperative	
Reverse prosthesis (*n* = 30)	10	52	13	68	19	133	8	7	80
Total shoulder arthroplasty (*n* = 8)	15	60	19	67	39	130	17	40	100
Hemiarthroplasty (*n* = 6)	26	56	31	62	78	128	12	32	66

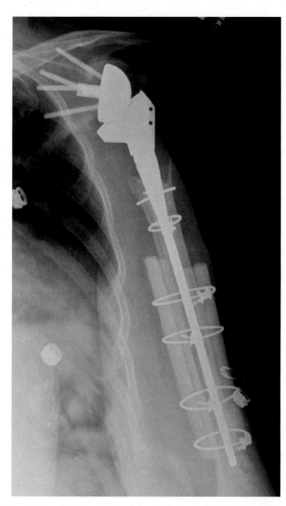

Figure 42-1 Radiograph of a patient with an intraoperative humeral shaft fracture incurred during revision arthroplasty that was treated with a long-stem humeral implant and allograft struts fixated with cerclage cables.

Glenoid

Intraoperative glenoid fractures at the time of revision shoulder arthroplasty occur during extraction of the glenoid component or during preparation (reaming) of the glenoid. Patients with osteopenia are most at risk. Fractures may involve only the peripheral glenoid rim or may extend significantly into the articular surface. Adequate capsular release helps minimize the risk for glenoid fracture. Additionally, a motorized reamer (not a drill) should be used for preparation of the glenoid surface. The reamer should be started before the surgeon applies force to engage the reamer onto the glenoid face. This avoids having the reamer "catch" an edge of the glenoid, which may cause a fracture.

When implanting an unconstrained glenoid component, fractures that involve only a small portion of the peripheral rim generally require no treatment and the glenoid component can be inserted as planned. Glenoid fractures that extend into the central portion of the glenoid (keel slot or peg holes) should be bone-grafted with autogenous iliac crest bone graft and placement of a glenoid component avoided. Placement of a glenoid component in the face of a fracture involving the central portion of the glenoid can result in early glenoid failure.

When implanting a reverse glenoid component, fractures that involve only a small portion of the peripheral rim generally require no treatment, and the glenoid component can be inserted as planned. Glenoid fractures that extend into the central portion of the glenoid should be bone-grafted with autogenous iliac crest bone graft. The reverse glenoid component can be placed to help secure the bone graft and internally fix the fracture. If the central post of the reverse component (a long-posted revision base plate can be used) is firmly seated within native glenoid bone, consideration can be given to placing the humeral component during the same surgical setting. If the glenoid component does not seem to be secure or the central post of the glenoid base plate is not firmly seated in unfractured native glenoid bone, insertion of the humeral component should be delayed for 6 months to allow the fracture to heal. After 6 months, a humeral component can be placed as the second part of a two-stage procedure. Alternatively, if an intraoperative glenoid fracture occurs, the fracture can be bone-grafted, and the humeral stem with a hemiarthroplasty adapter can be placed. After the fracture has healed and remodeled (around 6 months after the index attempt at reverse shoulder arthroplasty), the second stage of the procedure consisting of implantation of the glenoid component may be performed.

Rotator Cuff

Damage to the rotator cuff during revision shoulder arthroplasty usually occurs during the surgical approach and glenohumeral exposure. The anatomy is commonly distorted by the primary arthroplasty. Dissection should be slow and meticulous to avoid inadvertent damage to the rotator cuff. In the event that the rotator cuff is substantially compromised during the surgical procedure, consideration is given to implantation of a reverse prosthesis as the revision implant.

Neurovascular Structures

Catastrophic injury to the neurovascular structures around the shoulder is rare during revision shoulder arthroplasty. The neural structures most at risk during revision shoulder arthroplasty are the axillary and musculocutaneous nerves. If a humeral osteotomy is performed or if revision surgery is performed for a periprosthetic fracture, the radial nerve is also at risk. Nerve injury during revision shoulder arthroplasty can occur as a neuropraxic stretch injury or as a transection injury. Neuropraxic injury caused by stretch most commonly involves the axillary nerve but can involve any nerves within the brachial plexus. Care should be taken when positioning the patient to maintain the cervical spine in neutral alignment to avoid a stretch injury to the brachial plexus. When treating a periprosthetic fracture with revision arthroplasty or when a humeral osteotomy is anticipated for extraction of the humeral stem, the radial nerve should be carefully exposed to ensure its protection. Careful exposure of the radial nerve often results in transient neuropraxia. Patient education preoperatively is of paramount importance in dealing with neuropraxia inasmuch as patients are much more accepting if they have heard about the possibility of this complication before surgery. Axillary and radial nerve neuropraxia is treated by observation, with most patients recovering by 3 to 4 months postoperatively.

Neural transection injury is rare in revision shoulder arthroplasty. Careful identification of nerves at risk (axillary nerve and, in certain situations as outlined earlier, the radial nerve) is the best way to prevent this complication. If a transection injury does occur, the ends of the nerve are identified and consultation with a microvascular surgeon obtained.

Although tearing of the cephalic vein is common and largely without consequence, significant arterial and venous injuries do occur, though rarely, during revision reverse shoulder arthroplasty. The brachial artery is most at risk during revision surgery requiring an extensile exposure (periprosthetic fracture, humeral osteotomy). Should one of these injuries occur, after cross-clamping of the injured structure, emergency intraoperative consultation with a vascular surgeon is required.

POSTOPERATIVE COMPLICATIONS

Postoperative complications are more common after revision shoulder arthroplasty than after primary shoulder arthroplasty. The most frequent postoperative complications include wound problems (dehiscence, hematoma), glenoid problems, humeral problems, instability, rotator cuff problems, stiffness, infection, and when a reverse prosthesis is used as the revision implant, acromial problems and radiographic scapular notching.

Wound Problems

Wound problems occur early after revision shoulder arthroplasty. Hematoma is most easily avoided by extensive use of electrocautery during shoulder arthroplasty. When a reverse shoulder prosthesis is used for revision shoulder arthroplasty, closed suction drainage is maintained for 24 hours after surgery. When a hematoma occurs, it is managed by symptomatic nonoperative treatment (warm compresses, pain medication). Operative drainage is reserved for situations in which drainage persists beyond 1 week or infection is suspected (see later) but is rarely necessary.

In most revision cases, the skin is closed with stainless steel skin staples. Problems with skin staples are extremely infrequent. Rarely, susceptible patients have a reaction to dissolving subcutaneous sutures. The presence of minimal serous drainage distinguishes this complication from the more serious deep infection. Superficial wound dehiscence is treated by local wound care, including removal of any residual dissolving suture material and chemical cauterization of any granulating tissue with silver nitrate applicators.

Glenoid Problems

Glenoid complications after revision arthroplasty are related to the type of revision arthroplasty performed—hemiarthroplasty, unconstrained total shoulder arthroplasty, or reverse shoulder arthroplasty. As with primary hemiarthroplasty, erosion of the remaining glenoid articular cartilage and osseous glenoid can occur. Successful treatment of glenoid erosion usually requires further revision surgery during which the glenoid is resurfaced.

Glenoid component failure after revision to unconstrained total shoulder arthroplasty can occur as a result of loosening of the glenoid component from the host bone or mechanical breakage of the glenoid implant (Fig. 42-2). Glenoid component problems, when symptomatic, generally require further revision surgery.

Glenoid component failure after revision to reverse shoulder arthroplasty, as with primary reverse shoulder arthroplasty, has been associated in all cases of which we are aware with initial placement of the glenoid component in a superiorly oriented direction, implantation of the prosthesis in the presence of an intraoperative glenoid fracture, or insertion of the glenoid component with the central post anchored only in grafted bone. These complications are best avoided. As with primary reverse shoulder arthroplasty, we implant the reverse prosthesis for revision arthroplasty through a deltopectoral approach to avoid inadvertent placement of the glenoid component in a

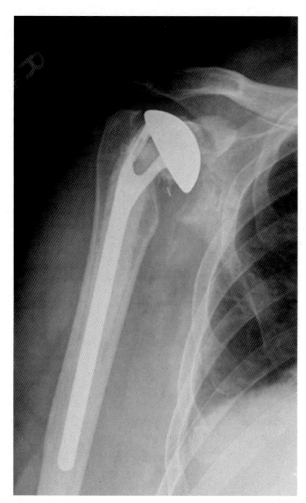

Figure 42-2 Unconstrained glenoid component loosening occurring 3 years after revision shoulder arthroplasty.

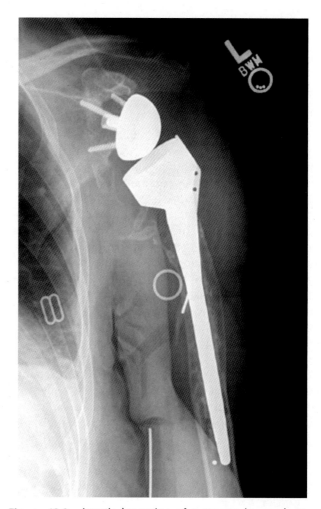

Figure 42-3 Aseptic loosening of a reverse humeral stem resulting from a fall.

superiorly oriented position, which can occur with use of the superior lateral approach. If an intraoperative glenoid fracture occurs, we treat it as described previously in this chapter. When glenoid failure occurs, further revision surgery consisting of glenoid reconstruction and conversion to a hemiarthroplasty is required.

Humeral Problems

Humeral problems after revision shoulder arthroplasty are rare and can be divided into loosening of the humeral component and periprosthetic humeral fracture. Most unconstrained humeral stems that we use for revision arthroplasty are cemented. Aseptic loosening of these stems is rare. Whenever loosening of a humeral stem occurs, infection must be ruled out (see later). In the rare instance of symptomatic aseptic loosening of an unconstrained humeral component,

treatment is further revision of the humeral stem.

Loosening of a reverse humeral stem after revision surgery is uncommon. The predominant risk factor for aseptic loosening of a revision reverse humeral stem is proximal humeral bone loss (Fig. 42-3). Whenever loosening of a revision reverse humeral stem occurs, infection must be ruled out, as with loosening of an unconstrained revision humeral stem (see later). In the rare instance of symptomatic aseptic loosening of a revision reverse humeral component, treatment is further revision of the humeral stem, usually combined with allograft reconstruction of the proximal humerus to provide osseous support of the proximal portion of the revision stem.

Mechanical problems of a revision reverse humeral component are exceedingly rare and related to the polyethylene liner. Incomplete seating of the polyethylene component at the revision arthroplasty can be responsible for dissociation of the polyethylene liner from the humeral stem. In this scenario, further revision surgery with replacement of the polyethylene liner is indicated. Polyethylene wear occurs medially on the rim of the polyethylene liner in many patients, as seen at the time of retrieval during revision surgery. It occurs as a result of scapular notching, as discussed later.

Periprosthetic humeral fractures after revision arthroplasty are more common than loosening of the humeral component and are almost always the result of a fall or similar low-energy trauma. The majority of these fractures occur just distal to the tip of the humeral stem, and most can be treated nonoperatively. Nonoperative treatment consists of fracture bracing, activity modification, pain medication, and frequent radiographic monitoring. If the fracture has not healed within 3 months, we will incorporate the use of an external bone stimulator (OL 1000 Bone Growth Stimulator, Donjoy Orthopedics, Vista, CA). Despite these measures, periprosthetic humeral fractures treated nonoperatively may take longer than 9 months to heal.[3] Our criteria for recommending operative treatment of periprosthetic fractures include complete displacement, angulation greater than 30 degrees, loosening of the humeral component, or failure of nonoperative treatment.

Instability

Instability after Unconstrained Revision Shoulder Arthroplasty

Instability after unconstrained revision shoulder arthroplasty is usually related to one or more of three factors, including the prosthesis (alignment, size), the capsule, and the rotator cuff. Cases in which prosthetic problems have led to dynamic or static shoulder instability require correction to resolve the instability. Prosthetic problems may be related to the humeral side (excessive retroversion, causing posterior instability; excessive anteversion, causing anterior instability; too small a prosthetic head, causing global instability) or the glenoid side (failure to correct posterior glenoid wear, causing posterior instability). Further revision arthroplasty is the treatment of instability related to a prosthetic problem.

Capsular problems resulting in instability occur very infrequently after unconstrained revision shoulder arthroplasty. In this rare situation, soft tissue procedures do not reliably restore stability to the glenohumeral joint, and we perform further revision surgery with a reverse prosthesis.

Rotator cuff problems can cause static and dynamic instability after unconstrained revision shoulder arthroplasty. Unconstrained revision arthroplasty in patients with a compromised rotator cuff often results in static instability. These patients should undergo further revision with a reverse-design prosthesis to resolve the complication. Rarely, in a patient with a previously intact rotator cuff who has undergone unconstrained revision shoulder arthroplasty, a massive rotator cuff tear will develop and contribute to static instability. These patients, when symptomatic, are best treated by further revision surgery with a reverse-design prosthesis.

Dynamic instability after unconstrained revision shoulder arthroplasty most commonly occurs as anterior instability resulting from failure of the subscapularis repair. It occurs more commonly after revision arthroplasty because the subscapularis has been violated on multiple occasions. In the revision scenario, if the patient is symptomatic, we opt for revision to a reverse-design prosthesis and do not attempt isolated repair of the compromised subscapularis.

Instability after Revision Surgery with a Reverse Shoulder Prosthesis

Instability after revision surgery with a reverse shoulder prosthesis is twice as common as that observed in the primary reverse arthroplasty scenario. Dislocations after revision arthroplasty with a reverse prosthesis occur early (within 6 weeks of revision surgery). Instability of a reverse prosthesis can be related to various factors. In revision cases, proximal humeral bone loss seems to be the greatest risk factor for dislocation of a reverse prosthesis. In this scenario, deltoid muscle tension is often solely responsible for the stability of the implant because no rotator cuff or joint capsule exists to provide stability. Even if the deltoid is properly tensioned initially, it can gradually lose its tension and result in dislocation. A second major risk factor for dislocation of a reverse prosthesis is subscapularis insufficiency, a common condition encountered when performing revision shoulder arthroplasty with a reverse prosthesis. A less common factor contributing to dislocation of a reverse prosthesis is mechanical impingement causing the prosthetic socket to be levered away from the glenoid component. This impingement usually occurs inferiorly as the arm is adducted and is often related to too superior positioning of the glenoid component on the glenoid face, as detailed schematically in Chapter 32. Finally, in the revision situation, the integrity and function of the axillary nerve should be ensured before performing revision arthroplasty with a reverse prosthesis because this neural deficit can result in prosthetic dislocation.

In most cases, as with dislocation of a primary reverse prosthesis, treatment initially consists of closed

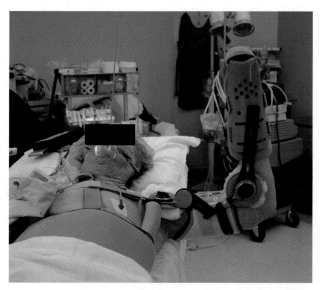

Figure 42-4 Placement of a brace used for the treatment of a dislocated revision reverse prosthesis after closed reduction.

reduction and a period of bracing. Closed reduction is performed in the operating room with the patient either heavily sedated or under general anesthesia. An attempt is made to reduce the dislocation under fluoroscopic guidance. If the prosthesis is successfully reduced, fluoroscopic examination is performed to ensure that mechanical impingement is not responsible for the instability. If the problem is not related to mechanical impingement and the prosthesis is successfully reduced, a brace is applied to maintain the arm with the humeral component centered on the glenoid component, usually in about 90 degrees of abduction and 30 degrees of forward flexion (Fig. 42-4). The patient maintains this brace at all times for 6 weeks, and radiographs are taken in the brace every 7 to 10 days to confirm that the prosthesis has remained located (Fig. 42-5). After 6 weeks the brace is discontinued and a normal rehabilitation regimen ensues.

If the prosthesis is not reducible by closed means, mechanical impingement causing dislocation exists,

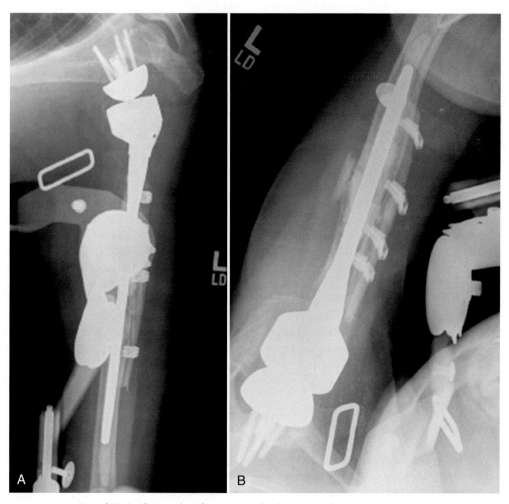

Figure 42-5 **A** and **B,** Radiographs obtained in the brace confirming maintenance of prosthetic reduction.

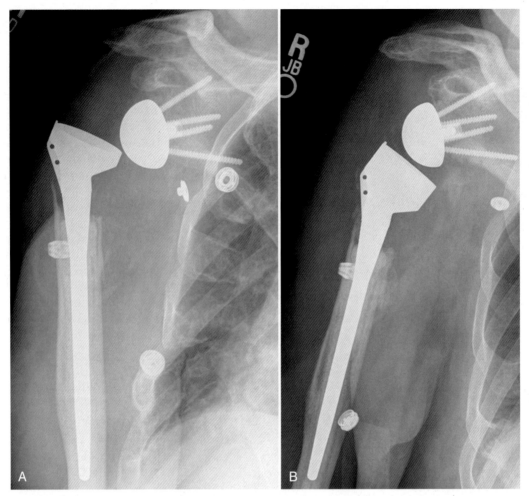

Figure 42-6   Treatment of a dislocated revision reverse prosthesis (**A**) with the addition of an augment to increase deltoid tension (**B**).

or closed reduction plus bracing has failed, open reduction with insertion of a thicker polyethylene spacer or metallic augment (or both) is performed (Fig. 42-6). Any mechanical impingement can simultaneously be addressed by careful removal of bone at the lateral aspect of the scapula just inferior to the glenoid component, if necessary. Postoperatively, the patient is treated with the same bracing protocol used after closed reduction of a dislocated reverse prosthesis.

Rotator Cuff Problems

Symptomatic problems of the rotator cuff after unconstrained revision shoulder arthroplasty often result in instability and were described earlier. Failure of the subscapularis repair is the most common postoperative rotator cuff problem that we observe. When subscapularis failure is minimally symptomatic or asymptomatic, no treatment is indicated. When symp-

tomatic, treatment is indicated as described previously in the "Instability" section of this chapter.

Isolated internal rotation weakness is not diagnostic of subscapularis failure after unconstrained revision shoulder arthroplasty. It is common for individuals to lose internal rotation strength after tenotomy and repair of the subscapularis during primary shoulder arthroplasty, and this finding becomes more pronounced after revision surgery. Subscapularis failure should be documented by computed tomographic arthrography before considering operative treatment of this complication.

Stiffness

Glenohumeral stiffness after revision shoulder arthroplasty is related to capsular contracture or the prosthesis, or both. It is much more commonly observed when using an unconstrained revision implant than when using a reverse revision implant. Prosthetic

Infection

Infection after revision shoulder arthroplasty is expectedly more common than infection after primary shoulder arthroplasty. Patients most at risk for infection are those with systemic illness (diabetes mellitus), those with compromised soft tissues (radiation-induced osteonecrosis, post-traumatic arthritis), and those with inflammatory arthropathy (rheumatoid arthritis). These infections are most commonly caused by *Staphylococcus aureus* or *Propionibacterium acnes*. Infections after revision shoulder arthroplasty can be divided into perioperative (within 6 weeks of surgery) and late (hematogenous) infections.

Early perioperative infections are initially treated with two or three irrigation and débridement procedures and retention of the components. At the last planned irrigation and débridement procedure, absorbable antibiotic-impregnated beads are placed in the soft tissues around the shoulder (Stimulan, Biocomposites, Inc., Staffordshire, England). Consultation with an infectious disease specialist is obtained, and a minimum of 6 weeks of intravenous antibiotics tailored to the specific organism causing the infection (or covering the most likely offending organisms, if cultures remain negative despite obvious infection) is usually recommended. If this regimen fails, the prosthesis is removed.

Late-appearing infections are treated by removal of the prosthesis and intravenous antibiotics. The decision whether to perform a repeat revision shoulder arthroplasty or continue with a resection arthroplasty is patient specific, with resection arthroplasty selected in most cases.

Acromial Problems

Occasionally, acromial stress fractures are seen after revision reverse shoulder arthroplasty, just as with primary reverse shoulder arthroplasty. These fractures result from deltoid tension applied to osteopenic bone. Frequently, these fractures exist preoperatively as a result of chronic superior migration of the humeral head with persistent acromiohumeral articulation (Fig. 42-8). Postoperatively, deltoid tension may cause the fracture fragment to tilt inferiorly. Despite these radiographic findings, no specific treatment is necessary for this complication. Additionally, patients obtain satisfactory results even with this radiographic finding.

Scapular Notching

Though debatable whether it should be considered a complication, notching of the scapula occurs within

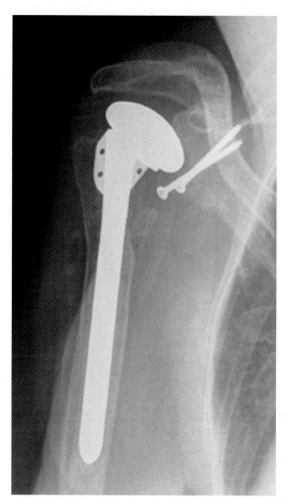

Figure 42-7 Malpositioned revision humeral stem contributing to glenohumeral stiffness.

problems resulting in stiffness are generally the result of implantation of too large an unconstrained humeral component or malpositioning of the revision component (Fig. 42-7). Rehabilitation with capsular stretching can be attempted in an effort to improve mobility. If this fails (no improvement over a 6-month period), revision surgery is indicated and consists of downsizing of the humeral head with open release of any capsular contractures that are present.

Stiffness related to capsular contracture almost always responds to nonoperative management involving aquatic-based rehabilitation (see Chapter 43). If the patient shows no improvement in mobility over a 6-month course of rehabilitation and has no obvious prosthetic problem, we will consider the patient a candidate for arthroscopic capsular contracture release if an unconstrained revision implant was used. We have no experience dealing with capsular contracture in a patient who has undergone revision shoulder arthroplasty with a reverse prosthesis.

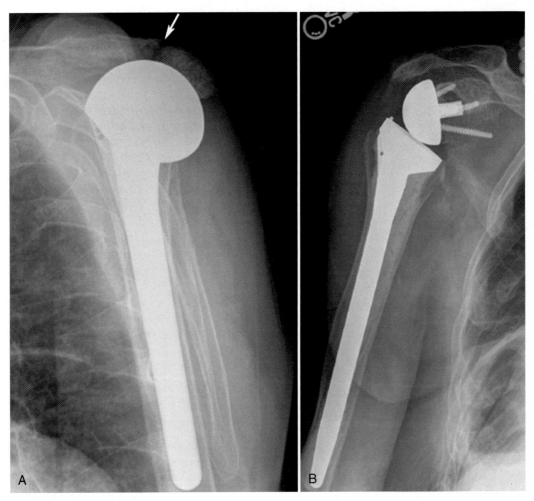

Figure 42-8 **A**, Acromial stress fracture (*arrow*) occurring after hemiarthroplasty for rotator cuff tear arthropathy. **B**, This patient underwent revision to a reverse prosthesis, with the stress fracture requiring no additional treatment.

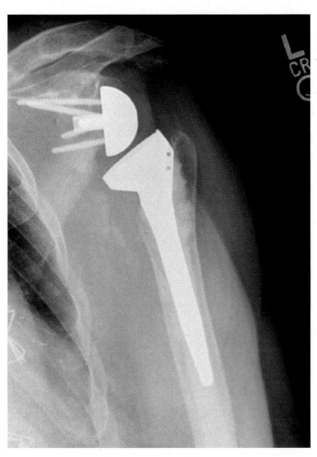

Figure 42-9 Scapular notching occurring after revision arthroplasty with a reverse prosthesis.

2 years of surgery in half the patients who have undergone reverse shoulder arthroplasty, both in the primary and in the revision situation (Fig. 42-9). This radiographic finding most likely occurs as a result of mechanical impingement of the medial aspect of the humeral component and the lateral aspect of the scapula just inferior to the glenoid. As the patient internally rotates the shoulder, the impingement is exacerbated. This mechanical impingement theory is further supported by the observation that patients' internal rotation seems to improve as the scapular notch progresses, thus suggesting that the prosthesis must "carve out" a portion of the scapula to maximize postoperative internal rotation. Another theory of the cause of scapular notching is polyethylene wear causing osteolysis, although this theory currently has less support than the mechanical impingement theory.

Scapular notching is commonly accompanied by a scapular osteophyte just medial to the notch. The degree of scapular notching has also been graded by severity.[4] The best way to avoid scapular notching seems to be by initially placing the glenoid component inferiorly on the glenoid face and by introducing slight inferior tilt during glenoid reaming, as discussed in Chapter 29. Despite the concerning appearance of this scapular notch, its clinical implications are unclear, with most of the evidence suggesting no adverse consequence. As long as the glenoid component remains stable, no treatment of an asymptomatic scapular notch is indicated.

REFERENCES

1. Constant CR, Murley AH: A clinical method of functional assessment of the shoulder. Clin Orthop Relat Res 1987;214:160-164.
2. Constant CR: Assessment of shoulder function. In Gazielly D, Gleyze P, Thomas T (eds): The Cuff. New York, Elsevier, 1997, pp 39-44.
3. Kumar S, Sperling JW, Haidukewych GH, Cofield RH: Periprosthetic humeral fractures after shoulder arthroplasty. J Bone Joint Surg Am 2004;86:680-689.
4. Valenti P, Boutens D, Nerot C: Delta 3 reversed prosthesis for osteoarthritis with massive rotator cuff tear: Long term results (>5 years). In Walch G, Boileau P, Molé D (eds): 2000 Prosthèses d'Epaule . . . Recul de 2 à 10 Ans. Paris, Sauramps Medical, 2001, pp 253-259.

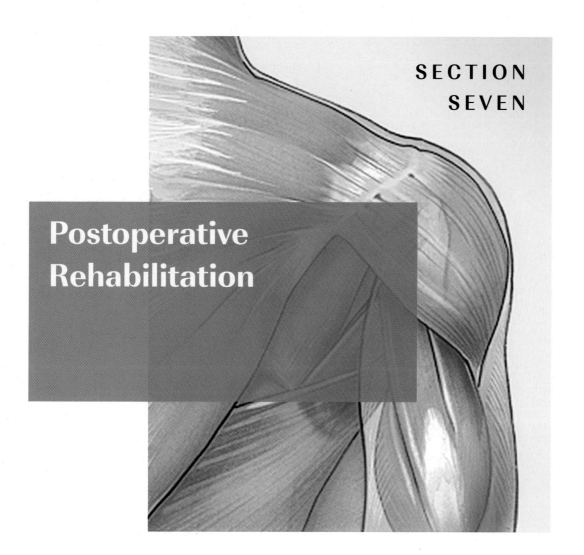

SECTION SEVEN

Postoperative Rehabilitation

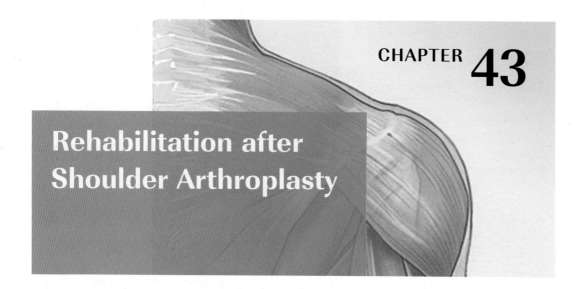

CHAPTER 43

Rehabilitation after Shoulder Arthroplasty

The goal of rehabilitation after shoulder arthroplasty is restoration of functional shoulder mobility in timely fashion. Biologic factors impose limitations in achieving mobility after shoulder arthroplasty. Histologically, collagenous connective tissues in the shoulder (tendons, ligaments, capsule) contract after shoulder arthroplasty. These connective tissues are subject to the biomechanical properties and limitations of collagen, including plasticity, stretching, and temperature sensitivity. The plasticity of collagen allows connective tissues to adapt to physiologic and pathologic conditions. Rehabilitation is designed to maximize these adaptations and provide functional recovery of mobility after shoulder arthroplasty. We use a hydrotherapy-based rehabilitation regimen after shoulder arthroplasty to regain shoulder mobility.[1]

PRINCIPLES OF HYDROTHERAPY

Rehabilitation in a warm-water pool facilitates gain of mobility after shoulder arthroplasty. Rehabilitation with the shoulder submerged or partially submerged in warm water provides a "weightless" environment. This "weightlessness" allows the arm to find the best path to achieve a specific movement. Additionally, a warm-water environment provides comfort and improves proprioception while minimizing pain. Whereas thermal neutrality is obtained with water heated to 34°C, a water temperature of 35°C increases skin comfort while increasing body temperature less than 1°C, thus minimizing the risk of development of a heat-induced inflammatory response.

REHABILITATION PROTOCOL

Rehabilitation starts with choosing the type of postoperative orthosis and its duration of use. This is based largely on the type of arthroplasty performed (unconstrained, fracture, reverse) and the performance of any associated procedures (posterior capsulorrhaphy). Table 43-1 summarizes the types of orthoses used and the duration of their use based on the procedure performed. All patients are instructed in hand, wrist, and elbow mobility exercises on postoperative day 1. Patients undergoing unconstrained shoulder arthroplasty for chronic conditions without performance of an associated posterior capsulorrhaphy are also instructed in pendulum exercises on postoperative day 1. These exercises are performed three to five times per day for approximately 15 minutes each time and are continued throughout the rehabilitative program. The time of initiation of hydrotherapy depends on the type of arthroplasty performed. Table 43-2 summarizes the time that hydrotherapy is instituted based on the procedure performed.

Hydrotherapy is performed in a warm (35°C) rehabilitation pool that is approximately 1.3 m in depth at its deepest point. The pool is fitted with supports that can accommodate the straps and harnesses used in the rehabilitation process. The surgical wound is covered with a waterproof, air-permeable hypoallergenic adhesive dressing. Patients are equipped with a mask and snorkel for use during hydrotherapy.

Hydrotherapy takes place daily (5 to 7 days per week, depending on availability) in a single 30- to 45-minute session. An abbreviated land-based verification

Table 43-1 TYPE OF POSTOPERATIVE ORTHOSIS USED AND DURATION OF USE

Procedure	Type	Duration (wk)
Unconstrained arthroplasty	Simple sling	2 to 4
Unconstrained arthroplasty + posterior capsulorrhaphy	Neutral rotation sling	4
Fracture prosthesis	Neutral rotation sling	4 to 6
Reverse prosthesis	Neutral rotation sling	3 to 4

Table 43-2 TIME FOR INITIATION OF HYDROTHERAPY

Procedure	Hydrotherapy Initiated (Postoperative Week)
Unconstrained arthroplasty	1
Unconstrained arthroplasty + posterior capsulorrhaphy	1
Fracture prosthesis	4 to 6
Reverse prosthesis	3 to 4

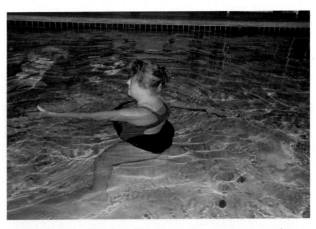

Figure 43-1   Shoulder flexion and extension exercises.

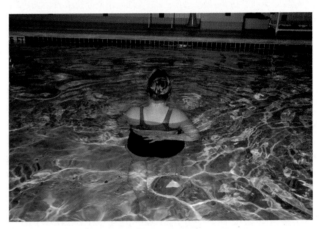

Figure 43-2   Internal rotation exercises.

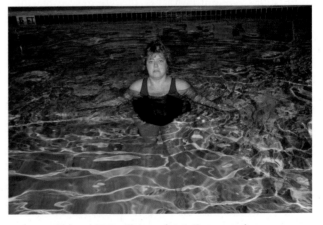

Figure 43-3   External rotation exercises.

session follows to affirm gains in mobility achieved in the pool. Various exercises designed to gain elevation, extension, horizontal adduction, internal rotation, and external rotation are performed in sets of 10 repetitions (Figs. 43-1 through 43-4). The unaffected extremity is used to help power the movement. Active mobility of the operated extremity is allowed in the form of a slow, gentle breaststroke motion with the palms placed horizontally (to not invoke resistance from the water), which is performed with the patient supported by a harness and the shoulders submerged (Fig. 43-5). In patients who have undergone unconstrained shoulder arthroplasty, external rotation beyond neutral is not allowed until 4 weeks postoperatively in patients with primary osteoarthritis or osteonecrosis and 6 weeks in patients with compromised

soft tissues (inflammatory arthropathies, revision surgery) to protect the subscapularis repair. In patients who have undergone an associated posterior capsulorrhaphy, internal rotation and horizontal adduction are avoided until 4 weeks postoperatively. With the exception of these cases, no limitations on mobility are imposed.

Mobility exercises with total body immersion are advised for all patients; however, it is not forced on anyone. Patients who wish to try such exercises are

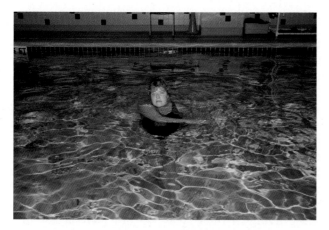

Figure 43-4   Horizontal adduction exercises.

fitted with a weighted belt and instructed to hold their breath as they kneel or recline supine on the bottom of the pool (Fig. 43-6). The same mobility exercises are then performed in the more insulated underwater environment. This technique is very helpful in accelerating gains in mobility.

As soon as the patient has achieved 140 degrees of elevation, the hands can be clasped behind the head in the "siesta" position (Fig. 43-7). Additional stretching exercises for the anterior capsule (Fig. 43-8) and posterior capsule (Fig. 43-9) can be performed in this position. From this position, motion is advanced until the "triple-locking" position is achieved, which stretches the inferior capsule (Fig. 43-10). Both the siesta and triple-locking positions are used extensively in a self-rehabilitation program implemented after the patient has been discharged from formal physical therapy.

An abbreviated session of land-based rehabilitation is used after the hydrotherapy session. The land-based session is performed principally to affirm the gains

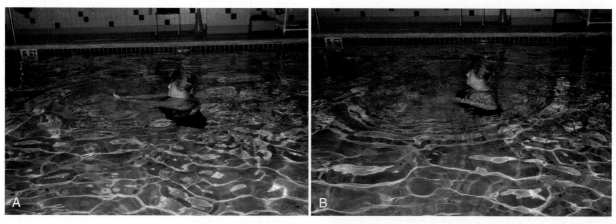

Figure 43-5   **A** and **B,** Breaststroke exercise.

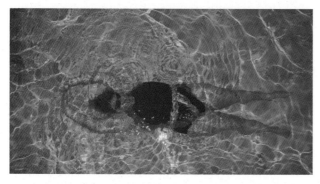

Figure 43-6   Total body immersion exercises.

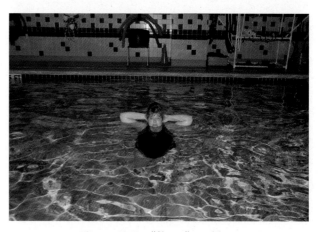

Figure 43-7   "Siesta" position.

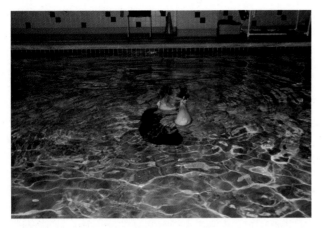

Figure 43-8 Anterior capsule stretching from the siesta position.

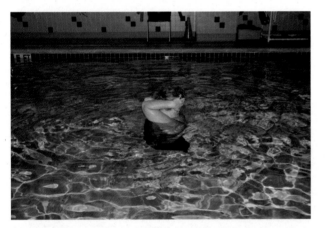

Figure 43-9 Posterior capsule stretching from the siesta position.

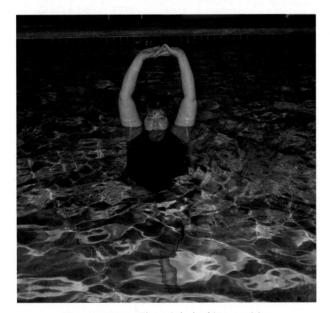

Figure 43-10 The triple-locking position.

that the patient has made during the hydrotherapy sessions. The same exercises are used, but with fewer repetitions. Modality treatment (i.e., cryotherapy) is used on an as-needed basis. Analgesic pain medication is provided to patients for the first 6 postoperative weeks to alleviate the discomfort associated with surgery and subsequent rehabilitation.

All patients participate in at least 5 weeks of hydrotherapy, after which they are re-evaluated. If acceptable active mobility has been achieved, hydrotherapy is discontinued and the patient is graduated to a land-based self-rehabilitation regimen incorporating the siesta and triple-locking stretches performed several times per day indefinitely. If it is determined that the patient would benefit from continued hydrotherapy, 6 additional weeks of hydrotherapy is prescribed. Most patients are able to discontinue hydrotherapy and graduate to the self-rehabilitation program by 3 months postoperatively. Some patients, particularly those living in rural areas, do not have access to a physical therapist with a rehabilitation pool. In these circumstances, patients learn the program from an experienced therapist in a more urban location and perform the program in any public or private pool that they may have available on their own. Additionally, any patients who prove adept at performing the exercises in the hydrotherapy program are allowed to complete the program independently with periodic monitoring by a physical therapist.

Rarely, we encounter a patient with a true fear of water. Although an inability to swim is not a contraindication to hydrotherapy rehabilitation, anxiety or fearfulness at the prospect of aquatic-based rehabilitation is a contraindication. In these patients, we prescribe a land-based program incorporating the same exercises that are used in the rehabilitation pool. In general, the land-based program is effective in obtaining an end result similar to that achieved with hydrotherapy, but it usually takes longer to achieve this result and patients tend to have more pain during rehabilitation.

RETURN TO ACTIVITY

With this protocol, patients can be expected to resume activities of daily living on a normal basis before 3 months postoperatively. No specific strengthening exercises are performed in this protocol. Gradual resumption of normal activities is all that is required to regain strength, and it presents minimal risk to the patient.

We allow our patients to pursue most activities and sports after shoulder arthroplasty. We do limit patients to noncontact sports. The majority of our arthroplasty patients with athletic interests participate in golf and tennis. Restrictions placed on golfers and tennis players are designed to protect the subscapularis repair. Putting is allowed as soon as the patient can tolerate it postoperatively, usually within 6 weeks. At 3 months, half swings with a seven iron off a tee are allowed. This is advanced until the patient is allowed to hit a full swing with all clubs off a tee 4 to 5 months postoperatively. At 6 months after surgery, unrestricted golf is allowed. Tennis players are permitted to begin gentle ground strokes 3 months postoperatively. The intensity of the ground strokes is increased 4 to 5 months after surgery. Unrestricted tennis, including serves and overhead shots, is allowed 6 months postoperatively.

Although we do not recommend any specific strengthening exercises as part of the rehabilitation program, some of our younger patients enjoy weightlifting as part of their fitness regimen. Upper extremity weightlifting is allowed starting 6 months postoperatively. Patients are encouraged to use weightlifting for muscle toning only and not to engage in any type of power-lifting exercises. We have had patients participate in sports such as trap shooting, water skiing, snow skiing, and mountain climbing 6 months after undergoing shoulder arthroplasty.

REFERENCE

1. Liotard JP, Edwards TB, Padey A, et al: Hydrotherapy rehabilitation after shoulder surgery. Tech Shoulder Elbow Surg 2003;4:44-49.

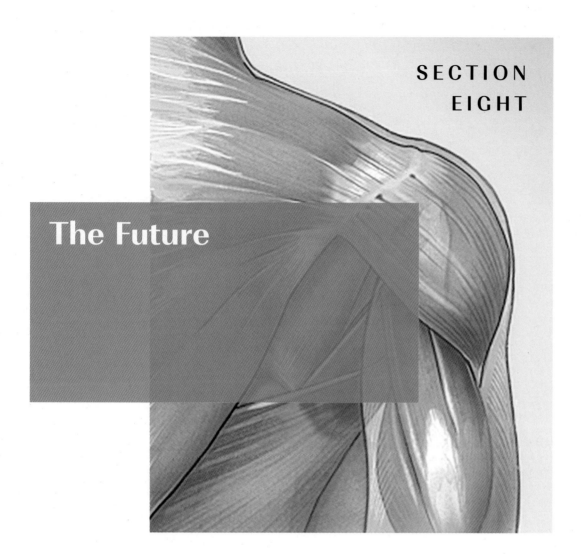

SECTION
EIGHT

The Future

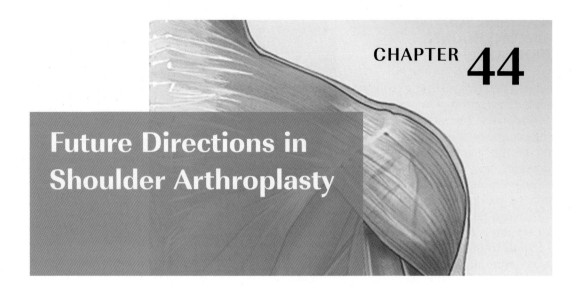

Future Directions in Shoulder Arthroplasty

Shoulder arthroplasty has advanced immeasurably since the first shoulder replacement was implanted by Péan in 1893.[1] Implant designs continue to evolve and improve, as do the materials from which these designs are constructed. The reverse prosthesis has gained widespread use in the United States since 2004 and continues to evolve, with minor design changes introduced by many companies that manufacture a version of this semiconstrained device.

Our personal interest in the future of shoulder arthroplasty has focused largely on computer-assisted navigation.[2,3] Computer-assisted navigation has been used successfully to improve implant alignment in hip and knee arthroplasty.[4,5] We have used similar technology involving an image-free system to monitor and improve implant alignment during shoulder arthroplasty.

Computer-assisted navigation can be used for both the humeral and glenoid portions of shoulder arthroplasty. For the humeral component, the primary usefulness of navigation in most cases is in allowing confirmation of appropriate humeral head resection. In cases of severe proximal humeral deformity (i.e., post-traumatic arthropathy after a previous proximal humeral fracture), computer-assisted navigation can help in achieving proper component positioning in the absence of reliable anatomic landmarks.

For the glenoid component, computer-assisted navigation permits precise correction of pathologic glenoid version and inclination caused by osseous glenoid wear. Without computer-assisted navigation, correction of pathologic glenoid version and inclination through reaming is largely dependent on surgeon

experience. Unfortunately, most surgeons performing shoulder arthroplasty do fewer than 10 cases per year. Of patients with primary osteoarthritis, only 25% to 35% have posterior glenoid wear with biconcave glenoid morphology. If the average surgeon performed replacements only for primary osteoarthritis (which is of course untrue), fewer than three of these cases would be encountered per year, thus making it extremely difficult to gain experience in treating this difficult situation. The use of computer-assisted navigation for correction of these glenoid deformities eliminates a large portion of the learning curve. In the current climate of health care reimbursement, minimizing extremely expensive revision arthroplasty has taken on a critical role.

Another potential use of computed-assisted navigation during shoulder arthroplasty involves positioning of the humeral stem when performing shoulder arthroplasty for a proximal humeral fracture. At the time of writing of this textbook, this application is being developed. Ultimately, the computer system will assist the surgeon in positioning the humeral stem at the correct height and in the correct humeral version.

Although the computer-assisted navigation system that we use (Kinamed, Inc., Camarillo, CA) is approved by the Food and Drug Administration, it is not readily available at most hospitals. As computer-assisted surgery continues to advance, these systems will undoubtedly become more readily available and their use more commonplace. This chapter discusses our use of computer-assisted surgical navigation in unconstrained shoulder arthroplasty.

PREOPERATIVE PLANNING FOR NAVIGATION IN UNCONSTRAINED SHOULDER ARTHROPLASTY

Although no additional preoperative planning is necessary for computer-assisted navigation of the humeral portion of shoulder arthroplasty, preoperative planning is essential in using computer-assisted navigation for proper positioning of the glenoid component. Axial computed tomograms are used to evaluate glenoid morphology and version preoperatively to allow precise correction of pathologic morphology with computed-assisted navigation.

The angle of glenoid version is determined relative to the long axis of the scapula from an axial computed tomogram.[6] The plane of section needed for this measurement is located in approximately the middle of the glenoid cavity and is estimated by using the first section inferior to the tip of the coracoid process. The long axis of the scapula is determined by taking the center point of the anteroposterior diameter of the glenoid and constructing a line from this point to the medial aspect of the scapula (Fig. 44-1). A reference neutral axis (0-degree version) is drawn perpendicular to the long axis of the scapula (Fig. 44-2). A line is drawn tangential to the anterior and posterior rims of the glenoid cavity (Fig. 44-3). The acute angle formed by these two lines is the angle of glenoid version (Fig. 44-4). Once version is measured, the amount of correction may be determined. Normal glenoid version ranges from 2 degrees of anteversion to 9 degrees of retroversion.[6] For the example in Figures 44-1 to 44-4, the retroversion measures 23 degrees.

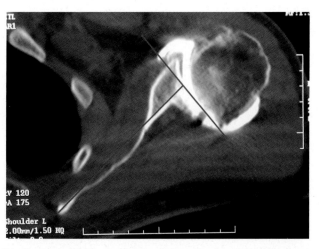

Figure 44-2   A line is drawn perpendicular to the long axis of the scapula.

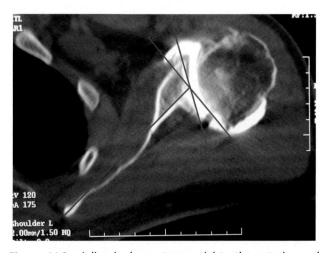

Figure 44-3   A line is drawn tangential to the anterior and posterior rims of the glenoid.

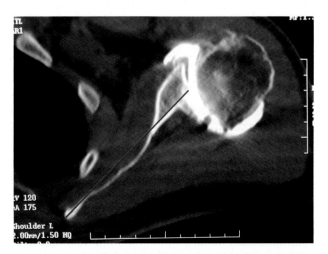

Figure 44-1   The long axis of the scapula is determined by taking the center point of the anteroposterior diameter of the glenoid and constructing a line from this point to the medial aspect of the scapula.

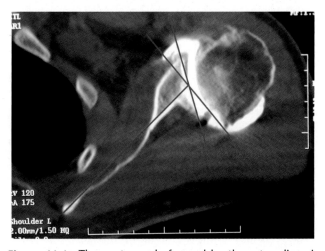

Figure 44-4   The acute angle formed by these two lines is the angle of glenoid version.

Chapter 44 • *Future Directions in Shoulder Arthroplasty* **505**

SURGICAL TECHNIQUE FOR NAVIGATION OF THE HUMERAL COMPONENT DURING SHOULDER ARTHROPLASTY

When we use computer-assisted navigation for the humeral portion of unconstrained shoulder arthroplasty, we follow the same steps as in non-navigated shoulder arthroplasty (see Section Two). The proper steps for surgical navigation are merely added to the existing procedure.

Room Setup

The operating room is initially set up as for non-navigated shoulder arthroplasty. A cart containing the navigational computer with two cameras is placed at the foot of the operating table slightly on the patient's operative side (Fig. 44-5). The camera holder is equipped with an alignment laser to ensure that the cameras are directed properly toward the operative field (Fig. 44-6). The patient is then prepared and draped as per standard technique with exception of the humeral epicondyles' being draped free to allow use of the epicondyles as referencing points (Fig. 44-7). The three tracking instruments—a probe, a large black tracker, and a small green tracker—are placed in front of the navigational cameras and their identification by the computer verified (Fig. 44-8).

Surgical Technique

The deltopectoral surgical approach, glenoid exposure, and humeral exposure are performed in the manner previously described throughout this textbook. A clamp to hold the humeral optical tracking device (small green tracker) is secured to the anterolateral humerus with two unicortical threaded pins just distal to the humeral metaphysis (Fig. 44-9). Alternatively, a

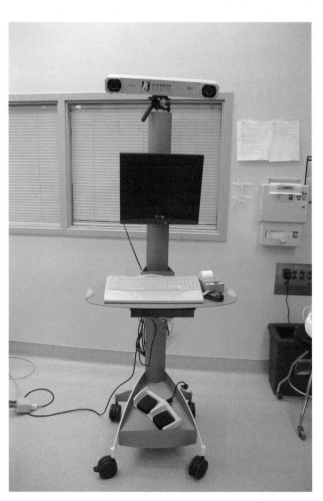

Figure 44-5 Cart containing the navigational computer and data input cameras.

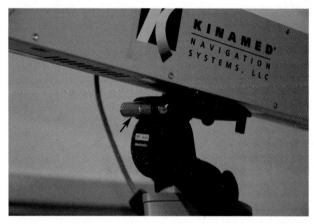

Figure 44-6 Laser pointer (*arrow*) to assist in directing the input cameras.

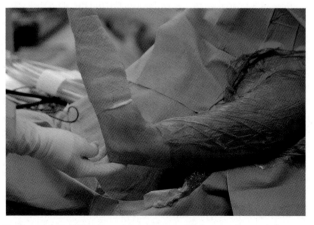

Figure 44-7 The humeral epicondyles are draped free to allow palpation with the computer probe.

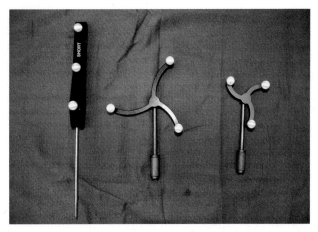

Figure 44-8 The three different navigational trackers used in computer-assisted navigation during shoulder arthroplasty.

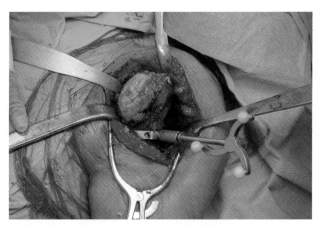

Figure 44-10 Alternative C-clamp jig for holding the humeral navigational tracker.

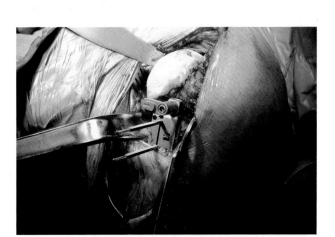

Figure 44-9 The clamp for the humeral tracker is secured to the proximal humerus with two unicortical pins.

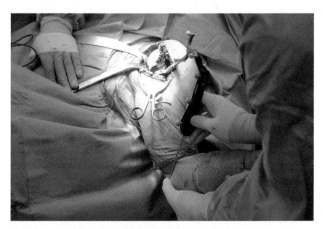

Figure 44-11 The probe is used to palpate the medial and lateral epicondyles.

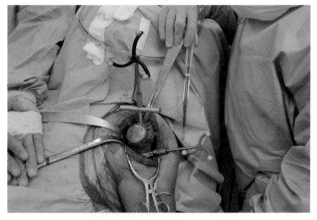

Figure 44-12 The navigated canal finder is introduced into the humeral canal.

C-clamp jig can be used to hold the humeral tracking device (Fig. 44-10). After attachment of the tracking device, the probe is used to palpate the medial and lateral humeral epicondyles to create a reference line for humeral version (Fig. 44-11). The surgeon uses a foot pedal to input each data point. A navigated canal finder with the large black tracker attached is inserted into the humeral canal to create a reference axis for humeral inclination (Fig. 44-12). The humeral canal finder is removed after the axis is entered into the navigational computer. Osteophytes around the native humeral anatomic neck are removed to identify the anatomic neck of the humerus. Before resection of the humeral head, the anatomic neck axis (inclination, retroversion) and diameter are measured with the navigation system by palpating six points around the perimeter of the native humeral neck with the probe (Fig. 44-13). The humeral head is resected, and the

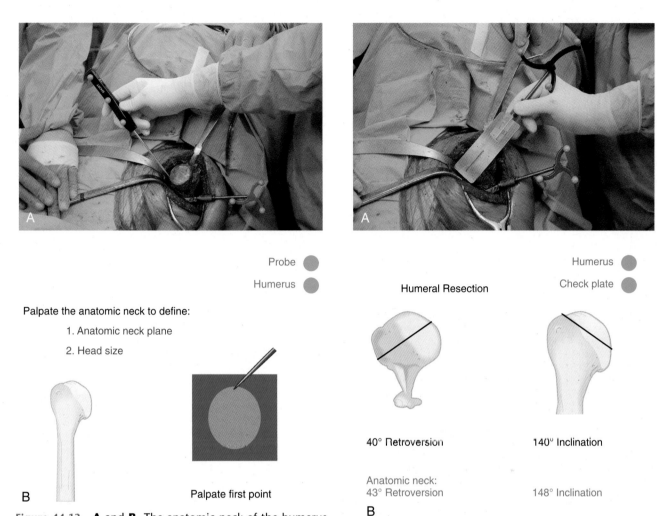

Probe ●
Humerus ●

Palpate the anatomic neck to define:

1. Anatomic neck plane

2. Head size

B   Palpate first point

Figure 44-13   A and **B,** The anatomic neck of the humerus is input into the navigational computer via the probe.

Humerus ●
Check plate ●

Humeral Resection

40° Retroversion   140° Inclination

Anatomic neck:
43° Retroversion   148° Inclination

B

Figure 44-14   A and **B,** The navigational check plate is used to record inclination and version of the humeral resection.

navigation system with the large black tracker attached to a check plate is used to record inclination and retroversion of the resected plane (Fig. 44-14). The humeral tracking device is removed and humeral preparation is performed by following the technique described in Chapter 11.

SURGICAL TECHNIQUE FOR NAVIGATION OF THE GLENOID COMPONENT DURING SHOULDER ARTHROPLASTY

After humeral preparation, the coracoid process is exposed by placing the tip of a Hohmann-type retractor behind the base of the coracoid (Fig. 44-15). The clamp for the scapula tracker is secured to the coracoid process with two orthogonal screws (Fig. 44-16). The large black tracker is attached to the coracoid clamp (Fig. 44-17). The posterior glenoid rim retractor is

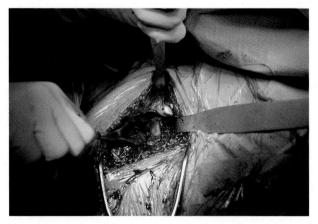

Figure 44-15   Exposure of the coracoid process.

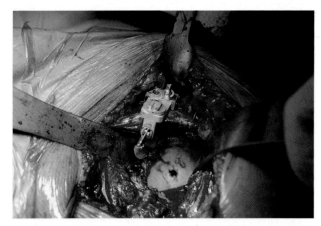

Figure 44-16 The clamp for the scapula tracker is secured to the coracoid process with two orthogonal screws.

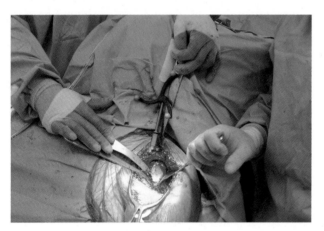

Figure 44-17 The large black tracker is attached to the coracoid clamp.

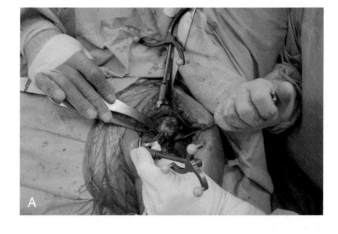

Scapula
Glenoid plate ●

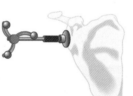

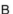

1. Attach humerus tracker to glenoid plate

2. Align with native glenoid or in a desired position

3. Press right pedal to capture glenoid plate orientation

Figure 44-18 **A** and **B,** The glenoid referencing instrument with the small green tracker attached is used to register version and inclination of the native glenoid surface.

placed to obtain exposure of the glenoid. A glenoid referencing instrument with the small green tracker attached is used to register version and inclination of the native glenoid surface (Fig. 44-18). In certain situations, such as excessively obese patients and those with severe glenoid deformity, it can be difficult to place the instrument flush with the glenoid surface because of limitations in exposure. To assist in these situations, the glenoid referencing instrument has a variable-angle linkage that allows the glenoid faceplate to be positioned in full contact with the native glenoid and facilitate visualization of the small green tracker by the cameras (Fig. 44-19). Once the glenoid faceplate is placed on the glenoid surface, the data are entered into the navigational computer.

A centering hole is placed on the glenoid face as described in Chapter 12. The glenoid reamer is inserted and the small green tracker is attached to the shaft of the reamer with a special clamp (Fig. 44-20). The

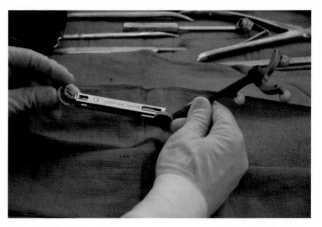

Figure 44-19 Details of the glenoid referencing instrument.

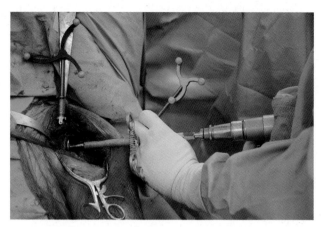

Figure 44-20 Glenoid reamer with attached tracking device.

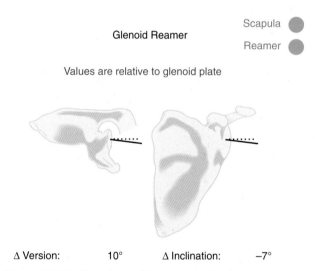

Glenoid Reamer

Scapula ●
Reamer ●

Values are relative to glenoid plate

Δ Version: 10°   Δ Inclination: −7°

Figure 44-21 Reaming with real-time feedback on correction of glenoid version and inclination.

glenoid is reamed while the surgeon receives real-time feedback on the change in version and inclination relative to the native glenoid (Fig. 44-21). This allows the surgeon to ream the exact amount of glenoid for correction as determined from preoperative planning. For the example in Figures 44-1 to 44-4, the glenoid is corrected 20 degrees with guidance from the navigational computer. Once reaming is complete, the coracoid clamp is removed, and the remainder of the arthroplasty is completed as described in Section Two.

REFERENCES

1. Lugli T: Artificial shoulder joint by Péan (1893). The facts of an exceptional intervention and the prosthetic method. Clin Orthop 1978;133:215-218.
2. Sarin VK, Gartsman GM, Edwards TB: Computer-aided navigation for shoulder arthroplasty—a cadaver study. Paper presented at the 6th Annual Meeting of the International Society for Computer Assisted Orthopaedic Surgery, June 2006, Montreal.
3. Sarin VK, Pilgeram KC, Gartsman GM, Edwards TB: Computer-assisted total shoulder arthroplasty—a cadaver study. Paper presented at the 18th Annual Symposium of the International Society for Technology in Arthroplasty, September 2005, Kyoto, Japan.
4. Digioia AM 3rd, Jaramaz B, Plakseychuk AY, et al: Comparison of a mechanical acetabular alignment guide with computer placement of the socket. J Arthroplasty 2002;17:359-364.
5. Haaker RG, Stockheim M, Kamp M, et al: Computer-assisted navigation increases precision of component placement in total knee arthroplasty. Clin Orthop Relat Res 2005;433:152-159.
6. Friedman RJ, Hawthorne KB, Genez BM: The use of computerized tomography in the measurement of glenoid version. J Bone Joint Surg Am 1992;74:1032-1037.

Index

Note: Page numbers followed by the letter f refer to figures; those followed by the letter t refer to tables.